Current Issues in Platelet Transfusion Therapy and Platelet Alloimmunity

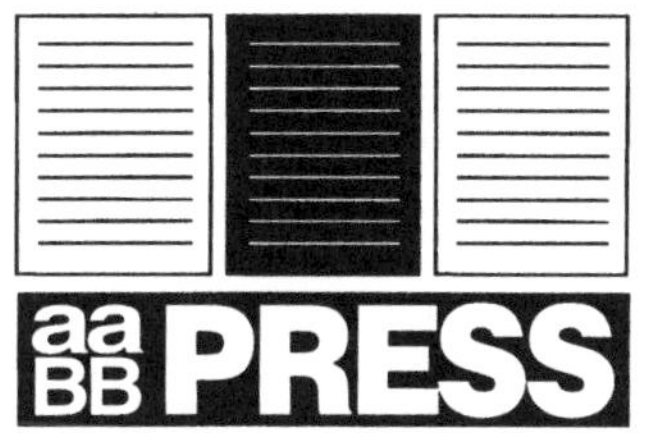

Other related publications available from the AABB:

Blood Components and Pharmocologic Agents in the Treatment of Congenital and Acquired Bleeding Disorders
Edited by Barbara M. Alving, MD

Transfusion Therapy: Clinical Principles and Practice
Edited by Paul D. Mintz, MD

Apheresis: Principles and Practice
Edited by Bruce C. McLeod, MD; Thomas H. Price, MD; and Mary Jo Drew, MD

Cytokines in Transfusion Medicine: A Primer
Edited by Robertson D. Davenport, MD, and Edward L. Snyder, MD

Transfusion Reactions
Edited by Mark A. Popovsky, MD

Platelet Transfusion: New Approaches to Old Topics
Edited by Estre Culotta, MHS, MT(ASCP)SBB, and Antonio Ordinas, MD, PhD
(also available in Spanish)

Platelet Transfusions: Problems and Solutions
Edited by Glenn Ramsey, MD

Current Issues in Platelet Transfusion Therapy and Platelet Alloimmunity

Thomas S. Kickler, MD
Johns Hopkins University School of Medicine
Baltimore, Maryland

Jay H. Herman, MD
Temple University School of Medicine
Philadelphia, Pennsylvania

AABB Press
Bethesda, Maryland
1999

Mention of specific products or equipment by contributors to this AABB Press publication does not represent an endorsement of such products by the AABB Press nor does it necessarily indicate a preference for those products over other similar competitive products.

Efforts are made to have publications of the AABB Press consistent in regard to acceptable practices. However, for several reasons, they may not be. First, as new developments in the practice of blood banking occur, changes may be recommended to the AABB *Standards for Blood Banks and Transfusion Services.* It is not possible, however, to revise each publication at the time such a change is adopted. Thus, it is essential that the most recent edition of the *Standards* be consulted as a reference in regard to current acceptable practices. Second, the views expressed in this publication represent the opinions of authors. The publication of this book does not constitute an endorsement by the AABB Press of any view expressed herein, and the AABB Press expressly disclaims any liability arising from any inaccuracy or misstatement.

American Association of Blood Banks
8101 Glenbrook Road
Bethesda, Maryland 20814-2749

ISBN NO. 1-56395-105-3
Printed in the United States

AABB Press Editorial Board

Contributors

Clarence B. Sarkodee-Adoo, MD
Marlene and Stewart Greenebaum Cancer Center
University of Maryland School of Medicine
Baltimore, Maryland

Kaaron Benson, MD
University of South Florida College of Medicine
H. Lee Moffitt Cancer Center
Tampa, Florida

Victor S. Blanchette, FRCP
The Hospital for Sick Children
Toronto, Ontario, Canada

James B. Bussel, MD
Weill Medical College of Cornell University
New York, New York

Manuel Carcao, MD, FRCP(c)
The Hospital for Sick Children
Toronto, Ontario, Canada

John Freedman, MD
St. Michael's Hospital
University of Toronto
The Toronto Platelet Immunobiology Group
Toronto, Ontario, Canada

Richard C. Friedberg, MD, PhD
University of Alabama at Birmingham
Birmingham Veterans Affairs Medical Center
Birmingham, Alabama

Brian Gaupp, MD, PhD
University of Alabama at Birmingham
Birmingham, Alabama

Jay H. Herman, MD
Temple University Hospital
Philadelphia, Pennsylvania

Meyer R. Heyman, MD
Marlene and Stewart Greenebaum Cancer Center
University of Maryland School of Medicine
Baltimore, Maryland

Christopher D. Hillyer, MD
Emory University School of Medicine
Atlanta, Georgia

Heather Hume, MD, FRCP(c)
Hôpital Sainte-Justine
Montreal, Quebec, Canada

K.J. Kao, MD, PhD
University of Florida
Gainesville, Florida

Maryann Keashen-Schnell
American Red Cross Blood Services, Penn-Jersey Region
Philadelphia, Pennsylvania

Thomas S. Kickler, MD
Temple University Hospital
Philadelphia, Pennsylvania

Scott Murphy, MD
American Red Cross Blood Services, Penn-Jersey Region
Philadelphia, Pennsylvania

Margaret L. Rand, PhD
The Hospital for Sick Children
Toronto, Ontario, Canada

John D. Roback, MD, PhD
Emory University School of Medicine
Atlanta, Georgia

Charles A. Schiffer, MD
Wayne State University School of Medicine
Harper Hospital
Detroit, Michigan

John W. Semple, PhD
St Michael's Hospital
University of Toronto
Toronto, Ontario, Canada

Table of Contents

Preface

IT MAY BE DIFFICULT FOR THE READERS OF THIS BOOK to imagine the time in the not-too-distant past (which we can still remember) when platelet concentrates for transfusion were not routinely produced, and fatal hemorrhagic consequences led the list of adverse outcomes for oncology and transplant patients. Large-scale platelet production from both whole blood donor collection as well as plateletpheresis expanded in the 1970s and 1980s to keep pace with the marked growth in the fields of oncology and transplantation. Thrombocytopenic patients have now benefited, as platelet transfusion products are readily available in most parts of the United States at any time. This is amazing given the fastidious storage needs of this short-lived component.

However, basic issues related to the correct dose, transfusion trigger, target platelet count, and expected response to transfusion have not been resolved, although recent evidence incorporated in the chapters of this book may shed light on these difficult problems. Platelet products are often the most expensive blood component used by a transfusion service, and in the absence of rigorous study, conventional practices have been adapted to accommodate both economic realities as well as the constraints imposed by storage and availability requirements.

Whenever possible, the friends and colleagues we asked to summarize each particular area covered by a chapter in this book were urged to include both key historical developments in the particular topic as well as the most recent synthesis of transfusion medicine information. Suggestions for practical application to the transfusion decisions made in the care of patients are also included. These decisions must often balance realistic concerns related to the leukocyte reduction process, adverse transfusion reactions, and declining health-care reimbursements, as well as the traditional blood banking issues of ABO compatibility and component storage. Lively discussions regarding the proper role of apheresis platelet concentrates versus whole-blood-derived platelets still abound in most transfusion services, and each author was asked to comment on this issue where it applies to the topic.

Along with the growth in platelet transfusion medicine as a field of interest, there has been an explosion in the base of knowledge related to platelet membrane antigens, platelet serology, and alloimmunity. This has led to the possibility of preventing or treating antibody-mediated platelet destruction. Because many of our views in this area have been clearly stated in numerous past publications, we enlisted other experts in the field to shed new light in the matters of identifying and treating platelet refractoriness, preventing alloimmunization, providing alternatives to platelet transfusion, and addressing matched platelet support. Patients who are refractory to platelet transfusion are still widely encountered and are often extremely frustrating to support. Since universal leukocyte reduction is fast becoming a reality, chapters on the basic immunologic principles of leukocyte reduction and the clinical response in human trials of leukocyte reduction have also been included.

Also included in the text are chapters relating specifically to both pediatric and neonatal platelet transfusion and alloimmunization. Although most clinicians only infrequently are involved in providing care and support to both adult and pediatric patients, transfusion medicine practitioners as well as those involved in blood centers and platelet collection activities frequently overlap both age groups. Recognized authorities in these fields were therefore invited to add to this work. The case discussion format adopted for the neonatal chapter provides treatment paradigms that should prove useful to those who care for these infants.

The concluding chapter seeks to put the entire field of platelet transfusion and alloimmunity into proper prospective. Dr. Charles Schiffer is widely regarded as one of the leaders in the development of modern platelet transfusion practice, and he and his colleagues have contributed many of the seminal studies in this field. We are fortunate that he accepted our offer to share his perspective on what he sees ahead for the field of platelet transfusion.

Undertaking this project at the request of the American Association of Blood Banks, we were both delighted to be able to deliver what we feel is a highly focused and clinically relevant book that will be useful to a diverse audience of those involved in the care of thrombocytopenic patients. We would like to thank the publication staff at the AABB for their support and patience, the chapter authors for their perseverance, numerous colleagues and coworkers for their understanding when editorial duties conflicted with our real jobs, the teachers and mentors we have had over the years, and all of the patients we have cared for over the past 25 years who have taught us so much.

Thomas S. Kickler, MD
Jay H. Herman, MD
Editors

About the Editors

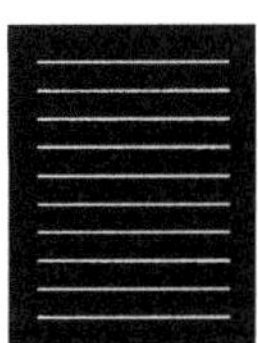

Thomas S. Kickler, MD, is a professor of pathology, medicine, and oncology at the Johns Hopkins University School of Medicine. He is also executive director of the Eugene and Mary B. Meyer Center for Advanced Transfusion Practices and Blood Research at the Johns Hopkins University. Dr. Kickler received his medical degree from the University of West Virginia and did his postgraduate work at the University of Wisconsin, the Johns Hopkins University School of Medicine, the Mayo Graduate School of Medicine, and the University of Rochester.

Dr. Kickler has published almost 100 articles in medical journals and many chapters in medical textbooks. He is on the editorial boards of *TRANSFUSION* and the *Journal of Transfusion Alternatives* and a member of the AABB, the American Society of Hematology, the College of American Pathologists, and the International Society of Hemostatis and Thrombosis.

Jay H. Herman, MD, is professor of medicine and oncology at Temple University School of Medicine and the medical director of the Stem Cell Processing Laboratory at Temple University Hospital, where he was previously director of transfusion medicine. Prior to that he was director of transfusion medicine at St. Christopher's Hospital for Children and medical director of the Penn-Jersey Regional Blood Services of the American Red Cross.

Dr. Herman received his medical degree from Harvard Medical School and continued his medical training at Grady Memorial Hospital in Atlanta, the University of Virginia Medical Center, and the Johns Hopkins School of Medicine. He has published 57 papers and 46 abstracts related to blood banking and hematology. His areas of interest include platelet transfusion practice, platelet and granuloctye immunobiology, neonatal alloimmune disorders, apheresis technology, and posttransplant immune cytopenias. Dr. Herman is a member of the AABB, the American Society of Hematology, the American Society of Pediatric Hematology/Oncology, and the American Society for Apheresis.

In: Kickler TS, and Herman JH, eds.
Current Issues in Platelet Transfusion Therapy and Platelet Alloimmunity
Bethesda, MD: AABB Press, 1999

1

Platelet Transfusion: Indications, Considerations, and Specific Clinical Settings

RICHARD C. FRIEDBERG, MD, PhD, AND
BRIAN GAUPP, MD, PhD

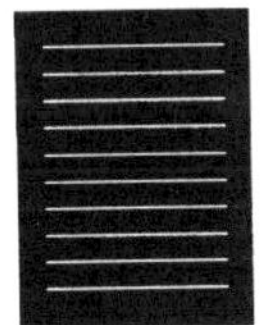

EARLY DESCRIPTIONS OF WHOLE BLOOD TRANSFUSION generally present the goal not as one related to hemostasis, but rather as an attempt to restore an ebbing life force. With the recognition of blood as a complex mixture of independent components and interrelated functions, however, the goal of blood transfusion changed. As the role of red corpuscles in oxygen trans-

Richard C. Friedberg, MD, PhD, Associate Professor of Pathology, Associate Head, Transfusion Medicine, Associate Medical Director, Blood Bank, Division of Laboratory Medicine, Department of Pathology, University of Alabama at Birmingham; and Chief, Pathology and Laboratory Medicine Service, Birmingham Veteran's Affairs Medical Center, Birmingham, Alabama; and Brian Gaupp, MD, PhD, Fellow, Division of Hematology/Oncology, Department of Medicine, University of Alabama at Birmingham, Birmingham, Alabama

port became evident early in the 20th century, the goal of whole blood transfusion became one of maintaining tissue oxygenation.

Unlike whole blood or red blood cells (RBCs), platelets do not have a transfusion history dating back centuries. Rather, the indications and considerations for platelet transfusion are much more recent, having evolved significantly over the past 35 years. In the 1960s, platelet concentrates were increasingly being produced by the fractionation of whole blood. At this time, the primary limiting factor for platelet transfusion was availability. As transfusion practice matured from whole blood to component therapy, the availability of platelet concentrates improved. Coincident with this was the advent of improved and increasingly myelotoxic chemotherapy regimens. Once the limitation of marrow toxicity had been circumvented, oncologists could go after cancerous cells more aggressively. Indeed, platelet consumption increased from 410,000 units in 1970 to approximately 8.3 million equivalent units in 1992.[1] Taking into consideration the increased reliance on platelets collected by apheresis, the United States now consumes more platelets than RBCs (in terms of whole-blood-derived units).

The nation's blood centers have done an impressive job of providing platelets for transfusion; however, demand continues to outstrip supply. Part of the reason for this supply-demand disparity lies in technical and biological limitations on platelet acquisition, handling, and storage. Yet a key element in the disparity is inappropriate usage. This deep-seated problem stems from two different sources: the frightening picture of a potentially preventable hemorrhagic death and historically poor data to help determine the circumstances under which such a fatality is indeed preventable.

Like the indications for RBC transfusion, those for platelet transfusion cannot be dictated solely on the basis of quantitative criteria. Indeed, there are only a few studies to help guide the ever-growing practice of platelet transfusion. But whereas the appropriate indications for RBC or Fresh Frozen Plasma (FFP) transfusion are familiar to many medical practitioners, those for platelet transfusion are less familiar.

Indications and Considerations

The history of platelet transfusion begins with the association of hemorrhage with low platelet counts. The relationship between the need to achieve a sustained rise in platelet count and the hemostatic effect of platelet transfusion has been known since the early 1960s. A review of the causes of death among acute leukemia patients at the National Cancer Institute from 1954 to 1963 noted, "A striking finding...is the decline in fatal hemorrhage subsequent to platelet transfusion therapy. All hemorrhage declined from 66.8% to 37.2%."[2(p102)] Seeking to identify a quantitative relationship between platelet count and hemorrhage, Gaydos et al[3] identified 92 consecutive adult (40) and pediatric (52) patients with acute myeloid (34) or lymphoid (57) leukemia, and followed 85 patients throughout their clinical course until death. Hemorrhage was associated with low or falling platelet counts below 20,000/μL, but clinically significant hemorrhage was associated only with platelet counts below 5,000/μL. The authors noted that "the lower the platelet count, the greater the frequency of hemorrhage," yet there was no threshold—only a linear relationship of bleeding to platelet count. Both the frequency and the severity of hemorrhage increased as platelet counts decreased. Sixteen of 92 patients—8 with intracerebral leukemia (median platelet count = 10,000/μL) and 8 without (median platelet count = 1-3,000/μL)—died from intracranial hemorrhage. Other factors also influenced bleeding: "The quantitative relation observed indicates that other, more proximate causes interact with low platelets to produce hemorrhage. . . . Precipitating events that alone would also fail to cause hemorrhage regularly result in hemorrhage when coupled with thrombocytopenia."[3(p909)] In an often overlooked part of data interpretation, these authors have subsequently reminded us of an unwritten confounding component of the study—namely, that most of the patients were receiving aspirin in accord with the common practice of the day—and the data need to be viewed with that caveat in mind.

A 1974 study supported the notion that prophylactic platelet transfusions prevent hemorrhage in leukemia patients while also noting that fever preceded "substantial hemorrhage" in 77% of patients.[4] This association led to the concept of prophylactic platelet transfusion to prevent instead of treat hemorrhage. A 1978 study by Slichter and Harker selected 20 aplastic anemia patients to undergo ^{51}Cr-labeled autologous RBC survival studies to detect spontaneous occult fecal blood loss at various platelet counts in the absence of transfusion.[5] Normal blood loss of less than 5 mL per day was seen at platelet counts greater than 10,000/μL. An increase in blood loss to 9 mL per day was noted at platelet counts of 5-10,000/μL, and marked blood loss (greater than 50 mL/day) was seen at platelet counts of less than 5,000/μL. A 1979 study of children with acute lymphoblastic leukemia found that transfusions for platelet counts below 20,000/μL were necessary only in the setting of coincident clinically significant bleeding.[6] A 1982 randomized study by Murphy et al followed 56 children with leukemia who received platelet transfusion either when their platelet counts fell below 20,000/μL (prophylactic) or when significant hemorrhage was noted (therapeutic).[7] Three of 25 patients had 1 bleed each in the prophylactic group vs 8 of 21 patients with a total of 27 bleeds in the therapeutic group ($p<0.00001$). Even though survival was not directly improved, it was found that hemorrhage could be controlled with platelet transfusions. In the last month of life, however, bleeding episodes were more difficult to control in the prophylactic group. Patients receiving prophylactic transfusion had twice the number of transfusions, yet survival was unaffected. Nevertheless, although the authors "would have liked to be able to make firm recommendations concerning the indications for platelet transfusion[,] . . . the data permit an adequate defense of either prophylactic or therapeutic platelet transfusion."[7(p353)] By 1987, 73% (55/75) of academic leukemia and stem cell transplantation services surveyed used prophylactic platelet transfusions to maintain platelet counts greater than 20,000/μL.[8]

More recently, several groups have advocated altering the common practice of prophylactic platelet transfusion to reflect both current understanding of a much lower baseline threshold platelet count and the presence of clinical risk factors for bleeding. Most of the arguments in favor of prophylactic transfusion center on the notions that there are often no warning signs prior to lethal intracerebral hemorrhage and that emergency platelet transfusions are not always immediately available. A 1991 study by Gmur et al of 102 acute leukemia patients identified constant clinical assessment for risk factors coupled with a sliding scale of platelet counts for the prophylactic platelet transfusion.[9] If the morning platelet count was 0-5,000/μL, platelets were transfused that same day regardless of the patient's condition. For counts of 6-10,000/μL, transfusions were indicated for fever (>38 C) or fresh minor hemorrhagic manifestations. For counts between 11,000 and 20,000/μL, prophylactic platelet transfusion was indicated for coagulation disorders or heparin therapy, or before such procedures as marrow biopsy or lumbar puncture. At counts greater than 20,000/μL, platelets were indicated for prophylaxis only in the presence of major bleeding complications or before surgical procedures. The incidence of bleeding at all triggers was lower among these patients than among a historical control group, while platelet use decreased. In 69% of the patient-days with platelet counts below 20,000/μL, platelet transfusion was withheld. Minor hemorrhage was common, but the incidence of major hemorrhage was low: 3% with lethal bleeds and 1% with significant central nervous system (CNS) sequelae; most major bleeds were due to immune refractoriness or profound thrombocytopenia with numerous clinical risk factors.

Use of the transfusion threshold platelet count of 20-30,000/μL has been a commonly accepted practice, although one without factual basis.[10,11] Recent studies have validated and reviews have supported lower transfusion thresholds with significant reductions in platelet consumption and associated risks.[9,10,12-17] Generally, if the platelet count is less than 5,000/μL, prophylactic transfusion is reasonable. If it is less than 10,000/μL, platelet transfusion is reasonable if the patient is febrile, hemorrhagic, or perceived to be at significant risk. For many patients, and for stem cell transplantation patients in particular, the rate of reduction in the platelet count may be more significant than the specific count at a given point in time.[18] For "coverage" prior to minor invasive procedures, a threshold of 50,000/μL is commonly used. In the postoperative setting, prophylactic transfusion is reasonable if the platelet count is less than 50,000/μL. Considerations should include that platelet transfusion will not limit hemorrhage that is unrelated to quantitative or qualitative platelet dysfunction.

In 1992, Schiffer advocated a consensus practical approach to prophylactic transfusion.[19] He correctly noted that many of the oft-cited early studies of platelet transfusion were statistically underpowered and methodologically weak. In addition, many of these studies suffered from numerous unacknowledged confounding factors. Some studies included patients on aspirin therapy, as was the standard of the day. Others included patients on antifungal or antibiotic treatment regimens that would be considered inadequate by today's standards, let alone the fact that the underlying infection is now known to be closely related to likelihood of hemorrhage. Such confounding factors could have had a tremendous impact on both the functionality of the transfused platelets and the hemorrhagic tendency of the recipients. Moreover, advances in platelet storage and collection technology have dramatically improved the quality of platelets for transfusion. Schiffer also noted that experienced oncologists can identify most patients at risk of hemorrhage without stringent criteria, given the subjective nature of the assessment of risk factors. Much of the concern for prophylactic vs therapeutic platelet transfusion practices arises when the notion of automatically transfusing platelets on the basis of platelet counts and arbitrary transfusion triggers is abandoned. Some patients may need platelet counts maintained at high levels whereas others may safely avoid any transfusions even at counts of 5,000/μL. Most patients, however, fall in between and need to have their threshold and target increment individualized. Moreover, factors such as lack of readily available physician assessment in hospitals without house staff, lack of accessible platelet inventories, and scheduling problems inherent in outpatient treatment can interfere with the application of such a scale. Indeed, "it is clear that it is inappropriate to automatically administer platelet transfusion at a given platelet count and that the number of platelet transfusions administered to many patients can be decreased with proper physician and patient education."[19(p297)]

Dosage

Given all the discussion and investigation into the indications for platelet transfusion (ie, when and why), one would imagine that a similar amount of thought had been given to the dosage (ie, how much). However, there have been relatively few studies of platelet dosage. Part of the problem lies in the origins of product itself. Platelets for transfusion were initially obtained as a by-product of the fractionation of whole blood into packed RBCs, platelet-rich plasma, and platelet-poor plasma. The common "random-donor platelet concentrate" is the platelet-rich plasma portion. Since a unit of whole blood could vary significantly in total volume (±10%), hematocrit (±20%), and platelet count (±50%), and since the processing steps also add a significant degree of variation, the ultimate platelet count in the platelet-rich plasma could easily vary by a factor of 2 or more. Each whole-blood-derived platelet unit (concentrate) contains $4\text{-}8 \times 10^{10}$ platelets; one platelet dose is generally considered to be a pool of 4-8 of these random units, totaling $3\text{-}6 \times 10^{11}$ platelets. Alternatively, the entire dose can also be obtained by apheresis collection from a single donor. Moreover, variations in unit processing, storage, handling, and counting, coupled with variations in recipient size, age, splenomegaly, and clinical condition, further cloud the attempt to define a correlation between dosage and posttransfusion platelet increment.

Consequently, a number of common platelet dosing algorithms, all expected to achieve an "adequate" transfusion response, have been advanced to make ordering easier. The traditional dose of one whole-blood-derived unit of platelets per 10 kg (IU/10 kg) was initially calculated to add 100,000/µL to the peripheral platelet count; then the complication of splenic sequestration became evident. Later, one unit of platelets was estimated to raise the platelet count between 10 and 20,000/µL per square meter of body surface area, acknowledging the wide biologic variation in the transfusion response. This evolved into a standard of 6, 8, or 10 units as an adult "dose" containing approximately $3\text{-}6 \times 10^{11}$ platelets. Curiously, adult dosing schemes are typically even numbers and independent of body weight, and regimens are independent of platelet count in either the recipient or the product. Other common rules of thumb include 10 mL/kg for infants and neonates, and IU/10 kg for children and smaller adults. In some regions, the higher platelet yield from whole-blood-derived platelets has led to "standard" pools of five or four units, again given to patients regardless of body size. For single-donor platelets collected by apheresis, the old "unit" terminology is irrelevant as the standard apheresis dose became one unit of approximately 3-6 × 10^{11} platelets.

Recently, many centers have sought to collect higher-yield ("double-dose") platelets so that they can "split" that single collection into two or more products containing the traditional quantity of 3-6 × 10^{11} platelets. This has led to a reduction in the platelet content of many apheresis platelets, since the "fatter" units are split into "thinner" units. The motivation for splitting is less for equivalency of dose than it is for availability and effective use of resources. In addition to split platelet products, newer apheresis collection techniques may also affect platelet quality. For example, addition of an in-line collection chamber to minimize white blood cell spillover into the platelet product has been promoted as a cost-effective method to remove leukocyctes from the platelet product efficiently and theoretically gain the benefits associated with established methods of leukocyte reduction. However, the same chamber may also result in collections of smaller platelets. If this were confirmed, the total active surface area could be significantly different for two platelet products collected by different methods, even though each contained the same quantity of platelets. Indeed, perhaps the most technically correct measure for platelet dosage is total functional platelet surface area.

A number of early studies tried to define platelet dose and expected response to transfusion, but differences in transfusion products and clinical settings may lead to questions of applicability. In 1963, Freirich et al used fresh (less than 6-hour-old) platelet-rich plasma prepared by plateletpheresis to transfuse a median platelet dose of 2.6 × $10^{11}/m^2$ to 28 pediatric leukemia patients with median pretransfusion platelet counts of 6,000/µL.[20] Increments were directly related to dose given: for doses of less than 1.25 × $10^{11}/m^2$, the median increment was 12,000/µL, whereas for doses greater than 4.5 × $10^{11}/m^2$, the median increment was 60,000/µL. Posttransfusion platelet survival was curvilinear, depending on how high the platelet transfusion increment raised the platelet count as well as the presence of fever or sepsis. The incidence of hemorrhage was linear, from less than 20% at platelet counts above 40,000/µL to more than 80% at platelet counts of 2,000/µL, while transfusion reduced bleeding significantly, especially major hemorrhage.

In a 1963 study, Djerassi et al used fresh (less than 3-hour-old) platelet concentrates with doses calculated by body weight.[21] Despite the calculated goal of increasing the platelet count by 100,000/µL, only 3 of 34 platelet transfusions to 18 leukemia patients resulted in the expected platelet increments. Nonetheless, the platelet transfusions resulted in an increase from a pretransfusion median of 25,000/µL to a 2-hour posttransfusion median of 40,000/µL. A dose of 0.08 U/lb (2 U/10 kg) was more likely to yield an increment of 20,000/µL than a dose of 0.04 U/lb (1 U/10 kg, $p<0.01$). Looking at the data in another way, the double dose resulted in a posttransfusion increment of more than twice that of the single dose. Hemostasis correlated with the posttransfusion increments (not absolute platelet counts) of greater than 20,000/µL, with 84% of bleeds stopping when this increment was achieved (vs 33% stopping at lower increments, $p<0.01$). Overall, survival of transfused platelets to bleeding patients was shorter (2-3 days) than that of normal platelets. A later study by Roy et al found no difference in the incidence of bleeding among children with acute leukemia treated with prophylactic platelet transfusion at doses of either 0.03 or 0.06 U/lb (1 or 2 U/15 kg).[22] These early studies all suffer from the previously mentioned high variability in the quantity of platelets in a unit.

Given the fact that platelet transfusion therapy is a significant cost component in the treatment of malignancy, one would expect that the appropriate dose would be better defined. Recently, more researchers have begun to address the lack of data regarding the effect of platelet dose on transfusion outcome. Kiss et al noted that higher sustained increments were achieved with higher-dose apheresis platelets (median = 7.7×10^{11}) than with standard-dose products (median = 4.1×10^{11}).[23] Of interest is that the 48-hour posttransfusion increment for the higher-dose product was twice that of the standard dose (or split high-yield) product, implying that fewer transfusions might be necessary with large up-front doses. As expected, however, higher-dose platelets were as ineffective as standard doses in correcting nonalloimmune refractoriness. Norol et al found that larger-dose platelet transfusions increased the interval between transfusions, resulting in fewer transfusions and donor exposures.[24] Benson et al found that split apheresis platelets had lower normalized increments 14 hours after transfusion than did "whole" apheresis platelets, although the difference was not statistically significant.[25] Taking a cost-containment approach, Menitove et al reduced the standard dose from 1 U/10 kg to 1 U/12 kg but were concerned that the lower dose may decrease the mean transfusion interval.[26] In fact, they found that the mean number of platelet units transfused to hematology, oncology, and other patients did diminish but that the mean interval between transfusions did not.

In a prospective, randomized, double-blinded study to investigate the economic and clinical consequences of increased platelet dose for prophylactic transfusion in stem cell transplant recipients, Herman et al segregated apheresis platelets according to platelet content into low-dose (range

= 2.5-3.5 × 10^{11}, median = 3.1 × 10^{11}) and high-dose (range = 4.5-6.1 × 10^{11}, median = 4.9 × 10^{11}) cohorts.[27] Low-dose and high-dose platelets were transfused in random sequential pairs to the same patient. The multiple crossover design controlled for clinical risk factors and patient variables while no changes were made in transfusion parameters (threshold of 15,000/µL). Only sequential prophylactic transfusions were studied, and refractory patients were excluded. The results of 79 paired transfusions to 46 patients revealed that high-dose platelets had a median time to next transfusion of 3.0 days compared with 2.0 days for low-dose platelets in the same patient (p=0.0005), with disproportionate differences in median platelet increments: 32,000/µL for high-dose platelets compared with 17,000/µL for low-dose (p=0.0001) platelets. Multiple regression analysis of 74 patient variables identified no other patient factors aside from bilirubin and creatinine as having an independent effect on platelet response. A related study by the same group noted that the use of higher-dose apheresis platelets can reduce the costs associated with platelet transfusions for stem cell transplant patients.[28]

Most of the focus on appropriate platelet dosing has been lost amid the attention to specific platelet counts and increments. Strauss summarized this in 1995 by mathematically demonstrating that the posttransfusion platelet count depends on the platelet dose, assuming a standardized response to platelet transfusion.[29] If the particular platelet count is determined to be a clinically appropriate goal of platelet transfusion, the dose of platelets transfused must be adjusted for patient size and pretransfusion platelet count. If only the posttransfusion increment is determined to be relevant, the pretransfusion platelet count may not matter but the platelet dosage must.

Assessing the Efficacy of Platelet Transfusion

If platelets were transfused in a given clinical circumstance solely for reasons of prophylaxis (ie, prevention of some complication), assessing the efficacy of the transfusion could be quantified by measuring the decrement in that complication. If, however, that complication is rare even without platelet transfusion, assessment of efficacy could be difficult. In addition, if the potential complication that the transfusion is hoped to prevent is as frightening and severe as a fatal hemorrhage, the assessment of efficacy is made even more difficult by ethical and clinical considerations. On the other hand, if the goal of platelet transfusion is to increase the circulating platelet count quantitatively, assessment of efficacy could be based on the posttransfusion platelet count. It may not be possible, however, to correlate that goal absolutely with the true goal of preventing a complication. In practice, the rationale for platelet transfusion is multifaceted, and the assessment of efficacy is both difficult and infrequent.

For those situations in which a quantitative assessment of efficacy is desired, a number of formulas have been developed. Simply measuring the difference between pre- and posttransfusion platelet counts is inadequate. Appropriate evaluation must take into account the facts that 1) a "dose" of platelets is actually a range as opposed to a specific quantity, 2) interindividual intravascular volume varies markedly, and 3) total body platelet count is difficult to estimate based on peripheral compartment sampling. The corrected count increment (CCI), maximal platelet increment, and percent platelet recovery are measures commonly used to adjust the observed increment to reflect dose variation and correct for body surface area or calculated blood volume. The platelet increment is the difference between pre- and posttransfusion platelet counts. The CCI is designed to normalize the platelet increment for the patient size and the dose of platelets transfused. Similarly, the maximal platelet increment adjusts the platelet increment to account for the dose of platelets transfused, splenic sequestration, and the blood volume. The percent platelet recovery is determined either by the ratio of the platelet increment to the maximal platelet increment or by the use of ^{111}indium-radiolabeled platelets. (See Fig 1-1 for formulas.)

Interpretation of these calculations must take into account a number of factors. First of all, the wide biologic variation of platelet transfusion response observed makes "failure" difficult to define. Sequestration of transfused platelets in the spleen and other organs is said to account for 30-40% of the platelets in commonly used doses. This sequestration of platelets may be increased, sometimes without overt splenomegaly. Moreover, sequestered platelets may return to the peripheral circulation, resulting in a peripheral platelet increment that does not reflect the increase in total body platelets. Therefore, the failure threshold has typically been set to 50% of whatever value was "expected," but other definitions of refractoriness to platelet transfusion have been set forth.

Second, peripheral platelet counts assess only the large venous peripheral vascular compartment. Third, the timing of the pre- and posttransfusion platelet counts relative to the transfusion directly affects the measured increment. There appears to be a baseline daily platelet requirement of 7,000/μL, perhaps to fix the leaks of everyday existence and maintain vascular integrity.[30] This figure corresponds to 18% of the normal rate of platelet turnover, yet median platelet survival is diminished (ie, the turnover percentage is greater) when the peripheral platelet count is less than 50,000/μL.[30] Mechanisms that affect the 1-hour posttransfusion incre-

$$\text{CCI} = \frac{(\text{Platelet increment}) \times (\text{Body surface area})}{\text{Platelets transfused} \times 10^{11}}$$

$$\text{MPI} = \frac{(\text{Platelets transfused} \times 10^{11}) \times (\text{Sequestration factor})}{\text{Blood volume}}$$

$$\text{PPR} = \frac{\text{Platelet increment}}{\text{MPI}} \text{ or } \frac{\text{Total peripheral radioactivity identifiable}}{\text{Total radioactivity infused}}$$

Figure 1-1. Formulas used to compare quantitative responses with platelet transfusions; see text for details.
CCI = corrected count increment; MPI = maximal platelet increment; PPR = percent platelet recovery

ment may differ significantly from those that affect the 24-hour posttransfusion increment.

Finally, countable platelets are not necessarily functional platelets, and vice versa. Platelets in a uremic environment are countable but dysfunctional, whereas the platelet-derived microparticles that make up a significant proportion (25%) of the total platelet surface area in a dose of platelets are functional but not countable.[31] Recently, platelet membrane microvesicles have been shown to limit bleeding in cardiopulmonary bypass patients as well as in animals.[32,33] For all these reasons, simply evaluating the quantitative response to platelet transfusion does not fully assess the efficacy of the transfusion. Strauss notes that "the calculated CCI value can be excellent and convey the appearance of a desirable response, despite a very poor posttransfusion platelet count."[29(p126)] Yet, that value may fail "to accurately reflect the magnitude of risk for thrombocytopenic bleeding." Achieving hemostasis during hemorrhage is a direct way to measure response to transfusion. The prevention of hemorrhage can be directly measured, but this requires controlled study for meaningful data. Assessment of platelet transfusion efficacy is usually limited to laboratory testing and utilization review activities.

Platelet refractoriness is one of the more common and difficult clinical conditions in which to assess the efficacy of platelet transfusion. In this condition, the posttransfusion survival of donor platelets is insufficient to provide the adequate levels perceived necessary for prophylaxis against hemorrhage, and additional platelet doses do not significantly increase the circulating platelet count. Platelet refractoriness can be the net result of a variety of independent and coincident factors.[34,35] In most centers, patients can be readily identified who exhibit poor CCIs despite no definable risk factors, but who can achieve higher raw increments and also higher CCIs with higher doses of platelets. Perhaps the baseline platelet loss to "fix the leaks of everyday existence" is increased in these patients, or else there is a greater degree of sequestration.

One of the many reasons for refractoriness is alloimmunization; other reasons include clinical factors (eg, fever, sepsis, neutropenia, splenomegaly, disseminated intravascular coagulation [DIC]), blood bank factors (eg, ABO mismatch, HLA mismatch, storage conditions), and patient-related factors (eg, age, gender, marrow transplantion, administration of amphotericin or intravenous immune globulin [IVIG]). Yet the simple presence or absence of these factors does not necessarily equate with refractoriness. The distinction between refractoriness and alloimmunization is important because, unlike refractoriness based on some clinical condition, true alloimmunization in the absence of relevant clinical factors can often be circumvented by the appropriate selection of platelets.[34,36] For example, platelet crossmatching is of benefit only when antibody-mediated clearance is the cause of the refractoriness; it provides no benefit in circumventing alloimmunization when refractoriness is due to splenomegaly or DIC. Indeed, the effective management of clinically important refractoriness requires the identification of the significant causative etiologic factors, recognizing that those factors can be multiple and independent.[34] Heddle and Blajchman point out that there are no formal studies to validate the correlation of bleeding with platelet refractoriness.[37] Many stable oncology patients maintain platelet counts below 20,000µL without either significant bleeding or adequate posttransfusion increments.[9,16-18] If these patients do not need to be transfused with platelets, the problem of refractoriness for them may be moot. Indeed, given that most platelets are transfused for prophylaxis, a large part of the platelet refractoriness problem may simply be an attempt to treat a number rather than a clinical condition.[2,38] If the goal of platelet transfusion is to prevent or correct hemorrhage, the relevant clinical outcome metric should relate to days of hemorrhage or fatalities due to hemorrhage and not simply to platelet count or posttransfusion platelet increment.

Specific Clinical Settings

Platelet transfusion therapy has proven itself of great benefit in reducing the mortality associated with hemorrhage from thrombocytopenia. There are risks associated with this therapy, however, as well as controversies regarding its appropriate use. Because of the requisite collection, storage, and processing conditions and the associated risk of bacterial contamination, platelets can involve considerable risk for the transfusion recipient. Moreover, the role of prophylactic platelet transfusion is made less clear by the lack of a well-defined correlation between platelet levels and the risk of hemorrhage. A true consensus has yet to be reached regarding the appropriate indications for platelet transfusion. Guidelines should guide (not dictate) practice, and specific clinical situations will always demand consideration of the immediate clinical circumstances. For example, the specific platelet dysfunction needs to be considered in order to understand the role of platelet transfusion. Platelet disorders can be qualitative (thrombocytopathy) or quantitative (thrombocytopenia). Thrombocytopathy can be congenital or acquired. Congenital causes include von Willebrand disease, Bernard-Soulier syndrome, and Glanzmann's thrombasthenia. Acquired causes can be pharmacologic (eg, heparin, aspirin), mechanical (eg, cardiopulmonary bypass), or clinical (eg, uremia). Thrombocytopenia can be due to increased destruction, decreased production, sequestration, or dilution of platelets. Increased platelet destruction may be immune [eg, idiopathic thrombocytopenic purpura (ITP), neonatal alloimmune thrombocytopenia (NAIT)] or nonimmune [eg, DIC, thrombotic thrombocytopenic purpura (TTP), hemolytic-uremic syndrome (HUS)]. The literature provides some assistance in determining the appropriate indications for platelet transfusion in each of these clinical settings.

Cardiopulmonary Bypass

Patients undergoing cardiopulmonary bypass have a number of stresses placed on both the formed elements and the free components of their blood. The extracorporeal circuit is composed of tubing that carries the venous blood to the system, an oxygenator, a pump to assist in blood flow, and further tubing that returns the blood to the arterial circulation. In addition, other devices, such as counterpulsation balloons and ventricular assist devices, are often used to assist in circulation. All such devices have thrombogenic synthetic surfaces, which require systemic anticoagulation to control thrombus generation and the consequent risk of thromboembolization. The mechanical effects of pumps and the effects of flow and surface interaction also have an impact on formed elements in the blood, especially platelets. Altogether, these stresses may lead to intra- and postoperative hemorrhage, with the potential for significant clinical and fiscal consequences.

For those patients undergoing their first cardiac surgery, the frequency of postoperative bleeding is 3-5%.[39] Patients undergoing complex surgery with prolonged extracorporeal circuit time may be at increased risk for postoperative bleeding. A number of factors are responsible for postoperative bleeding, including consumption of coagulation factors, initiation of fibrinolysis, and a reduction in both platelet number and function.[39] Platelet-related coagulopathies can be divided into effects on platelet number and effects on platelet function. Hemodilution and consumption are primarily responsible for the intra- and postoperative reduction in platelet number. Hemodilution occurs when the patient's blood is diluted with the priming fluid necessary to complete the extracorporeal circuit. Platelets may adhere to the nonendothelial surfaces of the circuit, thereby also reducing the circulating number. Some platelets are lost as a result of mechanical damage or activation by the oxygenator or pump. All these factors contribute to the decrease in platelet count, which routinely occurs within minutes following initiation of extracorporeal bypass.[40] The actual decrease may be as much as 40-60%. After the initial drop, the platelet count commonly stabilizes in the range of 100,000/μL during the procedure. This postoperative thrombocytopenia can persist for days.[39,41,42]

The remaining platelets are often dysfunctional, at least in terms of aggregability, adenosine diphosphate (ADP) release, and adhesiveness. A number of factors may contribute to this platelet dysfunction.[40-51] Kestin et al have suggested factors extrinsic to the platelet are primarily responsible for platelet dysfunction.[43] The extracorporeal circulation requires high-dose heparinization, which has both proaggregatory and inhibitory effects.[45] Protamine sulfate neutralization of heparin anticoagulation can damage platelets.[39] Intraoperative hypothermia can also diminish platelet activity.[46-48] Other possible etiologies include alpha-granule secretion due to platelet activation from the mechanical effects of the extracorporeal circuit and plasmin-mediated degradation of platelet membrane receptors.[49] Circulating fibrin degradation products may also inhibit platelet function,[50] as do drugs commonly used in cardiac patients, such as aspirin, nonsteroidal anti-inflammatory drugs, and heparin.[51]

Controlled prospective studies have shown no correlation between platelet counts and bleeding following cardiopulmonary bypass. A 1986 consensus conference on platelet transfusion therapy concluded that there is no detectable benefit from prophylactic platelet transfusion and that thrombocytopenia alone is not a justification for the therapy.[52] A study by Simon et al noted that prophylactic administration of platelets at the end of cardiopulmonary bypass prevented the prolongation of bypass-related bleeding time but did not affect chest tube drainage, transfusion requirements, or clinical outcome.[53] Tobe et al found no added value to the postoperative prophylactic infusion of autologous platelet-rich plasma in a prospective, randomized, double-blind study.[54] Daszynski and Ciszewski concluded that platelet transfusions should be given for cardiopulmonary bypass patients for the same indications that are applied to any surgical or hemorrhagic situation.[41] They also felt that platelet support in these patients was indicated for excessive bleeding with a platelet count below 50-60,000/μL.

Alternative therapies exist in the case of postoperative bleeding. In a double-blind, prospective, randomized trial, (desamino-8-D-arginine vasopressin, or desmopressin acetate) significantly reduced mean intraoperative and early postoperative blood loss.[55] Other studies dispute the effectiveness of DDAVP and warn of its thrombogenic potential.[56,57] The bovine proteinase inhibitor aprotinin is a potent antifibrinolytic agent with high affinity for plasmin. Aprotinin may preserve platelet function and thus control postoperative bleeding by inhibiting plasmin-mediated platelet damage or kallikrein. It is especially useful in patients undergoing repeat or complex operations, who are more likely to develop postoperative bleeding.[58,59]

Overall, platelet transfusion therapy in the setting of cardiopulmonary bypass must take into consideration the evolving patient condition. Because dysfunctional platelets are still countable, the platelet count alone cannot serve as the sole indication for platelet transfusion. Cardiopulmonary bypass itself may induce a thrombocytopathy, as can many of the pharmacologic agents employed. Postcardiopulmonary bypass patients with platelet-deficient bleeding may require platelet transfusions to control hemorrhage; however, any thrombocytopathy-inducing agents can also render the transfused platelets dysfunctional. Transfused platelets are of little to no benefit when hemorrhage is not due to small vessel injury or oozing.

Massive Transfusion

Massive transfusion has been arbitrarily defined as replacement of one blood volume (8-10 units) in less than 24 hours. Alternative definitions include replacement of more than 50% of blood volume in less than 3 hours, or transfusion of more than 20 units of packed RBCs. Crosson has suggested that the term be used to describe blood replacement in any patient requiring four units of red cells within 1 hour, with anticipation of ongoing usage.[60] Massive transfusion is typically seen in the treatment of acute hypovolemia due to hemorrhage resulting from trauma or surgical, obstetric, or gastrointestinal complications. The initial priority in the management of these situations is to maintain intravascular volume and oxygen-carrying capacity in an effort to maintain tissue perfusion and oxygenation. The loss of up to 75% of a patient's red blood cells can be tolerated, but the loss of greater than 30% of intravascular volume usually is not well tolerated and can result in a significant decrease in tissue perfusion. Maintenance of hemostasis, electrolyte balance, and colloid osmotic pressure are next-level priorities.

Hemostatic abnormalities may occur as a result of tissue hypoperfusion and the subsequent effects of tissue damage such as DIC. Abnormal hemostasis may also be secondary to dilutional effects from the replacement of lost blood with RBCs and crystalloid. Ideally, and in keeping with the age-old surgeon's maxim "patients bleed whole blood," blood lost from acute hemorrhage would be replaced with fresh, warm whole blood as this would deliver coagulation factors as well as platelets. Stored whole blood is not functionally equivalent to fresh, warm whole blood. However, fresh, warm whole blood transfusion is hampered by coagulation factor and platelet storage instability, potentially severe hyperkalemia, and availability. Thus, blood component replacement is more commonly practiced today, with the usual products being packed RBCs to treat reduced oxygen-carrying capacity, crystalloid/colloid to replace volume, and FFP to replenish coagulation factors.

Thrombocytopenia is variable but may be the earliest and most severe coagulation abnormality detected, perhaps related to the effects of perfusion disturbances on the microvasculature. Thrombocytopenia can occur as a result of hemodilution with crystalloid, colloid, or RBCs, or secondarily through consumption. Faringer et al report the development of coagulopathy in more than 70% of trauma patients who have been given more than 10 units of packed RBCs.[61] The most common abnormality found was a platelet count of less than 100,000/μL. In a retrospective study, Wilson et al describe platelet counts below 50,000/μL in 50% of patients receiving more than 20 units of RBCs in 24 hours.[62] Harrigan et al report low platelet counts in addition to prolonged bleeding times in patients requiring more than 20 units of RBCs.[63] The platelet counts dropped through the second and third postoperative day, and began to rise by day 4. The identification of a prolonged bleeding time in thrombocytopenic patients is not by itself an indication to transfuse platelets. Indeed, the bleeding time is linearly correlated with the platelet count below 100,000/μL so that a "normal" bleeding time for a platelet count of 50,000/μL is 17.5 minutes.[64] A prolonged bleeding time in a thrombocytopenic massive transfusion patient only serves to confirm the low platelet count and does not add any clinical information. Patients with thrombocytopenia may also develop diffuse microvascular bleeding (DMB) as opposed to the frank bleeding that occurs at the initial site. To result in DMB, the platelet count is usually less than 50,000/μL, a level not usually seen until 1.5 to 2.0 blood volumes have been replaced.

Different recommendations have been made regarding platelet replacement in the patient receiving massive transfusion, but most feel that one standard "dose" should be given when the platelet count falls below 50,000/μL. Faringer et al recommend that, for those patients with severe penetrating trauma, platelet transfusion be delayed until there is evidence of DMB.[61] They do, however, recommend prophylactic transfusions in the event of blunt trauma or brain injury. Ciavarella et al recommend prophylactic transfusion when platelets are less than 50,000/μL in the absence of DMB as platelet counts correlate highly with DMB in trauma and surgical patients.[65] However, Reed et al indicate that prophylactic platelet transfusion is not warranted to prevent microvascular bleeding.[66] They report that a prospective randomized double-blind study of prophylactic transfusion of 6 platelet concentrates vs 2 units of FFP for every 12 RBC units transfused showed no additional hemostatic benefit for platelets and no difference in the incidence of DMB.[66] An often overlooked fact is that since platelets are stored and transfused in plasma, a 200- to 300-mL platelet transfusion also includes a unit of plasma. Contrary to widely held beliefs, coagulation factor levels are reasonably well-maintained in platelet concentrates. Thus, transfusion of a dose of platelets also transfuses much of the coagulation factor activity of a unit of plasma. Fibrinogen and Factors II, VII, IX, X, XI, and XII all remain at 85% or greater throughout 3 days of storage at standard room temperature. Factor VIII decreases only to 70% and Factor V to 50% over the same timespan.[67] Therefore, transfused platelets not only help maintain the circulating platelet level but also provide a significant source of coagulation factors. A common rule of thumb without solid scientific support is to transfuse with one dose of platelets for every 10-20 RBC units given. This may help to limit DMB; however, it is less useful for gross hemorrhage, which will likely require mechanical intervention.

Platelet levels may be followed by monitoring platelet counts, but transfusion should also be based on evidence of clinical microvascular bleeding. Counts et al report that platelet counts are the most useful screening test but recommend that platelets be transfused only if evidence of DMB is present.[68] After transfusion, platelet counts may not achieve the levels expected given the degree of dilution. This may be due to splenic sequestration secondary to cotransfused microaggregates. Newer therapeutic options include the use of prostaglandin E1, reported by Locker et al, to prevent a reduction in platelet count, possibly through decreased platelet aggregation.[69] Yet, as mentioned previously, platelet count is independent of function. Ferrara et al report that many patients who were hypothermic or acidotic developed clinically significant bleeding despite adequate replacement therapy.[47] Valeri et al report reversible platelet dysfunction in hypothermic baboons, which they believe was due to the temperature-dependent production of thromboxane B2.[48] Therefore, blood and patient warmers may be indicated. Additional laboratory studies that should be followed include prothrombin time, activated partial thromboplastin time, and the use of fibrinogen, as these will help to indicate the need for FFP or the advent of DIC.

Disseminated Intravascular Coagulation

DIC was first described by Landois in 1875 after hyalin thrombi were found in the mesentery of dogs injected with human blood (reviewed in Hardaway and Williams[70]). Schneider later described the presence of fibrin clots in the microcirculation of the lung as a result of placenta abruptio (reviewed in Hardaway and Williams[70]). DIC is not a disorder that stands alone but rather is a process associated with a number of disorders, including shock (notably septic and traumatic), hemolysis, late pregnancy complications, extracorporeal circulation, snake bite, hypothermia, hyperthermia, burns, infections, and malignancy. The basic pathophysiology is a consumptive coagulopathy with excessive concurrent fibrinolysis. The clotting cascade is activated, resulting in the formation of thrombin; this leads to further activation of the clotting cascade with deposition of fibrin in the microcirculation and consumption of hemostatic elements. Meanwhile, the fibrinolytic pathway is also activated, leading to further consumption of hemostatic and fibrinolytic factors as well as of the regulatory proteinase inhibitors. Bick defines the minimal acceptable criteria for DIC as a systemic thrombohemorrhagic disorder seen in well-defined clinical situations, with laboratory evidence for inhibitor consumption, fibrinolytic activation, procoagulant activation, and evidence of end-organ failure or damage.[71]

The clinical effects of DIC are quite variable. In some patients, a low-grade DIC can be detected by laboratory values but no clinical effects may be evident. In the more extreme clinical picture, frank hemorrhage, multiple organ failure, thrombosis, or hemolytic anemia may be present. In the presence of endotoxin, platelet adhesiveness may increase with subsequent clumping. Thrombocytopenia is commonly present, as is prolonged prothrombin time and activated partial thromboplastin time. Treatment is primarily targeted at the underlying disorder. Pharmacologic interventions that may be useful include vitamin K administration to replete stores lost as a result of increased consumption, folic acid administration to prevent acute folate deficiency with impaired platelet production, and, in certain specific circumstances, heparin.[72] Replacement of lost blood components is recommended only if the patient is bleeding or if an invasive procedure is required.[72,73] Staudinger et al suggest that a platelet count of less than 20,000/μL should result in platelet transfusion and that any count below 50,000/μL may warrant transfusion because of possible platelet dysfunction.[74] Platelet transfusions are generally considered safe in patients with ongoing DIC.[71] However, platelet transfusions alone will not correct DIC; for that, the underlying disorder must be corrected.

Uremia

Patients with renal failure have multiple factors that contribute to impaired hemostasis—namely, coagulation factor deficiencies and anemia, as well as thrombocytopenia and platelet dysfunction. Thrombocytopenia may be present, but platelet counts may also be normal. However, independent of any quantitative thrombocytopenia, uremic patients manifest a thrombocytopathy. Platelet function defects include decreased adhesion, decreased platelet membrane procoagulant activity, decreased dense granule serotonin and ADP content, decreased platelet thromboxane generation, increased endothelial cell prostacyclin generation, and increased endothelial-derived relaxing factor.[75-77] These defects are felt to be the result of reduced clearance of metabolites such as guanido-succinic acid and phenols.

As the presence of these compounds on the platelet is believed to be the cause of the platelet dysfunction, platelet transfusion would introduce healthy platelets into a poisonous environment and thus provide only limited benefits. However, it is not absolutely contraindicated. Hemodialysis may have the greatest effect on platelet function, but transfusion with packed RBCs to a hematocrit of 26-30% may also help to improve platelet adhesion by the mechanical effect of displacing platelets toward the vessel walls.[76,78,79] Hemodialysis is usually performed with heparin, which itself can result in thrombocytopenia[80]; to reduce this risk, hemodialysis can also be performed with citrate or prostacyclin.[81,82] DDAVP and cryoprecipitate can temporarily correct a uremia-induced prolonged bleeding time and may help correct surgical bleeding in uremic patients.[83] Conjugated estrogens have been shown to decrease bleeding time for a prolonged period.[76] As with DIC, correction of the underlying disorder is most beneficial in correcting the patient's coagulopathy.

Hepatopathy

Because the liver is responsible for producing a number of clotting factors and regulatory proteins, disorders of hemostasis are commonly seen in liver disease. Not only can hepatocellular disease result in quantitatively and qualitatively abnormal clotting factors, but also thrombocytopenia can occur as a result of DIC, decreased thrombocytopoiesis, or possibly immune-mediated destruction of platelets.[84,85] Viral effects on megakaryocytes or platelets and decreased synthesis of platelet maturation factors (eg, thrombopoietin) may be responsible for decreased thrombopoiesis. Besides the potential for hemorrhagic consequences, however, the clinical importance of thrombocytopenia in hepatocellular disease is minimal.[84,85]

Cirrhosis can result in both thrombocytopenia and thrombocytopathy. Portal hypertension can lead to splenomegaly with increased splenic sequestration of platelets. Platelet aggregation may be diminished as a result of impaired signal transmission across the platelet membrane or the effects of alcohol, high-density lipoprotein abnormalities, fibrin split products, or medications.[84] On the other hand, platelet aggregation may be enhanced by increased circulating von Willebrand factor, platelet membrane phospholipid alteration, and platelet activation. Thrombocytopenia, along with the quantitative and qualitative coagulation factor defects in liver disease, results in a severe hemorrhagic tendency in affected patients. If invasive procedures are planned in this patient population or if there is clinical evidence of bleeding, Pereira et al recommend platelet transfusion when platelet counts are less than 50,000/µL.[86] If surgery is planned, a prolonged prothrombin time is present, or there is evidence of a platelet-deficient bleeding,[75] Humphries suggests transfusion when platelets are less than 80,000/µL. As with DIC and uremia, correction of the underlying disorder is most beneficial in correcting the patient's coagulopathy.

Congenital Disorders of Platelet Function

Congenital disorders of platelet function can be categorized according to disorders within the platelet (secretion defects) or interactions with other platelets, vessel walls, platelet agonists, or coagulation factors. These disorders encompass a wide variety of clinical manifestations, with effects ranging from minimal to severe bleeding. When present, symptoms usually include easy bruisability and oozing from mucous membranes, but patients may also present with severe bleeding following minor invasive events such as dental or obstetric procedures. The bleeding time is usually prolonged because of platelet dysfunction but the platelet count is generally normal.[87-89] Treatment of these disorders requires supportive care and, if possible, the use of pharmacologic agents such as DDAVP to improve hemostasis.

Congenital disorders of platelet function may be thought of as having intrinsic or extrinsic defects. Disorders such as von Willebrand disease comprise extrinsic defects that involve humoral factors in the plasma. These disorders can be treated with plasma products, but platelet transfusions generally have little, if any, benefit as platelet function depends on these humoral factors. Intrinsic platelet disorders may benefit from platelet transfusions, however, as such transfusions provide functional platelets. The clinical severity of the bleeding determines the need for platelet transfusion. In instances where platelet surface factors may be deficient, such as in Bernard-Soulier syndrome or Glanzmann's thrombasthenia, transfusions should be limited to significant hemorrhagic events or surgical procedures. The absence of specific factors, especially the platelet-specific antigens, on the platelet surface may predispose the patient to alloimmunization upon repeated transfusions. Therefore, antigen-matched or limited donor transfusions are recommended if available to reduce the risk of alloimmunization.[88-91] Patients with Glanzmann's thrombasthenia may have the additional complication of endogenous platelets interfering with the aggregation of normal transfused platelets, thereby requiring a higher number of circulating platelets to correct the prolonged bleeding time.[90]

Autoimmune Thrombocytopenia

ITP, or autoimmune thrombocytopenic purpura, is a disorder of accelerated platelet destruction. This destruction is mediated by platelet antibodies that bind to platelet antigens by the F_{ab} portion of the antibody molecule, with subsequent destruction of the sensitized platelets believed to occur predominantly in the spleen. Most autoantibodies are IgG and bind platelets via GPIIb/IIIa. Childhood ITP is classically acute and spontaneously remits within 1-6 months. Most adult ITP, on the other hand, is chronic and predominantly affects females of childbearing potential. Treatment options typically include the use of corticosteroids and/or IVIG as a first-line treatment, with the use of vinca alkaloids such as vincristine or vinblastine, or more recently intravenous anti-D immunoglobulin IV, as subsequent agents in refractory patients. Should these measures bring no response, the alternative treatment usually consists of splenectomy.

Platelet transfusion has a limited role in the treatment of ITP as this is an autoimmune disorder manifesting itself through increased platelet destruction. Compensatory platelet production is typically increased, as demonstrated by the increase in marrow megakaryocytes. Platelet transfusions may be indicated in these patients, however, when clinically significant bleeding occurs and a response from immune modulating treatments has yet to be achieved. Carr et al retrospectively evaluated 11 ITP patients for response to platelet transfusion and found that immediate posttransfusion platelet count increments of 20,000/μL or more occurred in 13 of 31 (42%) platelet transfusions.[92] Seven of the 11 patients had at least one successful transfusion, success being defined as an increment increase of 20,000/μL or as recovery of at least 20% of the transfused platelets. Five of the 13 cases showed the count increments to persist at 24 hours. Three patients had active bleeding described as wet purpura (gingival bleeding, epistaxis, guaiac positive stools, hematuria, or menorrhagia), which responded to platelet transfusion, although only two of the three had increased platelet count increments. Baumann et al showed an immediate sustained increase in platelet count by giving a single 400-mg/kg dose of IVIG prior to platelet transfusion in six patients, and they concluded that this may be useful in patients who require urgent increases in platelet counts for surgical preparation or to control bleeding.[93] It should be noted that a firm diagnosis of ITP should be made before platelets are given in this setting. Thrombocytopenia secondary to thrombotic thrombocytopenic purpura (TTP) or heparin-induced purpura must be excluded as platelet transfusions are typically contraindicated in these settings.

Neonatal Alloimmune Thrombocytopenia

Neonatal alloimmune thrombocytopenia (NAIT) pathophysiologically resembles hemolytic disease of the newborn, with maternal alloimmunization against fetal platelet antigens [typically HPA-1a (Pl^{A1})]. The IgG antibodies that are produced transfer across the placenta, where they bind to fetal platelets and result in reticuloendothelial clearance. The incidence is approximately 1 in 3000-5000 live births, and firstborn infants can be affected. Mortality reaches 15%, with most of the morbidity due to CNS hemorrhage, which occurs in 20% of cases (half in utero).[94] Platelet transfusions are indicated for platelet counts of less than 30,000/μL and/or for clinically significant bleeding.[95] As antigen-typed platelets may be difficult to obtain, the mother is usually used as the donor (by definition antigen-negative). Platelets must be gamma irradiated to prevent graft-vs-host disease and must be washed to remove platelet antibody. If the mother is unable to donate platelets and type-specific platelets are not available, it may be necessary to give random-donor platelets with the concomitant administration of IVIG.

Posttransfusion Purpura

Posttransfusion purpura (PTP) is a rare and sudden acute thrombocytopenia (typically less than 10,000/μL) that occurs 7-10 days following the transfusion of plasma-containing blood products.[96,97] Most recipients are Pl^{A1} (HPA-1a)-negative individuals who mount an immune response to soluble Pl^{A1} antigen in the transfused plasma. Patients are predominantly parous females, indicating an anamnestic response to Pl^{A1} initially seen in pregnancy. In posttransfusion purpura, endogenous platelets are also destroyed even though they are Pl^{A1}-negative. The disorder usually resolves within 10-14 days if there is no fatal complication. When necessary, treatment options are limited to IVIG, plasmapheresis, and platelet transfusions if necessary. Transfusion practice is usually geared to limit repeat exposure to soluble Pl^{A1} antigen in plasma. Treatment is otherwise supportive.

Thrombotic Thrombocytopenic Purpura/Hemolytic-Uremic Syndrome (TTP/HUS)

TTP is an uncommon disorder that was initially described in 1924.[98] A 16-year-old female with no previous history presented with fever, anemia, weakness, and petechiae. Urinalysis noted trace albumin with granular and hyaline casts. Within the week, she developed hemiparesis and died. The disorder is characterized by intravascular platelet aggregation and consequent marked consumptive thrombocytopenia, with widespread thrombotic occlusion of arterioles and capillaries. The net result is a fluctuating ischemia or infarction of various end organs, especially the CNS and kidneys. The classic findings are often referred to as a pentad (only if end-organ ischemia counts as two), including 1) microangiopathic direct antibody test-negative (Coombs' negative) hemolytic anemia with schistocytosis and elevated lactate dehydrogenase, 2) moderate to severe thrombocytopenia, 3) fever, 4) CNS dysfunction, and 5) acute renal failure. Only 40% of patients will have all five findings at any one time.[99]

Whereas TTP is classically thought of as having CNS signs predominating, hemolytic uremic syndrome (HUS) is a related disorder with predominantly renal findings. The pathogenesis of TTP/HUS involves vascular occlusion of the microcirculation by platelet aggregates. Histologic findings include platelet and fibrin thrombi occluding small arteries and arterioles.

Thrombi are evident in glomerular capillaries with strong staining for von Willebrand factor but only weak staining for fibrinogen. Postulated pathological mechanisms result in platelet aggregation, endothelial adherence, microvascular obstruction, and mechanical hemolysis. Although it is not clear whether the initial event is platelet activation or endothelial cell injury, the end result is platelet consumption and widespread deposition of thrombi throughout the vasculature. These occlusions lead directly to capillary bed and end-organ damage. Untreated, TTP/HUS is highly fatal.

The principal treatment for TTP/HUS is plasmapheresis.[100-102] Bell et al showed a 90% survival rate when plasmapheresis was combined with corticosteroids.[101] Platelet transfusions are contraindicated, however. Harkness et al described a patient with TTP who was given platelets and rapidly had a CNS event. Autopsy revealed significant formation of platelet aggregates and multiple thrombi in the microcirculation, most notably in the brain.[103] Gordon et al described two patients with similar outcomes upon platelet transfusion.[104] The risk appears to be further generation of platelet aggregates, so platelet transfusion is contraindicated in platelet-mediated microangiopathy.[99]

Summary

Improvement in the quality of the scientific evidence begins with a conceptual change in the role of platelets. Platelets should be thought of not as hemostatic agents, but rather as human biologic products designed for deficit replacement therapy. Simply having more platelets does not necessarily mean having more hemostasis. For someone else's platelets to be of benefit, patients should be deficient in their own platelet number or function. There are a number of recognized indications for platelet transfusion; the principal indication is severe thrombocytopenia or thrombocytopathy.[11,12,14,19,52,105] The most frequently encountered uses are the treatment of thrombocytopenic bleeding, the prevention of spontaneous hemorrhage associated with low platelet counts, and the provision of "coverage" for invasive procedures during thrombocytopenia.[10] Platelets may also be indicated to correct thrombocytopathic conditions, which can be either congenital (eg, von Willebrand disease, Bernard-Soulier syndrome) or acquired (eg, iatrogenic, aspirin, uremia, drug-induced, mechanical, post-cardiopulmonary bypass). The chief difficulty for these indications, aside from the paucity of data in support of platelet transfusion efficacy, is that many of these conditions will affect the transfused platelets as well as the patient's own. Platelets may be used in the treatment of clinical conditions that are associated with a consumptive coagulopathy, such as DIC, liver disease, and liver transplantation. In these conditions, platelet transfusion has but a temporizing effect while control of hemorrhagic risk depends on correcting the underlying disorder. The effectiveness of prophylactic platelet transfusion in these settings has not been widely studied, and unless the patient is at a definable risk, it is difficult to support the continued transfusion of platelets to treat a purely quantitative disorder. Appropriate judgment is based on the individual patient's clinical condition and knowledge of the inherent risks. In and of itself, platelet transfusion is not without significant risk and, in some situations, may only serve to exacerbate the true problem.

References

1. Wallace EL, Churchill WH, Surgenor DM, et al. Collection and transfusion of blood and blood components in the United States, 1992. Transfusion 1995;35:802-12.
2. Hersh EM, Bodey GP, Nies BA, Freirich EJ. Causes of death in acute leukemia: A ten-year study of 414 patients from 1954-1963. JAMA 1965;193:99-103.
3. Gaydos LA, Freirich EJ, Mantel N. The quantitative relation between platelet count and hemorrhage in patients with acute leukemia. N Engl J Med 1962;266:905-9.
4. Higby DJ. The prophylactic treatment of thrombocytopenic leukemic patients with platelets: A double-blind study. Transfusion 1974; 14:440-6.
5. Slichter SJ, Harker LA. Thrombocytopenia: Mechanisms and management of defects in platelet production. Clin Haematol 1978; 7:523-39.
6. Ilet SJ, Lilleyman JS. Platelet transfusion requirements of children with newly diagnosed lymphoblastic leukemia. Acta Haematol 1979;62:86-9.
7. Murphy S, Litwin S, Herring LM, et al. Indications for platelet transfusion in children with acute leukemia. Am J Hematol 1982; 12:347-56.
8. Patten E, Toy P. Prophylactic platelet transfusion policies (abstract). Blood 1988;72(suppl 1):283a.
9. Gmur J, Burger J, Schanz U, et al. Safety of stringent prophylactic platelet transfusion policy for patients with acute leukemia. Lancet 1991;338:1223-6.

10. Pisciotto PT, Benson K, Hume H, et al. Prophylactic versus therapeutic platelet transfusion practices in hematology and/or oncology patients. Transfusion 1995;35:498-502.
11. Beutler E. Platelet transfusions: The 20,000/μL trigger. Blood 1993; 81:1411-3.
12. Baer MR, Bloomfield CD. Controversies in transfusion medicine. Prophylactic platelet transfusion therapy: Pro. Transfusion 1992; 32:377-80.
13. Bishop JF, Schiffer CA, Aisner J, et al. Surgery in acute leukemia: A review of 167 operations in thrombocytopenic patients. Am J Hematol 1987;26:147-55.
14. Belt RJ, Leite C, Haas CD, Stephens RL. Incidence of hemorrhagic complications in patients with cancer. JAMA 1978;239:2571-4.
15. Morrow JF, Braine HG, Kickler TS, et al. Septic reactions to platelet transfusions. JAMA 1991;266:555-8.
16. Solomon J, Bofenkamp T, Fahey JL, et al. Platelet prophylaxis in acute non-lymphoblastic leukemia (letter). Lancet 1978;1:267.
17. Rebulla P, Finazzi G, Marangoni F, et al. The threshold for prophylactic platelet transfusions in adults with acute myeloid leukemia. N Engl J Med 1997;337:1870-5.
18. del Rosario MLU, Kao KJ. Determination of the rate of reduction in platelet counts in recipients of hematopoietic stem and progenitor cell transplant: Clinical implications for platelet transfusion therapy. Transfusion 1998;37:1163-8.
19. Schiffer CA. Prophylactic platelet transfusion. Transfusion 1992; 32:295-8.
20. Freirich EJ, Kliman A, Gaydos LA, et al. Response to repeated platelet transfusion from the same donor. Ann Intern Med 1963; 59:277-87.
21. Djerassi I, Farber S, Evans AE. Transfusions of fresh platelet concentrates to patients with secondary thrombocytopenia. N Engl J Med 1963;268:221-6.
22. Roy AJ, Jaffe N, Djerassi I. Prophylactic platelet transfusion in children with acute leukemia: A dose response survey. Transfusion 1973;13:283-90.
23. Kiss JE, Steer K, Triulzi DJ, Winkelstein A. Transfusion response to "standard" dose and high yield single donor platelets (abstract). Transfusion 1993;33(suppl):45.

24. Norol F, Duedari N, Kuentz CM, Vernant JP. Comparison of different doses of platelet transfusion (abstract). Blood 1995;86:353a.
25. Benson K, Martinez S, Tolzmann L, Leparc G. Split vs whole apheresis platelets: Clinical response in thrombocytopenic patients (abstract). Transfusion 1996;36(suppl):45.
26. Menitove JE, Hertenstein EG, Tse LC. Decreasing platelet concentrate dose: Impact on platelet transfusion interval (abstract). Blood 1996;88:333a.
27. Herman JH, Klumpp TR, Christman RA, et al. The effect of platelet dose on the outcome of prophylactic platelet transfusion (abstract). Transfusion. 1995;35(suppl):46S.
28. Ackerman SJ, Klumpp TR, Herman JH, et al. Cost analysis of higher-dose versus lower-dose single donor platelet transfusions in peripheral blood stem cell and bone marrow transplant (abstract). Blood 1996;88:333a.
29. Strauss RG. Clinical perspectives of platelet transfusions: Defining the optimal dose. J Clin Apheresis 1995;10:124-7.
30. Hanson SR, Slichter SJ. Platelet kinetics in patients with bone marrow hypoplasia: Evidence for a fixed platelet requirement. Blood 1985;66:1105-9.
31. Tans G, Rosing R, Christella M, et al. Comparison of anticoagulant and procoagulant activities of stimulated platelet and platelet-derived microparticles. Blood 1991;77:2641-8.
32. Sloand E, Alyono D, Yu M, Klein H. Platelet membrane glycoproteins and microvesicles in blood from postoperative salvage: A study in cardiac bypass patients. Transfusion 1995;35:738-44.
33. Chao FC, Kim BK, Houranieh AM, et al. Infusible platelet membrane microvesicles: A potential transfusion substitute for platelets. Transfusion 1996;36:536-42.
34. Friedberg RC, Donnelly SF, Boyd JC, et al. Clinical and blood bank factors in the management of platelet refractoriness and alloimmunization. Blood 1993;81:3428-34.
35. Friedberg RC. Clinical and laboratory factors underlying refractoriness to platelet transfusions. J Clin Apheresis 1996;11:143-8.
36. Friedberg RC, Donnelly SF, Mintz PD. Independent roles for platelet crossmatching and HLA in the selection of platelets for alloimmunized patients. Transfusion 1994;34:215-20.

37. Heddle NM, Blajchman MA. The leukodepletion of cellular blood products in the prevention of HLA-alloimmunization and refractoriness to allogeneic platelet transfusions. Blood 1995;85:603-6.
38. Friedberg RC, Mintz PD. Causes of refractoriness to platelet transfusion. Curr Opin Hematol 1995;2:193-8.
39. Woodman RC, Harker LA. Bleeding complications associated with cardiopulmonary bypass. Blood 1990;76:1680-97.
40. Harker LA, Malpass TW, Branson HE, et al. Mechanism of abnormal bleeding in patients undergoing cardiopulmonary bypass: Acquired transient platelet dysfunction associated with selective a-granule release. Blood 1980;56:824-34.
41. Daszynski J, Ciszewski T. Blood component therapy in open heart surgery. Materia Medica Polona 1989;3:207-11.
42. Moriau M, Masure R, Hurlet A, et al. Haemostasis disorders in open heart surgery with extracorporeal circulation. Vox Sang 1977;32: 41-51.
43. Kestin AS, Valeri CR, Khuri SF, et al. The platelet function defect of cardiopulmonary bypass. Blood 1993;82:107-17.
44. Michelson AD, Benoit SE, Barnard MR, et al. Platelet aggregation abnormalities after cardiopulmonary bypass. Blood 1994;83:299-306.
45. John LCH, Rees GM, Kovacs IB. Inhibition of platelet function by heparin. An etiologic factor in postbypass hemorrhage. J Thorac Cardiovasc Surg 1993;105:816-22.
46. Boldt J, Knothe C, Zickmann B, et al. Platelet function in cardiac surgery: Influence of temperature and aprotinin. Ann Thorac Surg 1993;55:652-8.
47. Ferrara A, MacArthur JD, Wright HK, et al. Hypothermia and acidosis worsen coagulopathy in the patient requiring massive transfusion. Am J Surg 1990;160:515-8.
48. Valeri CR, Cassidy G, Khuri S, et al. Hypothermia-induced reversible platelet dysfunction. Ann Surg 1987;205:175-81.
49. Addonizio VP. Platelet function in cardiopulmonary bypass and artificial organs. Hematol Oncol Clin North Am 1990;4:145-55.
50. Khuri SF, Wolfe JA, Josa M, et al. Hematologic changes during and after cardiopulmonary bypass and their relationship to the bleeding time and nonsurgical blood loss. J Thorac Cardiovasc Surg 1992; 104:94-107.
51. Ferraris VA, Ferraris SP, Lough FC, Berry WR. Preoperative aspirin ingestion increases operative blood loss after coronary artery bypass grafting. Ann Thorac Surg 1988;45:71-4.

52. NIH Consensus Conference. Platelet transfusion therapy. JAMA 1987;257:1777-80.
53. Simon TL, Akl BF, Murphy W. Controlled trial of routine administration of platelet concentrates in cardiopulmonary bypass surgery. Ann Thorac Surg 1984;37:359-64.
54. Tobe CE, Vocelka C, Sepulveda R, et al. Infusion of autologous platelet rich plasma does not reduce blood loss and product use after coronary artery bypass. A prospective, randomized, blinded study. J Thorac Cardiovasc Surg 1993;105:1008-13.
55. Salzman EW, Weinstein MJ, Weintraub RM, et al. Treatment with desmopressin acetate to reduce blood loss after cardiac surgery: A double-blind randomized trial. N Engl J Med 1996;314:1402-6.
56. de Prost D, Barbier-Boehm G, Hazebroucq J, et al. Desmopressin has no beneficial effect on excessive postoperative bleeding or blood product requirements associated with cardiopulmonary bypass. Thromb Haemost 1992;68:106-10.
57. Hackmann T, Gascoyne RD, Naiman SC, et al. A trial of desmopressin (1-desamino-8-D-arginine vasopressin) to reduce blood lose in uncomplicated cardiac surgery. N Engl J Med 1989;321: 1437-43.
58. Blauhut B, Gross C, Necek S, et al. Effects of high-dose aprotinin on blood loss, platelet function, fibrinolysis, complement, and renal function after cardiopulmonary bypass. J Thorac Cardiovasc Surg 1991;101:958-67.
59. Havel M, Teufelsbauer H, Knobl P, et al. Effect of intraoperative aprotinin administration on postoperative bleeding in patients undergoing cardiopulmonary bypass operation. J Thorac Cardiovasc Surg 1991;101:968-72.
60. Crosson JT. Massive transfusion. Clin Lab Med 1996;16:873-82.
61. Faringer PD, Mullins RJ, Johnson RL, Trunkey DD. Blood component supplementation during massive transfusion of AS-1 red cells in trauma patients. J Trauma 1993;34:481-7.
62. Wilson RF, Dulchavsky SA, Soullier G, Beckman B. Problems with 20 or more blood transfusions in 24 hours. Am Surg 1987;53: 410-17.
63. Harrigan C, Lucas CE, Ledgerwood AM, et al. Serial changes in primary hemostasis after massive transfusion. Surg 1985;98:836-43.
64. Harker LA, Slichter SJ. Bleeding time as a screening test for evaluating platelet function. N Engl J Med 1972;287:155-9.

65. Ciavarella D, Reed RL, Counts RB, et al. Clotting factor levels and the risk of diffuse microvascular bleeding in the massively transfused patient. Br J Haematol 1987;67:365-8.
66. Reed RL II, Ciavarella D, Heimbach DM, et al. Prophylactic platelet administration during massive transfusion. A prospective, randomized, double-blind clinical study. Ann Surg 1986;203:40-8.
67. Simon TL, Henderson R. Coagulation factor activity in platelet concentrates. Transfusion 1979;19:186-9.
68. Counts RB, Haisch C, Simon TL, et al. Hemostasis in massively transfused trauma patients. Ann Thorac Surg 1979;190:91-9.
69. Locker GJ, Staudinger T, Knapp S, et al. Prostaglandin E1 inhibits platelet decrease after massive blood transfusions during major surgery: Influence on coagulation cascade? J Trauma 1997;42:525-31.
70. Hardaway RM, Williams CH. Disseminated intravascular coagulation: An update. Compr Ther 1996;22:737-43.
71. Bick RL. Disseminated intravascular coagulation: Objective clinical and laboratory diagnosis, treatment, and assessment of therapeutic response. Semin Thromb Hemost 1996;22:69-88.
72. Baglin T. Disseminated intravascular coagulation: Diagnosis and treatment. Br Med J 1996;312:683-7.
73. Feinstein DI. Treatment of disseminated intravascular coagulation. Semin Thromb Hemost 1988;14:351-62.
74. Staudinger T, Locker GJ, Frass M. Management acquired coagulation disorders in emergency and intensive-care medicine. Semin Thromb Hemost 1996;22:93-104.
75. Humphries JE. Transfusion therapy in acquired coagulopathies. Hematol Oncol Clin North Am 1994;8:1181-201.
76. Carvalho A. Acquired platelet dysfunction in patients with uremia. Hematol Oncol Clin North Am 1990;4:129-43.
77. Remuzzi G. Bleeding in renal failure. Lancet 1988;1:1205-8.
78. Livio M, Marchesi D, Remuzzi G, et al. Uraemic bleeding: Role of anemia and beneficial effect of red cell transfusions. Lancet 1982; 2:1013-5.
79. Castillo R, Lozano T, Escolar G, et al. Defective platelet adhesion on vessel subendothelium in uremic patients. Blood 1986;68:337-42.
80. Chong BH. Heparin-induced thrombocytopenia. Aust N Z J Med 1992;22:145-52.
81. Eberst ME, Berkowitz LR. Hemostasis in renal disease: Pathophysiology and management. Am J Med 1994;96:169-79.

82. Zusman RM, Rubin RH, Cata AE, et al. Hemodialysis using prostacyclin instead of heparin as the sole antithrombotic agent. N Engl J Med 1981;304:934-9.
83. Mannucci PM, Remuzzi G, Pusineri F, et al. Deamino-8-D-arginine vasopressin shortens the bleeding time in uremia. N Engl J Med 1983;308:8-12.
84. Mammen EF. Coagulation abnormalities in liver disease. Hematol Oncol Clin North Am 1992;6:1247-57.
85. Kelly DA, Summerfield JA. Hemostasis in liver disease. Semin Liver Dis 1987;7:182-91.
86. Pereira SP, Langley PG, Williams R. The management of abnormalities of hemostasis in acute liver failure. Semin Liver Dis 1996;16: 403-14.
87. Rao AK. Congenital disorders of platelet function. Hematol Oncol Clin North Am 1990;4:65-86.
88. Bennett JS, Kolodziej MA. Disorders of platelet function. Dis Mon 1992;38:579-631.
89. George JN, Caen JP, Nurden AT. Glanzmann's thrombasthenia: The spectrum of clinical disease. Blood 1990;75:1383-95.
90. Jennings LK, Wang WC, Jackson CW, et al. Hemostasis in Glanzmann's thrombasthenia (GT): GT platelets interfere with the aggregation of normal platelets. Am J Pediatr Hematol Oncol 1991; 13:84-90.
91. Yamaguchi K, Kawakatsu T, Kido H, et al. Platelet transfusion for patients with Glanzmann's thrombasthenia. Vox Sang 1992;63:290.
92. Carr JM, Kruskall MS, Kaye JA, Robinson SH. Efficacy of platelet transfusions in immune thrombocytopenia. Am J Med 1986;80: 1051-4.
93. Baumann MA, Menitove JE, Aster RH, Anderson T. Urgent treatment of idiopathic thrombocytopenic purpura with single-dose gammaglobulin infusion followed by platelet transfusion. Ann Intern Med 1986;104:808-9.
94. Kickler TS. Neonatal alloimmune thrombocytopenia. Clin Lab Med 1992;12:577-86.
95. Blanchette VS, Kuhne T, Hume H, Hellmann J. Platelet transfusion therapy in newborn infants. Transfus Med Rev 1995;9:215-30.
96. Lau P, Sholtis CM, Aster RH. Post-transfusion purpura: An enigma of alloimmunization. Am J Hematol 1980;9:331-6.

97. Brecher ME, Moore SB, Letendre L. Posttransfusion purpura: The therapeutic value of Pl[1] negative platelets. Transfusion 1990;30: 433-5.
98. Moschowitz E. An acute febrile pleiochromic anemia with hyaline thrombosis of the terminal arterioles and capillaries. An undescribed disease. Arch Intern Med 1925;36:89-93.
99. Hussein MA, Hoeltge GA. Platelet transfusion therapy for medical and surgical patients. Cleve Clin J Med 1996;63:245-50.
100. Blitzer JB, Granfortuna JM, Gottlieb AJ, et al. Thrombotic thrombocytopenic purpura: Treatment with plasmapheresis. Am J Hematol 1987;24:329-39.
101. Bell WR, Braine HG, Ness PM, Kickler TS. Improved survival in thrombotic thrombocytopenic purpura—hemolytic uremic syndrome. Clinical experience with 108 patients. N Engl J Med 1991; 325:398-403.
102. Gilcher RO, Strauss RG, Ciavarella D, et al. Management of renal disorders. J Clin Apheresis 1993;8:258-69.
103. Harkness DR, Byrnes JJ, Lian EC-Y, et al. Hazard of platelet transfusion in thrombotic thrombocytopenic purpura. JAMA 1981;246: 1931-3.
104. Gordon LI, Kwaan HC, Rossi EC. Deleterious effects of platelet transfusions and recovery thrombocytosis in patients with thrombotic microangiopathy. Semin Hematol 1987;24:194-201.
105. Patten E. Controversies in transfusion medicine. Prophylactic platelet transfusion revisited after 25 years: Con. Transfusion 1992; 32: 381-5.

In: Kickler TS, and Herman JH, eds.
Current Issues in Platelet Transfusion Therapy and Platelet Alloimmunity
Bethesda, MD: AABB Press, 1999

2

Criteria for Diagnosing Refractoriness to Platelet Transfusions

KAARON BENSON, MD

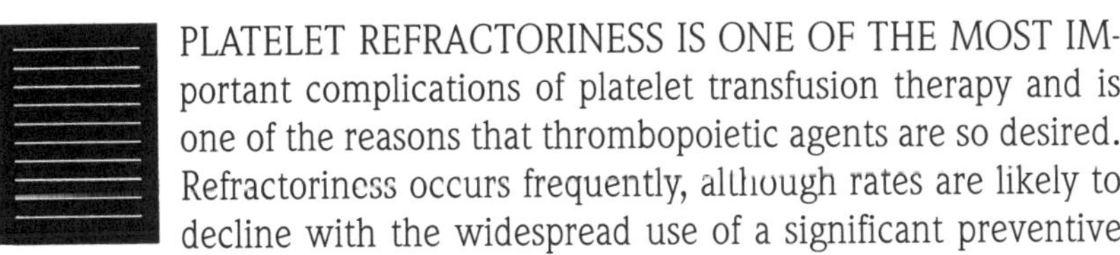

PLATELET REFRACTORINESS IS ONE OF THE MOST IMportant complications of platelet transfusion therapy and is one of the reasons that thrombopoietic agents are so desired. Refractoriness occurs frequently, although rates are likely to decline with the widespread use of a significant preventive measure: use of leukocyte-reduced cellular blood components. Patients with platelet refractoriness incur a significant financial burden, in part due to the additional tests, additional transfusions, and specialized platelet components that are often required.[1] They also pose a significant challenge

Kaaron Benson, MD, Associate Professor of Pathology and Laboratory Medicine, University of South Florida College of Medicine; Director, Blood Bank, H. Lee Moffitt Cancer Center, Tampa, Florida

to clinicians who are trying to prevent spontaneous, life-threatening hemorrhage or to control preexisting bleeding in a thrombocytopenic patient.

While much has been learned since platelet transfusion therapy first began, much remains unclear, especially concerning the issue of platelet refractoriness. Thus, this chapter reviews platelet refractoriness: what it is, how to diagnose it, what are the causes, and how to manage it.

Definition of Platelet Transfusion Refractoriness

Refractoriness is defined as a poor response to platelet transfusion. Platelet transfusions, as with all medical therapy, should be monitored to ensure that the patient has had the appropriate response. This response should be determined by both clinical and laboratory parameters—that is, by examining the patient for bleeding and measuring posttransfusion platelet counts. In a patient with bleeding primarily due to thrombocytopenia, the bleeding should slow or cease with the administration of platelets, and the posttransfusion platelet count should rise. With prophylactic platelet transfusions, the posttransfusion platelet count should increase sufficiently such that spontaneous, thrombocytopenic bleeding no longer presents a significant risk. In general, the average-sized patient should have the posttransfusion platelet count rise by at least 15,000/μL at 1 hour and by at least 9000/μL at 18-24 hours (see "Diagnosing Platelet Refractoriness" section).

Both posttransfusion platelet recovery and posttransfusion platelet survival are parameters that determine response to transfusion. The rise in the platelet count very soon—usually 1 hour—after transfusion determines platelet recovery, whereas platelet survival is measured in days. Because poor platelet survival can be dealt with by increasing the transfusion frequency, the most critical situation is a refractory patient who consistently fails to have an adequate platelet recovery.

An Algorithm for Evaluating Response to Platelet Transfusion

Platelets should be transfused when the need is indicated. In general, the average patient should receive at least 4-6 pooled random-donor platelet units or an apheresis platelet unit (Fig 2-1). (See Chapter 1 for the appropriate dose of platelets for various clinical settings.) A 1992 survey of American Association of Blood Banks institutions evaluated the average number of random-donor platelet units used per pool and found that the majority of primary teaching hospitals most commonly used a pool of 6 units.[2]

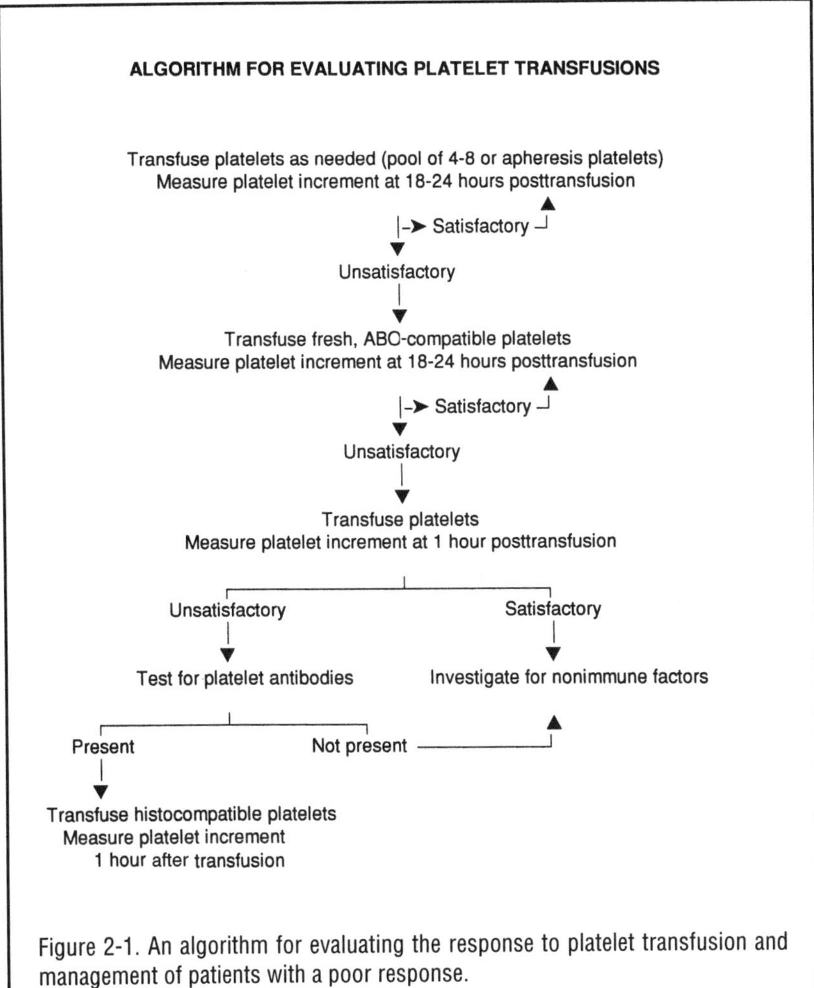

Figure 2-1. An algorithm for evaluating the response to platelet transfusion and management of patients with a poor response.

Platelet counts should be measured at 18-24 hours posttransfusion; samples can be collected the next morning when other laboratory samples are often obtained. Consideration should be given to performing Class I HLA-A, -B typing of the patient early, in the event that the patient ultimately requires HLA-matched platelets. Transfusions in the outpatient setting should still be monitored, and samples can be collected as soon as 10 minutes posttransfusion. Patients with satisfactory increments need no changes in their transfusion therapy.

When posttransfusion platelet increments are unsatisfactory, however, a trial of fresh, ABO-compatible platelets should be transfused on two occasions before any therapy changes are made.[3] A poor response to two consecutive platelet transfusions does not always predict subsequent refractoriness; some researchers have advocated delaying the diagnosis of refractoriness until three poor increments have occurred in a 2-week period.[4] There is no consensus on what constitutes fresh platelets, but for practical purposes the component should be no more than 2 days old. The pretransfusion platelet count should be obtained within a few hours of the transfusion. When a pretransfusion count is used from an early morning sample and the transfusion begins late in the day, the patient may appear refractory when the count may have actually dropped further during the day. To ensure that an adequate dose of platelets is used, the actual number of platelets used for the transfusion can be determined by obtaining a well-mixed unit, then measuring the platelet count (concentration) from a small sample and multiplying it by the unit's volume. This is preferable to using an estimate for the number of platelets transfused; while quality control data from the blood supplier are often used to make such an estimate, the actual number transfused may be far less and could be the source of poor increments. Posttransfusion platelet counts should be obtained at 1 hour to assess recovery and at 18-24 hours to assess platelet survival. "One-hour" posttransfusion counts can be obtained as soon as 10 minutes after the transfusion[5] and probably up to 4 hours after transfusion.

A satisfactory 1-hour posttransfusion platelet count indicates that the patient is unlikely to have immune causes for refractoriness[6,7] (Fig 2-2). Rather, the patient may have nonimmune factors responsible for the poor platelet recovery, and these factors should be investigated. One-hour posttransfusion counts should continue to be obtained as a patient may later develop immune factors. If the 1-hour posttransfusion increments are unsatisfactory, immune or nonimmune factors may be responsible, and tests for platelet antibodies should be performed. If platelet antibodies are identified, histocompatible platelets such as those from HLA-matched or crossmatch-compatible donors should be provided. HLA-alloimmunized patients should be retested periodically for platelet antibodies since levels may decline and these patients may again respond to unmatched platelets.[9,10] Other investigators have developed similar algorithms for evaluating patients' responses to platelet transfusion.[11-13]

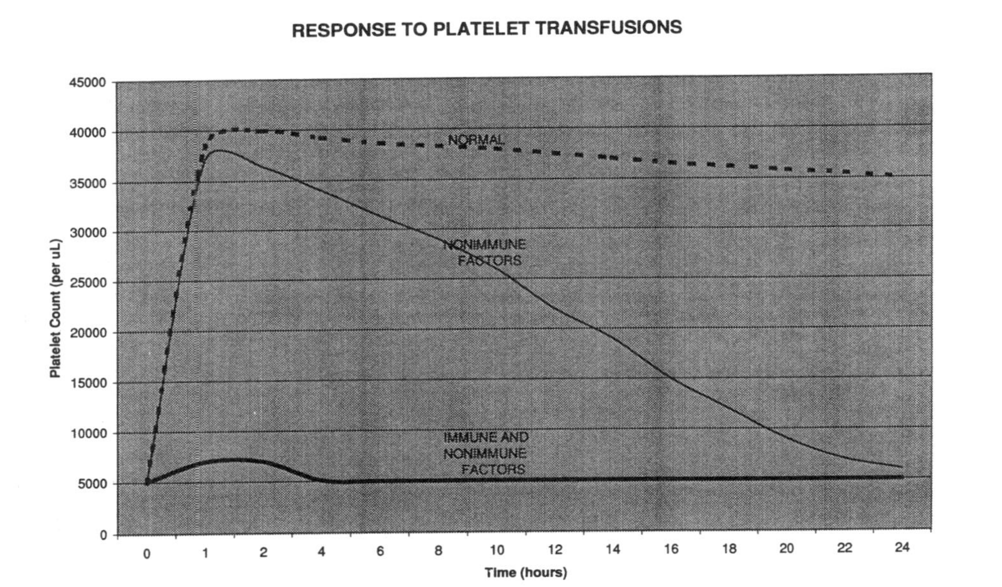

Figure 2-2. Prototype platelet counts following platelet transfusion for an average-sized patient receiving an average number of platelets. Normal response to transfusion shows good increments immediately after transfusion, with a slow, steady decline at 24 hours. Nonimmune factors may be associated with acceptable counts immediately posttransfusion, which soon decrease to pretransfusion levels. Immune factors can be anticipated to cause the rapid clearing of transfused platelets from the peripheral circulation, and nonimmune factors may also be capable of this poor response. (Modified from Simon TL.[8])

Diagnosing Platelet Refractoriness

What is the expected increase in the posttransfusion platelet count? For an average-sized patient, a rough approximation is a rise of about 5000-7000/µL per random-donor platelet unit transfused, or about 20,000 to 40,000/µL for a pool of 4-6 units, at 1 hour after transfusion. However, these numbers do not take into account a given patient's blood volume or the precise number of platelets transfused. Unexpectedly poor responses to platelet transfusion could be anticipated in larger patients and when the dose of platelets is less than expected (Fig 2-3). Therefore, a calculation to account for the patient's size (and blood volume) and the number of platelets transfused should be used before refractoriness is diagnosed. (Refer to Chapter 1 for a review of the corrected count increment [CCI], percent platelet recovery, and percent predicted platelet count increment formulas.)

There is no solid consensus on what threshold constitutes minimally acceptable posttransfusion platelet recovery. For those who use the CCI formula, a result of at least 7500 at 1 hour after transfusion is commonly accepted as successful (Fig 2-4), but values ranging from 2500 to 10,000 have also been used.[14] Platelet survival should also be assessed at 18-24 hours after transfusion, and a CCI of at least 4500 is generally considered successful; again, however, values from 2500 to 7500 have been reported. For those who prefer to calculate the percent platelet recovery, a 1-hour posttransfusion result of at least 20% or 30% is generally accepted.

The CCI formula can be used to calculate the average expected recovery for the average-sized patient. An average-sized patient (5'10", 160 lb, body surface area 1.9 m^2) transfused with an average number of platelets ($\sim 3.8 \times 10^{11}$) who has a CCI of 7500 must have had a posttransfusion platelet count increment of at least 15,000/µL. Therefore, for the above scenario, if this patient had a pretransfusion platelet count of 5000/µL, the 1-hour posttransfusion platelet count should be at least 20,000/µL for the transfusion to be considered successful at that point.

Incidence of Refractoriness

The incidence of refractoriness in patients appears to vary, largely because of differences in how refractoriness is defined. Some authors have considered a single episode of poor response to transfusion sufficient to label a patient refractory, whereas others require at least two or three such episodes. Rates of refractoriness may be declining as less immune refractoriness would be predicted with increasing routine use of leukocyte-reduced cellular blood components. Murphy and Waters[15] reported in 1991 that refrac-

Posttransfusion platelet count increment was 15,000 μL.
Was the platelet transfusion successful?

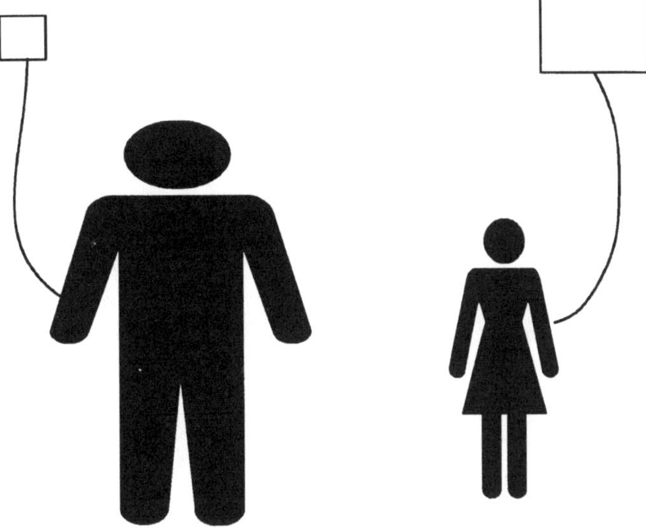

Large patient (BSA = 2.3 m^2)	Small patient (BSA = 1.6 m^2)
Height 6'4", weight 220 lb	Height 5'4", weight 125 lb
Small number of platelets (3.0×10^{11})	Large number of platelets (5.0×10^{11})
CCI = 11,500 SUCCESSFUL	CCI = 4,800 UNSUCCESSFUL

Figure 2-3. The posttransfusion platelet count increment is not sufficient information to determine the effectiveness of transfusion. The same increment for two different-sized patients receiving different numbers of platelets results in a successful transfusion for the larger patient and an unsuccessful transfusion for the smaller patient.

BSA = body surface area; CCI = correct count increment

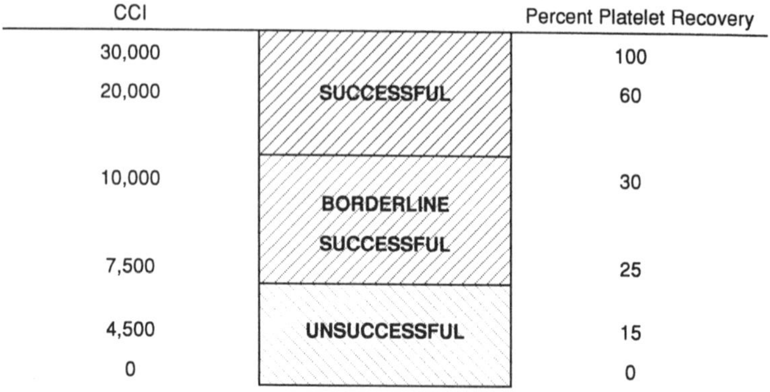

CCI		Percent Platelet Recovery
30,000		100
20,000	SUCCESSFUL	60
10,000	BORDERLINE SUCCESSFUL	30
7,500		25
4,500	UNSUCCESSFUL	15
0		0

Figure 2-4. Comparison of CCI and percent platelet recovery in the evaluation of the 1-hour posttransfusion platelet count. Unsuccessful transfusions are usually defined by a CCI less than 7500 or by platelet recovery below 25%.

CCI = corrected count increment

toriness occurs in about 50% of patients who are repeatedly transfused, while Slichter et al[16] reported in 1997 that only 16% of patients studied over an 8-week period became refractory.

The development of immune refractoriness may be based on a patient's immunocompetence; patients with aplastic anemia have higher rates of immune refractoriness than leukemia patients.[17] Whether refractoriness is due to immune or nonimmune factors or both may be related to how carefully one investigates. Immune factors, with or without nonimmune factors, have been reported in 31%[18] to 86%[19] of refractory patients.

Laboratory Testing

The immune factors responsible for refractoriness primarily include HLA and platelet-specific antibodies. Patients suspected of having immune refractoriness because of low 1-hour posttransfusion platelet counts should be tested for platelet antibodies. Once these antibodies are identified, appropriate platelet components can be provided. Clinicians treating refractory patients may inappropriately order HLA-matched platelets if the necessary tests to identify HLA antibodies are not performed.[20]

When clinicians are testing for platelet antibodies, it is advisable to use more than one test method. This is because false-positive and false-negative results can occur, and a second test method would provide verification of the original result.[21]

Tests for HLA Antibodies Only

The most common platelet antibodies responsible for refractoriness are HLA antibodies, and the most commonly used test to detect HLA antibodies is the lymphocytotoxicity test.[22-24] Either commercial kits or a small pool (10-30) of donor lymphocytes can be used with the patient's serum sample. While a positive test result has been defined by some as any reactivity identified, most agree that isolated, nonspecific reactivity may represent false positivity. Results are reported as a percentage of the panel that is reactive (panel reactive antibody). A PRA of at least 10% or 20% is generally correlated with immune refractoriness.[19] While this test would show positive results in most patients with immune refractoriness, it cannot identify platelet-specific antibodies, which may be present alone or in combination with HLA antibodies.

Tests for Platelet-Specific Antibodies

Antibodies may be directed against antigens that are present only on platelets. These antigens have been renamed on the basis of a new uniform nomenclature system. All are designated by the prefix "HPA" for human platelet antigen, followed by a number (in the order recognized), and then by the letter "a" for the high-incidence allele or "b" for the low-incidence allele. One test that is often used to identify platelet-specific antibodies is the monoclonal antibody immobilization of platelet antigen (MAIPA) test,[25] which enables platelet-specific antibodies to be identified in the presence of HLA antibodies. Other methods to identify platelet-specific antibodies have also been used.[26,27]

Tests for Both HLA and Platelet-Specific Antibodies

The solid-phase red-cell-adherence assay for platelet antibodies is widely used because it detects both HLA and platelet-specific antibodies consistently and with relative ease.[28] A commercial kit is available (Capture P, Immucor, Norcross, GA), and testing can be readily performed by both blood centers and hospital transfusion services. Additional test methods include enzyme immunoassay,[29] immunofluorescence,[30-33] latex agglutination,[34,35] and a radiolabeled antiglobulin test.[36] Tests capable of identifying both HLA and platelet-specific antibodies cannot distinguish between the

Table 2-1. Causes of Poor Response to Platelet Transfusions

Platelet Factors
- Low numbers
- Increased age
- Decreased viability
- ABO incompatibility

Patient Factors—Nonimmune
- Splenomegaly
- Severe infection/septicemia
- Fever
- Antibiotics
- Amphotericin B
- Disseminated intravascular coagulation
- Marrow transplantation
- Active bleeding

Patient Factors—Immune
- HLA alloimmunization
- Platelet-specific alloimmunization
- ABH alloimmunization
- Autoantibodies
- Drug-related antibodies

two, however, unless HLA antigens are first removed by pretreatment with chloroquine or acid.

Causes of a Poor Response to Platelet Transfusions

A poor response to platelet transfusions can be caused by either platelet or patient-related factors. Platelet factors include the number, age, viability, and ABO type of the platelets transfused (Table 2-1). Patient-related factors can be divided into nonimmune and immune causes. This classification is useful because it allows the readily correctable causes, platelet factors, to be quickly identified and managed.

There is not always a clear cause-and-effect relationship between the factors known to be associated with refractoriness and a poor response to transfusion. Patients may have immune or nonimmune factors known to cause refractoriness and yet still respond to transfusions. Conversely, refractory patients may have no identifiable cause of their refractoriness.

Platelet Factors

Number of Platelets Transfused

Platelets for transfusion do not have a precise, fixed number per unit. There is a wide range in the number of platelets that a patient may receive per transfusion episode; this is primarily because of the variability of donor platelet counts. This range in the platelet yield per unit emphasizes the need to correct for the exact number of platelets transfused by use of a calculation such as the CCI.

The number of platelets provided per transfusion may be declining. "Split" apheresis components—apheresis platelets originally containing at least 6.0×10^{11} platelets divided into two components for two different patients—are often made available from donors with high platelet counts. This practice may reduce the average number of platelets in an apheresis unit. The usual number of random-donor platelets used by many transfusion services per platelet pool has also declined from a high of 10 to four or six.

Age of the Platelets

While older platelets do result in lower average posttransfusion increments, the actual deterioration with storage is modest, and 5-day-old platelets still provide acceptable clinical results for the nonrefractory patient.[37,38] Data from Schiffer et al[37] reveal that for an average-sized patient receiving an average number of platelets, the platelet increment would be about 8000/μL lower for 5-day-old platelets than for 1-day-old platelets. Years ago the platelet storage lesion was more problematic, but with the improved quality of platelet storage bags and the use of anticoagulants with higher pH, the storage lesion has been minimized, and platelet age is a less important variable in transfusion practice for the clinically stable, thrombocytopenic patient.[38]

While the nonrefractory patient does not require fresh platelets, refractory patients have been shown to have better increments with fresh platelets to the point that they may no longer be classified as refractory.[39,40] Skodlar et al[39] found that 97% of 108 refractory patients without platelet antibodies had successful responses to fresh (36 hours old or less) platelets. Clinically ill patients may especially benefit from fresh platelets since these patients appear to clear transfused platelets at a more rapid rate and may have better posttransfusion platelet recovery and survival with fresh platelets.[38] However, not all investigators have found that platelet age affects increments in refractory patients.[41,42]

Factors other than age or prolonged storage may also adversely affect platelet viability and result in a poor response to transfusion.[43] For example, viability may decrease when platelet components are not properly processed and stored, or when platelets are volume-reduced and not transfused quickly.[11]

ABO Compatibility

Plasma-Incompatible Platelets. Donor platelets suspended in plasma that is ABO incompatible with the recipient's red cells—for example, group O platelets transfused to a group A recipient—may be referred to as plasma-incompatible platelets. While plasma-incompatible platelets should result in adequate platelet increments posttransfusion, they can cause a positive result on a direct antiglobulin test in the recipient and can—albeit rarely—cause acute hemolysis.[44,45] Typically, patients receiving plasma-incompatible platelets do not experience a decrease in their hemoglobin level, nor do they require more red cell transfusions.[45,46] It is prudent, though, to try to restrict the amount of ABO-incompatible plasma for small-sized patients, such as children or small adults. If plasma-incompatible platelets must be used in such patients, reducing the amount of plasma should be considered. The platelets can be centrifuged at a low speed ("soft-spin"), and most of the plasma can be expressed into a separate bag. The platelets must then be resuspended and, because of platelet activation, allowed to rest prior to the transfusion. Component manipulation such as volume reduction may be associated with minor loss of platelets.

Platelet-Incompatible Platelets. Platelets have ABH antigens on their surface; some are intrinsically present and some are adsorbed from the plasma.[47] When these antigens are incompatible with the recipient's ABH antibodies, the platelets may be referred to as platelet incompatible. While platelets are generally regarded to have only weak expression of A and B antigens, some donors may have strong A or B antigen expression, which may result in refractoriness to isolated units.[48] The importance of platelet ABH antigens in platelet recovery was clearly demonstrated in 1965 by Aster.[49] Group A platelets transfused to group O volunteers resulted in average recoveries of only 19%, while ABO-compatible platelets showed recoveries similar to autologous platelets with an average of 63%.

Generally, less striking differences in increments are seen in practice when ABO-compatible and ABO-incompatible platelets are compared; increments have been found to be only about 20% lower for ABO-incompatible units.[50,51]

Refractoriness due solely to ABO incompatibility has been reported,[52,53] although not all investigators have found these incompatible platelets to influence posttransfusion increments.[54] The lowest posttransfusion platelet recoveries appear to be in group O patients, particularly those with high-titer anti-A who receive group A platelets. Repeated ABO-incompatible platelet transfusions can result in increased A and B antibody titers, and refractoriness has been reported in association with these high titers.[52,55]

Refractory patients receiving ABO-incompatible platelets have been shown to have circulating immune complexes composed of ABO antigens and their corresponding antibodies, complexes that may account for the poor increments seen.[56] Patients who receive ABO-incompatible platelets have been found to develop refractoriness more often and more rapidly than patients who receive ABO-identical platelets[57,58] and may require more platelet transfusions.[58]

In summary, efforts should be made to provide ABO-compatible platelets whenever possible. In general, though, refractoriness due to ABO incompatibility is not common, and the reduction in platelet recovery associated with ABO incompatibility is not so great as to contraindicate the use of ABO-mismatched platelets. When consistently poor recoveries do occur in a patient receiving ABO-incompatible platelets, a trial of ABO-compatible platelets may resolve the apparent refractoriness.

Patient Factors—Nonimmune

The nonimmune clinical factors responsible for adverse posttransfusion platelet increments are not fully known or understood. In addition, as was pointed out by Schiffer,[59(p198)] "their [clinical factors'] effects may be somewhat exaggerated in many texts because excellent increments are often obtained in the sickest of patients in whom many of these clinical factors are present." It is often difficult to predict which factors may be significant for any given patient. Many of the studies performed to investigate nonimmune factors are retrospective, and refractory patients often have multiple factors simultaneously, making the assessment of any individual factor more difficult (Table 2-2). While much has been written about immune refractoriness and its pathophysiology, management, and prevention, comparatively little is known about nonimmune refractoriness. Management

Table 2-2. Key Selected Nonimmune Factors Found To Be Significantly Associated with Platelet Refractoriness

Investigator/ Reference	No. of Study Patients	No. of Platelet Transfusions	Splenomegaly	Infection/ Sepsis	Fever	Antibiotics	Amphotericin B	DIC	BMT	Bleeding
Alcorta[18]	52	52	(+)	(+)	++	0	0	0	+	0
Bishop[60]	133	941	+	0	(+)	(+)	++	+	++	0
Bishop[61]	108	623	++	0	0	+	++	(+)	++	0
Böck[54]	46	400	++	0	+	++	++	0	+	0
Enright[62]	538	6919	++	++	++	0	++	0	0	++
Friedberg[53]	71	962	0	+	+	0	0	0	0	+
McFarland[7]	29	334	(+)	+	++	0	0	0	0	0

++ = highly significant; + = significant; (+) = marginally significant; 0 = not significant or could not be evaluated; DIC = disseminated intravascular coagulation; BMT = bone marrow transplantation

of patients with nonimmune factors is limited, and preventive measures are virtually nonexistent.

Splenomegaly

In normal individuals, about one-third of the total body platelet mass is sequestered in the spleen. As the spleen enlarges, a greater percentage of the body's platelets remain within this organ, a situation referred to as splenic sequestration.[63,64] Splenomegaly or hypersplenism is usually identified on physical examination of the abdomen and defined as a palpable spleen or one that extends below the left costal margin.

Transfused platelets generally suffer the same fate as autologous platelets in hypersplenic patients. Posttransfusion platelet recovery is generally less in the patient with splenomegaly, possibly as low as 15-35%[38,54,64] (Fig 2-5). Splenomegaly has clearly been identified as a cause of refractoriness in several studies.[54,60,62,65,66] Platelet survival in hypersplenic patients has been reported as both shortened[66] and close to normal.[64] Patients with the biggest spleens may have the poorest posttransfusion increments.[66] Thus, it may be necessary to transfuse larger doses of platelets or to transfuse more frequently in these patients.

However, patients with palpable spleens may not have platelet refractoriness[18] or poor increments with all transfusions; Hussein et al[66] found that 42% of transfusions to hypersplenic patients were successful. Other investigators found that splenomegaly is not associated with increased transfusion requirements[67,68] or an increased risk of bleeding.[67]

Since the spleen is responsible for clearing dead and dying platelets, it is not surprising that asplenic patients have higher platelet counts and higher posttransfusion platelet increments[60,63]; posttransfusion platelet recovery among these patients may approach 100%. Among a group of allogeneic marrow transplant patients with chronic myelogenous leukemia, those with prior splenectomy required platelet transfusions for half as many days as did patients with intact spleens.[68] These asplenic patients also developed significantly less platelet refractoriness. In this study there was no difference in the posttransplantation survival of patients with or without splenectomy.[68] Asplenia is the one consistent factor that has been associated with increased posttransfusion platelet recoveries.

Severe Infection/Septicemia

Patients with severe infection and sepsis are often thrombocytopenic with shortened platelet survivals.[69,70] Platelet refractoriness has been independ-

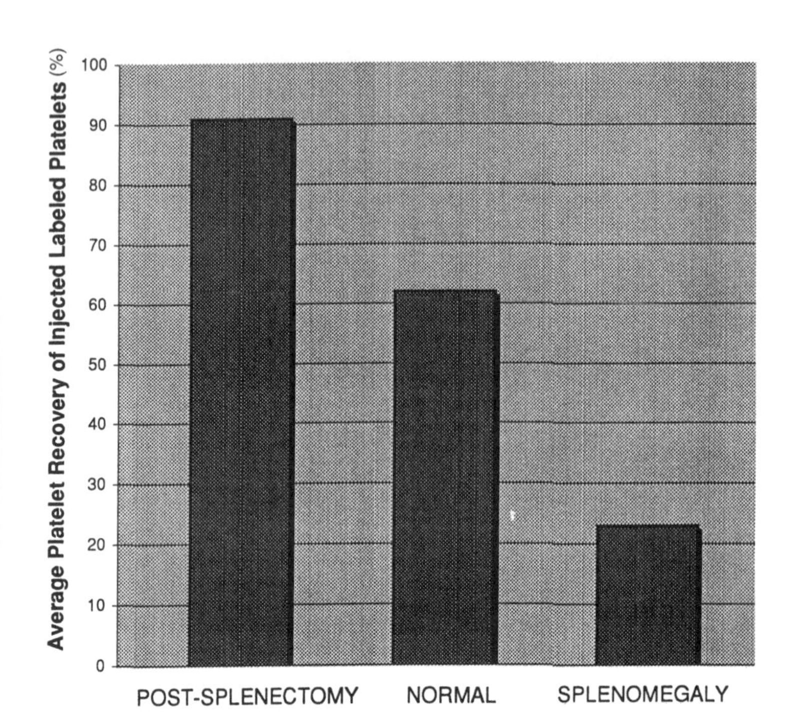

Figure 2-5. Platelet recovery: Effect of splenectomy and splenomegaly. Asplenic patients have high platelet recoveries, while patients with splenomegaly have reduced recoveries.[64]

ently associated with infection.[53,62] McFarland et al[7] found that septic patients had reduced 24-hour posttransfusion platelet recoveries.

Fever

Multiple investigators have found fever to be an independent factor associated with platelet refractoriness, and fever has been shown to lower posttransfusion platelet increments by as much as 20-40%.[7,53,54,60,62,65,71] A trend toward lower recoveries was seen in infected leukemia patients when the body temperature was greater than 39 C (102.2 F).[72] Not all investigators, though, have found fever to be associated with lower posttransfusion platelet increments.[61]

Fever is often a manifestation of infection, and infected patients are treated with antibiotics. Whether one or more of these factors (fever, infection, antibiotics) are responsible for refractoriness is unclear, and distinguishing between them proves difficult because many patients have all three factors simultaneously. It is also unknown whether it is necessary to attempt to lower the temperature of febrile patients with antipyretics prior to platelet transfusion. It is probable that the underlying cause of the fever, and not the fever itself, is responsible for the associated refractoriness.

Antibiotics

Concurrent use of antibiotics has been associated with poor responses to platelet transfusion. Although Bishop et al[60] found increased numbers of concurrent antibacterial antibiotics to be of only marginal importance in refractoriness, Böck et al[54] found posttransfusion CCIs to be reduced by an average of 36%. Vancomycin has been specifically identified as a clinical factor independently associated with platelet refractoriness.[73]

Drug-dependent immune thrombocytopenia has been described for a few drugs such as heparin[74] and certain antibiotics.[75] It is possible that a similar immune mechanism exists that is responsible for the refractoriness seen in patients receiving antibiotic therapy. In general, though, most drugs do not appear to be associated with platelet refractoriness.

Amphotericin B

Concurrent use of the antifungal agent amphotericin B has been shown to adversely affect posttransfusion platelet increments,[60,62,64,66,76,77] which have been found to be from about 30%[76] to as much as 78% lower[54] during amphotericin B therapy.

In-vitro studies have shown that amphotericin B does not affect platelet shape or the number of platelet pseudopodia, but it does enhance a normal storage lesion; surface membrane pitting.[77] Other in-vitro studies have shown that therapeutic levels of amphotericin B are associated with partial loss of total platelet glycoprotein 1b in both fresh and stored platelets and with decreased surface expression of the glycoprotein in stored platelets.[78] These effects on platelet membrane glycoproteins were not present in autologous platelets from patients on the antifungal agent. Other studies have suggested that amphotericin B may induce drug-dependent antibodies and cause lower posttransfusion increments through an immune mechanism.[11] Another proposed mechanism for refractoriness is a direct toxic effect of the drug that results in platelet dysfunction and abnormal platelet circulation.[76]

Not all patients receiving amphotericin B develop refractoriness.[18] This difference in response to platelet transfusion may be related to the timing of the amphotericin in relationship to the transfusion. Some institutions try to administer amphotericin B at least several hours apart from the platelet transfusion, which may produce less of an effect on the transfused platelets.[79,80] A second antifungal drug, fluconazole, has been found to have no in vitro effects on platelet membrane expression of glycoproteins and has not been associated with refractoriness.

Disseminated Intravascular Coagulation

Disseminated intravascular coagulation (DIC) is a consumptive process that results in the clearing of a patient's platelets and coagulation factors from the plasma.[81] Transfused allogeneic platelets are not exempt from the consumption and are also depleted. DIC has been found to be a significant independent factor associated with refractoriness.[60] While a number of pathologic conditions are associated with DIC, sepsis and malignancy are among the most common. Treatment of the underlying cause of DIC should correct the platelet refractoriness.

Marrow Transplantation

Patients who have received a marrow transplant have been shown to have lower posttransfusion platelet increments.[60,61] Alcorta et al[18] found that marrow transplantation for patients with chronic myelogenous leukemia was an independent factor associated with refractoriness but that allogeneic marrow transplantation for other diseases was not independently associated with refractoriness. Similarly, others have not found marrow transplantation to be an independent factor associated with refractoriness in adults[53] or children.[82]

The platelet refractoriness seen in some marrow transplant patients may be related to graft-vs-host disease (GVHD). Anasetti et al[83] found platelet-bound autoantibodies in allogeneic marrow transplant patients with either acute or chronic GVHD, and the presence of these antibodies correlated with lower peripheral platelet counts and lower survivals of transfused ^{51}Cr-labeled platelets. However, these researchers found no autoantibodies in a small group of allogeneic marrow transplant patients without GVHD.

Active Bleeding

Some studies have found that active bleeding, established either directly by clinical examination or indirectly by assessment of the number of recent red cell transfusions, is an independent factor associated with refractoriness.[42,53,62] Yet, several other studies[7,54,60,65] have found that bleeding does not significantly contribute to refractoriness. Patients who are massively transfused with red cells may develop a dilutional thrombocytopenia but would be expected to have relatively adequate recoveries posttransfusion. It is unclear whether active bleeding is truly associated with refractoriness, and if so, what amount of blood loss is significant and what mechanism is involved.

Patient Factors—Immune

The frequent use of leukocyte-reduced cellular blood components to prevent or delay the onset of HLA alloimmunization has benefited large numbers of multitransfused patients. Patients with poor posttransfusion platelet increments soon after transfusion should be suspected of having immune refractoriness and should be tested for platelet antibodies. When platelet antibodies are identified, a search for possible nonimmune factors should still be made because patients may have both immune and nonimmune factors; either or both could be responsible for adversely influencing the patient's response to platelets. Platelet antibodies may include HLA alloantibodies, platelet-specific alloantibodies, ABH antibodies, autoantibodies, and drug-related antibodies.

HLA Alloimmunization

HLA alloimmunization is one of the most important complications of platelet transfusion therapy. Rapid diagnosis of HLA alloimmunization allows for the appropriate use of histocompatible platelets. Exposure to allogeneic leukocytes via prior cellular blood transfusions or prior pregnancies incites the antibody formation. The immune response begins with exposure to Class I and II HLA alloantigens present on leukocytes, and antibodies form against Class I antigens. Platelets have Class I but not Class II antigens, and while they are not responsible for initiating the immune response, the platelets become the target of these alloantibodies.[38] Primary alloimmunization takes several weeks to occur, whereas secondary alloimmunization may be detected in hours to days after an antigenic challenge. The number of prior cellular blood transfusions does not appear to affect the development of alloimmunization.[84] Once a patient is exposed to allogeneic Class I and II HLA antigens, the immune response may have been initiated.

Immunocompetent recipients develop these antibodies more readily than recipients with weakened immune systems. These HLA alloantibodies not only are associated with the rapid destruction of transfused platelets but have also been implicated in febrile transfusion reactions, transfusion-related acute lung injury, and other deleterious events. The incidence of HLA alloimmunization varies but, in general, has decreased considerably with the increasing use of leukocyte-reduced cellular blood components.

Platelet-Specific Alloimmunization

Platelet-specific alloimmunization is a process whereby alloantibodies directed against antigens unique to platelets form after exposure to allogeneic platelets. The first three platelet-specific antigen systems recognized were HPA-1, HPA-2, and HPA-3. Since the platelet-specific antigens have a high gene frequency for one allele, antigen-negative patients are rare. This form of immune refractoriness appears clinically similar to HLA alloimmunization. Platelet-specific alloimmunization should be suspected when 1) there is a low 1-hour posttransfusion platelet count, HLA antibodies are not identified, and the patient is platelet crossmatch-incompatible with most donors, or 2) the patient with HLA antibodies fails to respond to HLA-matched platelets that are well-matched and nonimmune factors are not present.

Posttransfusion purpura is an uncommon transfusion reaction and should be suspected in the patient who suddenly develops severe thrombocytopenia and platelet refractoriness following recent red cell transfusion. Unlike most patients with platelet-specific alloimmunization, patients with posttransfusion purpura rapidly clear both allogeneic and autologous platelets.

ABH Alloimmunization

ABH alloimmunization was discussed previously under platelet factors responsible for a poor response to platelet transfusion. The platelet increment posttransfusion may be affected by the patient's ABH titer and/or the number of A and B antigens present on donor platelets.[38] While platelet recoveries may be lower with ABO-mismatched platelets, survivals are the same as with ABO-matched platelets. Increased levels of circulating immune complexes have been correlated with lower posttransfusion increments; immune complexes may be responsible for refractoriness in some patients.[38]

Autoantibodies

Patients with autoimmune thrombocytopenia have platelet antibodies capable of binding to both autologous and allogeneic platelets. These autoantibodies are associated with immune refractoriness and make platelet transfusion ineffective. Tests to detect platelet-associated immunoglobulin can be used when platelet autoantibodies are suspected. These tests have a high negative predictive value; when results are negative, a patient generally does not have autoantibody. When results are positive, the test's predictive value is much less and a patient may or may not truly have autoantibodies.

The presence of platelet autoantibodies is not always correlated with thrombocytopenia. These antibodies have been described in patients with a variety of diseases, and some patients may be capable of compensating despite a shortened platelet survival.[38] Similarly, transfused allogeneic platelets may have a relatively normal survival in these patients.

Drug-Related Antibodies

The role of drug-related platelet antibodies in platelet refractoriness remains unclear. Drugs such as amphotericin B and vancomycin have been implicated as causative factors.[73,76] The possible mechanisms for the poor posttransfusion recoveries may be immune mediated.[11,73] A number of therapeutic drugs, particularly heparin, have been associated with immune-mediated thrombocytopenia.[38] A review of current medications for a refractory patient with thrombocytopenia may identify a drug associated with thrombocytopenia. Discontinuation of an implicated drug may resolve both the refractoriness and thrombocytopenia.

Other Patient Factors

Other factors that have been studied and found to significantly influence refractoriness in isolated reports include hepatic veno-occlusive disease,[85] hepatomegaly,[54] male gender,[42] patient body surface area greater than 1.7 m^2,[42] concurrent steroid administration,[42] patient neutrophil count less than $1 \times 10^9/L$,[53] and increasing numbers of prior platelet transfusions.[62]

Additional factors that have been studied and not found to significantly influence refractoriness include concurrent chemotherapy,[54] concurrent intravenous immunoglobulin,[42,53] number of previous platelet transfusions,[54] hemoglobin concentration,[54] patient white cell count,[54] patient absolute neutrophil count,[42] patient gender.[53]

Management of Nonimmune Refractoriness

Fresh, ABO-compatible platelets should be tried in a patient with poor posttransfusion platelet increments. This approach appears to be especially useful in clinically unstable patients—for example, patients receiving amphotericin B or patients with GVHD, sepsis, splenomegaly, or veno-occlusive disease.[38,86]

In platelet-refractory patients with splenomegaly, the number of platelets transfused will probably need to be increased.[87] Although splenectomy would eliminate the sequestration of platelets, it is generally not recommended since most patients experience transient thrombocytopenia and the spleen serves important immune functions. Surgical removal of the spleen can be considered in patients with persistent thrombocytopenia and platelet refractoriness due to splenomegaly.[88]

In febrile, severely infected patients receiving antibiotics, platelet refractoriness may complicate their medical care. It is unknown whether reducing a patient's fever is necessary, yet many clinicians do use antipyretics prior to platelet transfusion in febrile patients. The refractoriness may be a result of the infection and/or therapy, and when the infection resolves and medication is discontinued, adequate posttransfusion platelet increments may return.

For patients receiving amphotericin B, many centers will use at least a 4-hour, and perhaps even an 8- to 12-hour, interval between administration of the antifungal agent and infusion of the platelets, whenever possible. Patients with DIC are often platelet refractory, and treatment of the underlying cause of the coagulopathy will resolve both the DIC and the refractory state. Managing marrow transplant recipients with platelet refractoriness can prove challenging. Regular monitoring for platelet antibodies is essential.

When platelet-refractory patients remain unresponsive to transfusions and are receiving platelet transfusions prophylactically, consideration should be given to discontinuing the transfusions and carefully monitoring the patient for evidence of bleeding. Invasive procedures should be avoided or delayed whenever possible, and medication that would adversely affect platelet function must be avoided. When these same patients require therapeutic platelet transfusions because of bleeding, large doses or more frequent transfusions, perhaps up to three or four daily, may be needed. Antifibrinolytic agents, such as epsilon aminocaproic acid, may prove useful for uncontrollable bleeding episodes.[89]

For patients who are persistently refractory, clinicians should continue to investigate for both new immune and/or nonimmune factors that may be responsible. While no immune factors may have been identified during the initial evaluation of a refractory patient, platelet antibodies may develop later.[84] The converse is also possible in that immune-refractory patients may no longer have detectable antibody over time[84,90]; Dutcher et al[84] reported that about one-fifth of HLA-alloimmunized acute leukemia patients subsequently had no detectable antibody despite repeated transfusions, and these patients did respond to standard platelet transfusions.

Platelet-refractory patients present a substantial challenge to medical staff; careful evaluation and appropriate management are critical. While leukocyte-reduced blood components prevent or delay the onset of HLA alloimmunization in substantial numbers of multitransfused patients, there are no known methods to prevent refractoriness due to nonimmune factors. We can only try to be vigilant for evidence of refractoriness, investigate for the underlying causes, and provide the appropriate management.

References

1. Lill M, Snider C, Calhoun L, et al. Analysis of utilization and cost of platelet transfusions in refractory hematology/oncology patients (abstract). Transfusion 1997;37(suppl):26S.
2. Pisciotto PT, Benson K, Hume H, et al. Prophylactic versus therapeutic platelet transfusion practices in hematology and/or oncology patients. Transfusion 1995;35:498-502.
3. Lee EJ, Schiffer CA. ABO compatibility can influence the results of platelet transfusion. Results of a randomized trial. Transfusion 1989; 29:384-9.
4. Petz LD. Platelet transfusions. In: Petz LD, Swisher SN, Kleinman S, et al, eds. Clinical practice of transfusion medicine. 3rd ed. New York: Churchill Livingstone Inc, 1996:359-412.
5. O'Connell B, Lee EJ, Schiffer CA. The value of 10-minute posttransfusion platelet counts. Transfusion 1988;28:66-7.
6. Daly PA, Schiffer CA, Aisner J, Wiernik PH. Platelet transfusion therapy: 1-hour posttransfusion increments are valuable in predicting the need for HLA initial preparation. JAMA 1980;243:435-8.
7. McFarland JG, Anderson AJ, Slichter SJ. Factors influencing the transfusion response to HLA-selected apheresis donor platelets in patients refractory to random platelet concentrates. Br J Haematol 1989; 73:380-6.
8. Simon TL. Platelets: Uses, abuses and indications. In: Kolins J, McCarthy LJ, eds. Contemporary transfusion practice. Arlington, VA: American Association of Blood Banks, 1987:47-63.
9. Lee EJ, Schiffer CA. Serial measurement of lymphocytotoxic antibody and response to nonmatched platelet transfusions in alloimmunized patients. Blood 1987;70:1727-9.

10. Murphy MF, Metcalfe P, Ord J, et al. Disappearance of HLA and platelet-specific antibodies in acute leukemia patients alloimmunized by multiple transfusions. Br J Haematol 1987;67:255-60.
11. Weiner RS, Kao K-J. Clinical and laboratory diagnosis of the refractory state. In: Kurtz SR, Brubaker DB, eds. Clinical decisions in platelet therapy. Bethesda, MD: American Association of Blood Banks, 1992: 73-85.
12. Slichter SJ. Algorithm for managing the platelet refractory patient. J Clin Apheresis 1997;12:4-9.
13. British Committee for Standards in Haematology. Guidelines for platelet transfusions. Transfus Med 1992;2:311-8.
14. Bishop JF, Matthews JP, Yuen K, et al. The definition of refractoriness to platelet transfusion. Transfus Med 1992;2:35-41.
15. Murphy MF, Waters AH. Clinical aspects of platelet transfusions. Blood Coagul Fibrinolysis 1991;2:389-96.
16. Slichter SJ and the Trial to Reduce Alloimmunization to Platelets Study Group. Leukocyte reduction and ultraviolet B irradiation of platelets to prevent alloimmunization and refractoriness to platelet transfusions. N Engl J Med 1997;337:1861-9.
17. Schiffer CA, Slichter SJ. Platelet transfusions from single donors. N Engl J Med 1982;307:245-8.
18. Alcorta I, Pereira A, Ordinas A. Clinical and laboratory factors associated with platelet transfusion refractoriness: A case-control study. Br J Haematol 1996;93:220-4.
19. Hogge DE, Dutcher JP, Aisner J, Schiffer CA. Lymphocytotoxic antibody is a predictor of response to random donor platelet transfusion. Am J Hematol 1983;14:363-9.
20. Phekoo KJ, Hambley H, Schey SA, et al. Audit of practice in platelet refractoriness. Vox Sang 1997;73:81-6.
21. Wernet D, Schnaidt M, Mayer G, Northoff H. Serological screening, using three different test systems of platelet-transfused patients with hematologic-oncologic disorders. Vox Sang 1993;65:108-13.
22. Mittal KD, Michey MR, Singal DP, Terasaki PI. Serotyping for homotransplantation, XVIII: Refinement of the microdroplet lymphocyte cytotoxicity test. Transplantation 1968;6:913-27.
23. Mittal KK. Standardization of the HLA typing method and reagents. Vox Sang 1978;34:58-63.
24. Terasaki PI, Bernoco D, Park MS, et al. Microdroplet testing for HLA-A, -B, -C, and -D antigens: The Phillip Levine Award Lecture. Am J Clin Pathol 1978;69:103-20.

25. Kiefel V, Santoso S, Weisheit M, Mueller-Eckhardt C. Monoclonal antibody-specific immobilization of platelet antigens (MAIPA): A new tool for the identification of platelet-reactive antibodies. Blood 1987; 70:1722-6.
26. von dem Borne AEGKr, Vergheught FWA, Oosterhof F, et al. A simple immunofluorescence test for the detection of platelet antibodies. Br J Haematol 1978;39:195-207.
27. Lucas GF, Hadley AG, Hoburn AM. Anti-platelet opsonic activity in alloimmune and autoimmune thrombocytopenia. Clin Lab Haematol 1987;9:59-66.
28. Rachel JM, Summers TC, Sinor LT, Plapp FV. Use of a solid phase red blood cell adherence method for pretransfusion platelet compatibility testing. Am J Clin Pathol 1989;90:63-8.
29. Brubaker DB, Duke JC, Romine M. Predictive value of enzyme-linked immunossay platelet crossmatching for transfusion of platelet concentrates to alloimmunized recipients. Am J Hematol 1987;24:375-87.
30. Sintnicolaas K, deVries W, van der Linden R, et al. Simultaneous flow cytometric detection of antibodies against platelets, granulocytes and lymphocytes. J Immunol Methods 1991;142:215-22.
31. Sintnicolaas K, Lowenberg B. A flow cytometric platelet immunofluorescence crossmatch for predicting successful HLA matched platelet transfusions. Br J Haematol 1996;92:1005-10.
32. Friedberg RC, Donnelly FF, Mintz PD. Independent roles for platelet crossmatching and HLA in the selection of platelets for alloimmunized patients. Transfusion 1994;34:215-20.
33. Skogen B, Christiansen D, Husebekk A. Flow cytometric analysis in platelet crossmatching using a platelet suspension immunofluorescence test. Transfusion 1995;35:832-6.
34. Ramos RR, Curtis BR, Chaplin H. A latex particle assay for platelet-associated IgG. Transfusion 1992;32:235-8.
35. Ogden PM, Asfour A, Kohler C, et al. Platelet crossmatches of single donor platelet concentrates using a latex agglutination assay. Transfusion 1993;33:644-50.
36. Kickler TS, Braine HG, Ness PM, et al. A radiolabeled antiglobulin test for crossmatching platelet transfusions. Blood 1983;61:238-42.
37. Schiffer CA, Lee EJ, Ness PM, Reilly J. Clinical evaluation of platelet concentrates stored for one to five days. Blood 1986;67:1591-4.
38. Slichter SJ. Mechanisms and management of platelet refractoriness. In: Nance SJ, ed. Transfusion medicine in the 1990's. Arlington, VA: American Association of Blood Banks, 1990:95-179.

39. Skodlar J, Bolgiano D, Teramura G, Slichter SJ. Distinguishing between mechanisms of platelet refractoriness: Abnormal post-storage platelet viability vs. immune destruction (abstract). Blood 1992; 80:260a.
40. Peter-Salonen K, Bucher V, Nydegger U. Comparison of post-transfusion recoveries achieved with either fresh or stored platelet concentrates. Blut 1987;54:207-12.
41. Murphy WG, Palmer JP, Green RHA. The management of haemorrhage in the refractory non-alloimmunized thrombocytopenic patient. Vox Sang 1994;67(suppl 3):99-103.
42. Klumpp TR, Herman JH, Innis S, et al. Factors associated with response to platelet transfusion following hematopoietic stem cell transplantation. Bone Marrow Transplant 1996;17:1035-41.
43. Kickler TS. Improving the quality of stored platelets. Transfusion 1991;31:1-3.
44. Zoes C, Dube VE, Miller HJ, et al. Anti-A1 in the plasma of platelet concentrates causing a hemolytic reaction. Transfusion 1977;17:29-32.
45. Mair B, Benson K. Evaluation of changes in hemoglobin levels associated with ABO-incompatible plasma in apheresis platelets. Transfusion 1998;38:51-5.
46. Shanwell A, Ringden O, Wiechel B, et al. A study of the effect of ABO incompatible plasma in platelet concentrates transfused to bone marrow transplant recipients. Vox Sang 1991;60:23-7.
47. Dunstan RA, Simpson MB, Knowles RW, Rosse WF. The origin of ABH antigens on human platelets. Blood 1985;65:615-9.
48. Ogasawara K, Ueki J, Takenaka M, Furihata K. Study on the expression of ABH antigens on platelets. Blood 1993;82:993-9.
49. Aster RH. Effect of anticoagulant and ABO incompatibility on recovery of transfused human platelets. Blood 1965;26:732-43.
50. Duquesnoy RJ, Anderson AJ, Tomasulo PA, Aster RH. ABO compatibility and platelet transfusions of alloimmunized thrombocytopenic patients. Blood 1979;54:595-9.
51. Tosato G, Applebaum FR, Deisseroth AB. HLA-matched platelet transfusion therapy of severe aplastic anemia. Blood 1978;52:846-54.
52. Brand A, Sintnicolaas K, Claas FHJ, Eernisse JG. ABH antibodies causing platelet transfusion refractoriness. Transfusion 1986;26:463-6.
53. Friedberg RC, Donnelly SF, Boyd JC, et al. Clinical and blood bank factors in the management of platelet refractoriness and alloimmunization. Blood 1993;81:3428-34.

54. Böck M, Muggenthaler K-H, Schmidt U, Heim MU. Influence of antibiotics on posttransfusion platelet increment. Transfusion 1996;36: 952-4.
55. Skogen B, Hansen R, Husebekk A, et al. Minimal expression of blood group A antigen on thrombocytes from A_2 individuals. Transfusion 1988;28:456-9.
56. Heal JM, Masel D, Rowe JM, Blumberg N. Circulating immune complexes involving the ABO system after platelet transfusion. Br J Haematol 1993;85:566-72.
57. Carr R, Hutton JL, Jenkins JA, et al. Transfusion of ABO-mismatched platelets leads to early platelet refractoriness. Br J Haematol 1990;75: 408-13.
58. Heal JM, Rowe JM, McMican A, et al. The role of ABO matching in platelet transfusion. Eur J Haematol 1993;50:110-7.
59. Schiffer CA. Untitled presentation. International Forum: Management of alloimmunized, refractory patients in need of platelet transfusions. Vox Sang 1997;73:198.
60. Bishop JF, McGrath K, Wolf MM, et al. Clinical factors influencing the efficacy of pooled platelet transfusions. Blood 1988;71:383-7.
61. Bishop JF, Matthews JP, McGrath K, et al. Factors influencing 20-hour increments after platelet transfusion. Transfusion 1991;31:392-6.
62. Enright H, Gernsheimer T, Woodson R, et al. Factors influencing the response to platelet transfusion (abstract). Blood 1997;90(suppl 1):268a.
63. Aster RH, Jandl JH. Platelet sequestration in man, II: Immunological and clinical studies. J Clin Invest 1964;43:856-69.
64. Aster RH. Pooling of platelets in the spleen: Role in the pathogenesis of "hypersplenic" thrombocytopenia. J Clin Invest 1966;45:645-57.
65. Parker RD, Yamamoto LA, Miller WR. Interaction effects analysis of platelet transfusion data. Transfusion 1974;14:567-73.
66. Hussein MA, Lee EJ, Schiffer CA. Platelet transfusions administered to patients with splenomegaly. Transfusion 1990;30:508-10.
67. Witzig TE, Ducatman BS, Wick MR, et al. Platelet transfusion therapy in acute leukemia: Lack of effect of splenomegaly on transfusion requirements and risk of hemorrhage. Am J Hematol 1985; 18:345-50.
68. Banaji M, Bearman SI, Buckner CD, et al. The effects of splenectomy on engraftment and platelet transfusion requirements in patients with chronic myelogenous leukemia undergoing marrow transplantation. Am J Hematol 1986;22:275-83.
69. Levin J. Bleeding with infectious diseases. In: Ratnoff OD, Forbes D, eds. Disorders of hemostasis. Orlando, FL: Grune & Stratton, 1984:339-55.

70. Poskitt TR, Poskitt PK. Thrombocytopenia of sepsis. The role of circulating IgG-containing immune complexes. Arch Intern Med 1985:145:891-4.
71. Freireich EJ, Kliman A, Gaydos LA, et al. Response to repeated platelet transfusions from the same donor. Ann Intern Med 1963;59:277-87.
72. Hocker P, Reizenstein P. Effect on platelet counts and fever of platelet transfusion in leukemia. Blut 1975;31:143-8.
73. Christie DJ, van Buren N, Lennon SS, Putnam JL. Vancomycin-dependent antibodies associated with thrombocytopenia and refractoriness to platelet transfusion in patients with leukemia. Blood 1990; 75:518-23.
74. Sheridan D, Carter C, Kelton JG. A diagnostic test for heparin-induced thrombocytopenia. Blood 1986;67:27-30.
75. Chong BH. Drug-induced immune thrombocytopenia. Platelets 1991;2: 173-81.
76. Kulpa J, Zaroulis CG, Good RA, Kutti J. Altered platelet function and circulation induced by amphotericin B in leukemic patients after platelet transfusion. Transfusion 1981;21:74-6.
77. McGrath K, Bertram JF, Houghton S, et al. Amphotericin B-induced injury in stored human platelets. Transfusion 1992;32:46-50.
78. Sloand EM, Kumar P, Yu M, Klein HG. Effect of amphotericin B and fluconazole on platelet membrane glycoproteins. Transfusion 1994; 34:415-20.
79. Hussein MA, Fletcher R, Long TJ, et al. Transfusing platelets 2 h after the completion of amphotericin-B decreases its detrimental effect on transfused platelet recovery and survival. Transfus Med 1998; 8:43-7.
80. Murphy S. Amphotericin B and platelet transfusion. Transfusion 1992;32:7-8.
81. Harker LA, Slichter SJ. Platelet and fibrinogen consumption in man. N Engl J Med 1972;287:999-1005.
82. Hogge DE, McConnell M, Jacobson C, et al. Platelet refractoriness and alloimmunization in pediatric oncology and bone marrow transplant patients. Transfusion 1995;35:645-52.
83. Anasetti C, Rybka W, Sullivan KM, et al. Graft-v-host disease is associated with autoimmune-like thrombocytopenia. Blood 1989;73: 1054-8.
84. Dutcher JP, Schiffer CA, Aisner J, Wiernik PH. Long-term followup of patients with leukemia receiving platelet transfusions: Identification of a large group of patients who do not become alloimmunized. Blood 1981;58:1007-11.

85. Rio B, Andreu G, Nicod A, et al. Thrombocytopenia in veno-occlusive disease after bone marrow transplantation or chemotherapy. Blood 1986;67:1773-6.
86. Norol F, Kuentz M, Cordonnier C, et al. Influence of clinical status on the efficiency of stored platelet transfusion. Br J Haematol 1994;86: 125-9.
87. Slichter SJ. Controversies in platelet transfusion therapy. Annu Rev Med 1980;31:509-40.
88. Hammersmith SM, Jacobson AF, Mankoff DA. Scintigraphy with indium-111-labeled homologous (donor) platelets in the platelet transfusion refractory bone marrow transplant patient. J Nucl Med 1997;38: 1135-8.
89. Benson K, Fields K, Hiemenz J, et al. The platelet-refractory bone marrow transplant patient: Prophylaxis and treatment of bleeding. Semin Oncol 1993;20:102-9.
90. McGrath K, Wolf M, Bishop J, et al. Transient platelet and HLA antibody formation in multitransfused patients with malignancy. Br J Haematol 1988;68:345-50.

In: Kickler TS, and Herman JH, eds.
Current Issues in Platelet Transfusion Therapy and Platelet Alloimmunity
Bethesda, MD: AABB Press, 1999

3

Issues in Platelet Storage

THOMAS S. KICKLER, MD, AND JAY H. HERMAN, MD

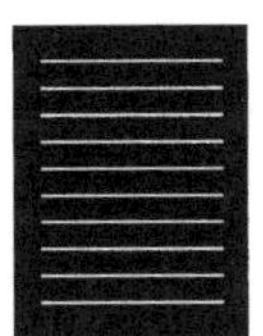

TWO DECADES AGO, PLATELET TRANSFUSION THERAPY was readily available only in specialized medical centers. The development of potentially curable chemotherapeutic regimens, which led to severe myelosuppression, necessitated intensive research into the biology of platelets, methods for their procurement and storage, and platelet transfusion practices. This research allowed the widespread availability of platelet transfusions for the treatment of both benign and malignant medical disorders, trauma cases, and complicated surgical procedures. This medical advance, which could only have happened with basic research into the properties of platelets that maintained their function and viability during preparation and storage, has revolutionized the practice of hematology and oncology.[1,2] The historical

---

Thomas S. Kickler, MD, Professor of Pathology, Medicine, and Oncology, John Hopkins University School of Medicine, Baltimore, Maryland; and Jay H. Herman, MD, Medical Director, Stem Cell Processing Laboratory, Temple University Hospital Bone Marrow Transplant Program, and Professor of Medicine and Associate Professor of Pediatrics, Temple University School of Medicine, Philadelphia, Pennsylvania

milestones leading to an effective and improved platelet product are listed in Table 3-1.

The usefulness of platelets is still limited by a relatively short storage period (5 days). Currently, the fundamental questions concerning platelet storage are as follows: 1) What are the molecular changes that determine loss of function and viability? 2) What degree of molecular damage is clinically significant and affects patient outcomes? 3) What in-vitro measurement is a good predictor of clinical hemostasis and can be used to evaluate platelet formulations? 4) How can platelets be sterilized? 5) Are there alternatives to liquid storage of platelets? The purpose of this chapter is to review these questions.

Platelet Preparations

Platelets and Platelets, Pheresis

Platelet transfusions are available as Platelets or Platelets, Pheresis. The volume and cellular composition of these components vary, leading to differences in storage requirements. Platelets are prepared from units of Whole Blood by centrifugation; Platelets, Pheresis are collected by apheresis devices.[2,3] Changes in platelet biology have been more widely studied in Platelets than in Platelets, Pheresis.[2,4,5]

In the United States, Platelets are separated from Whole Blood by first preparing platelet-rich plasma through centrifugation and then centrifuging the platelets a second time at a higher *g* force. The content of the platelet concentrates is highly variable, depending upon the technique; however, 50 mL of Platelets usually has at least 5.5×10^{10} platelets, with an

Table 3-1. Historical Milestones in Platelet Storage

- Demonstration that fresh blood transfusion corrects thrombocytopenia and simultaneously shortens bleeding time
- Development of plastic blood containers, permitting preparation of platelets from Whole Blood
- Development of platelet-rich plasma method of platelet preparation
- Elucidation of appropriate storage conditions
- Development of plasma-reduced platelets from crystalloid storage medium

average content of 7-9 × 10^{11} platelets. In Europe, platelets are most commonly prepared using the buffy coat method.[6] This involves centrifugation to prepare a buffy coat, from which platelets are separated by an additional centrifugation. For platelets prepared by the platelet-rich plasma method, the white cell concentration is approximately 10^8 per bag; for platelets prepared by the buffy-coat method, the white cell concentration is approximately 10^6 per bag. The relatively lower white cell content in platelets prepared by the latter method may be advantageous in reducing alloimmunization and febrile transfusion reactions. In addition, having fewer leukocytes could lead to a lower concentration of cytokines generated during storage.

Platelets, Pheresis are collected from donors by continuous centrifugation using a large intravenous catheter, which allows the processing of a large volume of blood and the removal of platelets by way of an automated system. Because the conventional transfusion dose of Platelets, Pheresis for an adult patient is approximately 6 units of pooled platelets, parameters have been used to collect this number of platelets from a donor. Modern apheresis devices are equipped to predict the yield from the donor's size, platelet count, and hematocrit, but actual platelet yields are still variable. The leukocyte content of this component also varies, depending on the technology used, but most devices leave a white cell content of less than 10^6 per bag.

Cryopreserved Platelets

In an attempt to increase inventory, cryopreserved platelets have been developed for long-term platelet storage using dimethyl sulfoxide (DMSO) or glycerol.[7] Both of these agents have been extensively researched. Hemostasis seems to be maintained with DMSO-preserved platelets. However, despite early promising results from glycerol-preserved platelets, glycerol has not been successfully adapted for clinical practice.

Cryopreserved platelets were especially developed for patients who become alloimmunized during induction chemotherapy for acute leukemia and who later require additional marrow suppressive therapy. Platelets can be collected during remission, frozen, and subsequently used when necessary. The average posttransfusion recovery of cryopreserved platelets is approximately 50%. Because the use of frozen platelets presents some logistical considerations, however, they are not widely used. Thus, there is relatively little research in progress on storing platelets in this form, especially for developing inventories for mass casualty use.

Lyophilized Platelets

The lyophilization of platelets may prove to be an alternative that circumvents the logistical concerns inherent in frozen stored platelets. Obviously, the storage of a stabilized platelet formulation such as this is relatively simple. In 1995, Read and coworkers[8] reported that lyophilized platelets may support hemostasis in an animal model. They showed that they could correct the bleeding time in thrombocytopenic animals and that the transfusion of reconstituted lyophilized platelets helped to form carotid arterial thrombus in a canine model. This form of platelets is currently undergoing human clinical trails and is not yet approved for routine use. Although these studies are provocative, additional studies are needed to substantiate the usefulness and safety of lyophilized platelets and to investigate other potential forms of platelet substitutes.

Platelet Storage Lesion

The guiding principle of platelet storage has been that preservation of platelet function is needed to maintain hemostasis.[9] It should be noted that the early success reported with lyophilized platelets is challenging this notion. Nonetheless, the long-term goal of liquid stored platelets should be to maintain the platelet's function and viability by preventing its activation and generation of the storage lesion.

The platelet storage lesion is multifactorial (see Table 3-2) and manifests as changes in morphology, function, and viability following transfusion. *Platelet activation*, a term that is widely used in reference to platelet stor-

Table 3-2. Causes of Storage Lesion

- Activated by centrifugation at preparation
- Activated by thrombin
- Activated by complement with microvesiculation and accelerated thrombin generation
- Activated by disruption of Ca^{+2} flux and signal transduction
- Degradation of glycoprotein Ib/IX by calpain, plasmin, and elastase
- Degradation of cytoskeleton by calpain
- Hypoxia, lactic acid generation, and acidification of storage medium

age, has been defined morphologically, biochemically, and functionally. However, as it relates to the platelet storage lesion, it is a rather imprecise term because there are no quantifiable limits that determine whether a platelet is "good" or "bad." Several studies have shown that the maintenance of normal morphology is the best predictor of the ability of stored platelets to survive after transfusion.[10-12] However, platelet activation results in changes in platelet morphology, including degranulation and the loss of discoid shape. Ultrastructurally, a circumferential band of microfilaments, the formation of pseudopodia, the loss of glycogen, vacuolization, and swelling can be observed.

A great deal of attention has been devoted to studying the changes that occur during storage in the major platelet receptors, platelet glycoproteins (Gp)Ib/IX and IIb-IIIa.[13-16] The adhesion of platelets depends on the functional GpIb-IX complex for thrombin generation. However, surface GpI has been shown to decrease with storage, and in-vitro testing has been correlated with defective adherence to damaged endothelium. The loss of GpIb appears related to plasmin generation; whether the loss that is seen at the maximum storage period of 5 days is enough to worry about is unclear. During storage, platelet GpIIb-IIIa is also altered in that it is changed to its active conformation. There have been reports of the loss of GpIIb-IIIa from the surface of the platelets. However, since there are at least 80,000 copies of this molecule on a platelet, it is not clear what percentage of decrease we should worry about, if any.

Several different kinds of molecules have been implicated as agents mediating the platelet storage lesion.[14-16] Although plasma provides a buffering capacity during storage, it also provides a variety of proteins, including plasmin, thrombin, and complement, that may be deleterious to platelets. Apparently, the anticoagulant properties of citrate are not sufficient to halt coagulation activation. Various approaches have been proposed to inhibit these troublesome biochemical interactions, but there is little enthusiasm for transfusing the inhibitory agents to patients.[16]

Assessing Platelet Quality

Initial results with platelet transfusions have shown that the function and viability of stored platelets correlate with a measurable posttransfusion increase in and survival of those platelets. A number of in-vitro tests have been used to estimate the function and viability of stored platelets (see Table 3-3). While the most clinically relevant outcome of these tests would be the prevention of morbidity and mortality from thrombocytopenia, this outcome measure is idealistic. The in-vivo function and viability can be es-

Table 3-3. Tests Used in the Laboratory Evaluation of Stored Platelets

- Platelet count
- Aggregation—single and dual agonists
- Recovery from hypotonic shock
- pH
- Morphology score by light microscopy
- Platelet reactivity with vessel wall subendothelium
- Measurement of platelet membrane glycoprotein
- Measurement of platelet activation markers, beta-thromboglobulin, p-selectin
- Platelet swirling

timated using the approaches shown in Table 3-4. This is because clinical factors in thrombocytopenic patients may confound the results of such studies of the storage lesion, making the prevention of morbidity and mortality difficult to determine and thus an impractical goal for experimental purposes. Therefore, other tests of platelet quality have used the infusion of radiolabeled autologous platelets in volunteers as an alternative approach.[17] Generally these studies have relied on radioactive forms of chromium and indium. Recently, biotin labeling of platelets has been used to perform platelet kinetic studies to avoid exposure of normal individuals to isotopes.[18]

Table 3-4. In-Vivo Evaluation of Stored Platelets

- Platelet count increment
- Radiolabeled platelet kinetics
- Correction of bleeding time
- Reduction in bleeding or red cell transfusions

Three in-vitro tests appear to offer reliable estimates of how well the platelet will survive posttransfusion.[2,19-21] These include 1) the osmotic reversal reaction, 2) the morphology score by phase microscopy, and 3) the visual assessment of platelet swirling. This last method is attractive because it does not involve sampling of the platelet container. Rather, it assesses the swirling or shimmering phenomenon exhibited by discoid platelets when they are placed in front of a light source and the container is gently rotated or squeezed with one thumb. Platelets that have lost their spherical shape do not demonstrate this swirling phenomenon.

Several animal models have been developed to test new platelet formulations by making the animal thrombocytopenic and then measuring bleeding times.[22] Whether these animal models are reliable for studying platelet transfusion efficacy needs further consideration. Given that bleeding times are notoriously unreliable even in cooperative patients, it would be valuable to determine in a controlled fashion what the reproducibility of the bleeding time is in a nervous rabbit with twitching ears or a mouse that has had its tail severed.

Storage Conditions

Platelet storage was first attempted when red cells were stored under refrigeration to avoid bacterial proliferation. However, it became evident that platelets became activated during storage, causing transfusion failures. This problem with cold storage was recognized early in the development of platelet transfusion therapy.[23] Since then, interest in cold storage has been revitalized by the realization that storage at 22 C brings increased risks of bacteremia. Table 3-5 lists the effects of cold exposure on liquid stored platelets. As can be seen from these numerous effects, cold-induced pathology encompasses all of the platelet's vital functions. A variety of new approaches, as shown in Table 3-6, are being applied to circumvent these effects.[24] Clearly, these approaches need vigorous proof of their safety in recipients.

Agitation

It appears that even after platelets leave the circulation where they are in constant motion, they continue to benefit from being in a nonstationary state.[5] Thus, whole blood-derived platelets must be agitated to maintain their viability. If they are kept stationary, on the shelf, lactate production accelerates and pH falls. Just as some forms of exercise are favorable for different body parts, the platelet also has its preferences. Agitation studies have revealed that either a flat bed rotator or face-on-face tumbling on an agita-

Table 3-5. Effects of Exposure to Cold Temperatures on Liquid-Stored Platelets

Morphology
- Loss of discoid shape
- Formation of platelet projections
- Decrease mean platelet volume and microparticle formation
- Loss of circumferential microtubules

Altered Physiologic Response on Recovering
- Decreased sensitivity to collagen in platelet aggregation
- Increased p-selectin expression
- Decreased adenosine triphosphate release

Biochemical Changes
- Decrease in actin-filament assembly
- Altered Ca^{++} flux
- Altered membrane lipid assembly
- Decreased fibrinogen binding

Table 3-6. New Preventive Approaches for Cold-Induced Platelet Alterations

Preventive Approach	Mechanism of Action
Physical method (Temperature recycling)	Maintains cytosolic calcium and reversal of cytoskeletal anomalies
Biochemical (Antifreeze glycoprotein)	Prevents lateral separation of membrane phospholipids
Signal transduction (Inhibitors)	Inhibits phospholipase A

tor is preferable to other types of motion.[25] Although these studies have been conducted with Platelets, presumably they apply to Platelets, Pheresis as well. However, experimental data in this regard are scant.

Metabolism

The liquid storage of platelets has been largely successful because it has benefited from systematic studies that have explained platelet metabolism. Early studies of platelets stored at 0 C based on knowledge of the metabolic needs of red cells proved unsuccessful since storage at 1-6 C resulted in the marked loss of viability.[26] Consequently, the challenges of platelet storage have been complicated by the need to nurture a metabolically active blood element. During storage at 22 C under aerobic conditions facilitated by gas exchange across the storage bag, platelet metabolism proceeds along two major metabolic pathways.

The first pathway is glycolysis, which occurs independent of oxygen. The second is the tricarboxylic pathway. Thus, in citrated plasma, platelets can use two substrates: glucose and fatty acids. In glycolysis, glucose is converted into lactate and hydrogen ion (H^+). Although this pathway generates pyruvate, very little of the pyruvate ends up being decarboxylated to acetyl coenzyme A. Instead, fatty acids metabolism is the primary source of acetyl coenzyme A. The production of carbon dioxide makes a second bag property necessary, permeability to this volatile acid.

The production of one lactate from glucose generates one molecule of adenosine triphosphate (ATP), while oxygen metabolism is more sustaining by producing six molecules of ATP. Were it not for the production of ATP, platelets would not be capable of maintaining their integrity during storage and certainly would not be able to secrete, contract, or adhere after transfusion. If there is cellular hypoxia, the rate of glycolysis increases (thc Pasteur effect), thus producing lactic acid. Lactic acid requires buffering by bicarbonate, a relatively scarce moiety sufficient in quantities only to buffer approximately 20mM of lactate. Exceeding this buffer limit, the pH may fall to 6.8 and progressively below that to 6.2, at which point cellular lysis ensues.

The challenge of platelet storage has been to produce conditions that permit gas exchange. One can readily see how, in the earliest days of blood component therapy, storing platelets in plastic instead of glass revolutionized the practice of transfusion therapy in a manner that was more significant than the avoidance of broken glass in a patient's room. Gases do not escape through microscopic pores in the plastic but rather make their exit by being solubilized in the plastic. When this barrier is saturated, gas diffusion occurs much like when an inflated balloon becomes flaccid.

Adequate gas exchange is affected by three determinants: 1) the number of platelets, 2) the surface area of the platelet container, and 3) the permeability properties of the plastic.[2,24] The situation for platelets is not particularly complicated. However, Platelets, Pheresis can have variable numbers and be in up to three contiguous containers. Because of this and the variability between different suppliers' bags, different storage recommendations are necessary, depending on volume and type of plastic. This situation may become more complicated as Platelets, Pheresis are being collected from thrombopoietin-stimulated donors.

Although platelets have been traditionally stored in citrated plasma, this practice is being reexamined. Much work is being done to develop alternative storage media.[27,28] This research has been stimulated by multiple considerations, including the need to 1) save plasma for other purposes, 2) reduce plasma-associated side effects, 3) improve the platelet storage conditions, and 4) increase the reliability of viral and bacterial sterilization. With these goals in mind, investigators have had to ensure that storage media maintain platelet function and viability. Rock and coworkers first applied an intravenous solution, Plasma Lyte A, to replace citrated plasma.[3] This solution contains acetate, a substrate that is oxidized, generating ATP. For each molecule of acetate that is metabolized, one hydrogen ion is consumed and two molecules of CO_2 and water are formed. This allows the maintenance of a stable pH and an unchanged concentration of bicarbonate during storage, even though some lactic acid is formed. Whether these synthetic storage media will be widely used appears to be unanswered at this time.

Adverse Effects of Transfusions Related to Platelet Storage

As extensively reviewed in a later chapter, platelet transfusions are associated with a significantly higher incidence of patient reactions than are red cell transfusions. It was thought for many years that leukocyte antibodies accounted for most febrile reactions to platelets. However, clinical observations on patients have suggested that this is not the complete answer. In nearly one-third of cases, reactions commonly occur with the first transfusion and are independent of the total number of transfusions. Furthermore, the majority of first reactions occur during the first three transfusions. While presensitization might account for some of these early reactions, other factors may also be involved.

It has been recognized that various can be generated during the in-vitro storage of platelets.[29] Chambers[30] reported in 1990 that the age of blood products predicts transfusion reactions. This was one of the first indications that some type of biomediator is present in platelets. Transfusion reactions were five times greater in platelets, and the older the platelet product and the higher the white cell count, the more likely it was that there would be a transfusion reaction,[30] including bronchospasm, wheezing, and dyspnea.

Cytokines in Platelet Concentrate

As noted above, several investigators have recently identified cytokines as possible important factors in certain transfusion reactions associated with the administration of platelet products.[29,31] Since all blood components contain leukocytes, which produce cytokines, it is not surprising that these hormone-like substances accumulate in products such as platelet concentrates during storage. Muylle and colleagues,[31] having investigated cytokine levels in stored platelet concentrates and the relationship between these levels and transfusion reactions, observed an increasing frequency and severity of transfusion reactions with increased platelet storage time. They found increasing amounts of such cytokines as tumor necrosis factor (TNF), interleukin 1 (IL-1), and IL-6 in the plasma of stored platelets. These authors speculated that these cytokines could be accounted for by damage to leukocytes in the platelets, which would lead to cytokine leakage and/or the activation of monocytes in the platelets.

Stack and Snyder[32] have also reported significant accumulations of IL-8, IL-1 beta, IL-6, and TNF-α in platelet concentrates during storage. Moreover, they found that leukocyte reduction by third-generation filters at day 1 of storage prevented the generation of IL-8 and IL-1 beta until day 5 of storage. Other investigators have also reported that leukocyte reduction of the platelets after processing and prior to storage would prevent the accumulation of the above substances.

Bacterial Contamination of Platelet Products

Because platelets are stored at room temperature, organisms that were introduced during phlebotomy or during transient donor bacteremia may proliferate. Bacterial contamination of platelet products can lead to transfusion-associated sepsis, the characteristic symptoms of which include chills, fever, hypotension, and hypoxia. Blood cultures drawn from the patient experiencing such reactions have been found to be positive in fewer than half the episodes. Estimates of the incidence of bacterial contamination in platelet products range from a high of 10% of all platelet pools to more conservative estimates of 4 in every 1000 pools.[33] It is not clear how this incidence of bacterial contamination can be prevented or reduced. While shortening the storage shelf life of platelet products to 3 days has been considered, studies have shown that this may be of little real value since bacteria can achieve log growth and relatively high concentrations by day 3 of storage. Various approaches have been considered to reduce the risk of transfusion-associated sepsis, including the addition of photoactive dyes that may bind to bacteria and, upon photoactivation, kill contaminating bacteria.[34] However, this approach so far as been problematic because bacterial inactivation also damages the platelets.

Conclusion

Numerous factors can contribute to poor platelet viability after transfusion if careful consideration is not given to their storage requirements. These factors must always be considered as contributing to poor platelet transfusion outcome, and investigation into these possible causes should be instituted whenever unexplained platelet refractoriness is encountered.

References

1. Hirsch EO, Gardner FH. The transfusion of human blood platelets. With a note on the transfusion of granulocytes. J Lab Clin Med 1952; 39:556-69.
2. Murphy S, Kahn RA, Holme S, et al. Improved storage of platelets for transfusion in a new container. Blood 1982;60:194-200.
3. Rock G, Senack E, Tittley P. Five-day storage of platelets collected on a blood cell separator. Transfusion 1989;29:626-8.
4. Slichter SJ, Harker L. Preparation and storage of platelet concentrates, II: Storage and variables influencing platelet function and viability. Br J Haematol 1976;34:403-19.
5. Fillip DJ, Aster RH. Relative hemostatic effectiveness of human platelets stored at 4 C and 22 C. J Lab Clin Med 1978;91:618-24.
6. Fijnher R, Pietersz RNI, Korte D, et al. Platelet activation during preparation of platelet concentrates: A comparison of the platelet rich plasma and the buffy coat methods. Transfusion 1990;30:634-8.
7. Valeri R, Feingold H, Marchionni LD. A simple method for freezing human platelets using 6 percent dimethylsulfoxide and storage at –80 degrees C. Blood 1974;43:131-6.

8. Read MS, Bode A, Brinkhouse K, et al. Preservation of hemostatic and structural properties or rehydrated lyophilized platelets. Proc Natl Acad Sci U S A 1995;92:397-401.
9. Murphy S. Platelet function, kinetics, and metabolism: Impact on quality, assessment, storage, and clinical use. In: McLeod BCC, Price TH, Drew MJ, eds. Apheresis: Principles and practice. Bethesda, MD: AABB Press, 1997:123-39.
10. Holme S, Murphy S. Quantitative measurements of platelet shape by light transmission studies: Application to storage of platelets for transfusion. J Lab Clin Med 1978;92:53-64.
11. Holme S, Vaidja K, Murphy S. Platelet storage at 22°C: Effect of type of agitation on morphology, viability, and function in-vitro. Blood 1978;52:425-35.
12. Murphy S, Gardner FH. Platelet storage at 22°C; metabolic, morphologic, and functional studies. J Clin Invest 1971;50:370-7.
13. Bode AP. Platelet activation may explain the storage lesion in platelet concentrates. Blood Cells 1990;16:109-26.
14. Holme S, Bode A, Heaton WAL, Swayer S. Improved maintenance of platelet in vivo viability during storage when using a synthetic medium with inhibitors. J Lab Clin Med 1992;119:144-50.
15. Seigl AM, Moroff G. Effect of forskolin on the maintenance of platelet properties during storage. J Lab Clin Med 1986;108:354-9.
16. Bode AP, Hole S, Heaton WA, Swanson MS. Extended storage of platelets in an artificial medium with the platelet activation inhibitors prostaglandin E1 and theophylline. Vox Sang 1991;60:105-12.
17. Snyder EL, Moroff G, Simon T. Symposium on radiolabeling of stored platelet concentrates. Transfusion 1986;26:1-42.
18. Heilman E, Friese P, Anderson S, et al. Biotinylated platelets: A new approach for the measurement of platelet lifespan. Br J Haematol 1993;85:729-35.
19. Valeri R, Feingold H, Marchionni LD. The relationship between the response to hypotonic stress and in vivo recovery of preserved platelets. Transfusion 1974;14:331-41.
20. Ross D, Holme S, Hartman P, et al. A quick visual method for quality control of platelet concentrates (abstract). Transfusion 1986; 26:550.
21. Bertolini F, Murphy S. A multicenter evaluation of reproducibility of swirling in platelet concentrates. Transfusion 1994;34:796-801.
22. Blajchman MA, Bardossy L, Carmen RA. An animal model of allogeneic donor platelet refractoriness. Blood 1992;79:1371-5.

23. Murphy S, Gardner FH. Platelet preservation. Effect of storage temperature on maintenance of platelet viability—deleterious effect of refrigerated storage. N Engl J Med 1969;280:1094-8.
24. Vostal JG, Mondoro TH. Liquid cold storage of platelets: A revitalized possible alternative for limiting bacterial contamination of platelet products. Transfus Med Rev 1997;11:286-95.
25. Mitchell SG, Hawker RJ, Turner VS. Effect of agitation on the quality of platelet concentrates. Vox Sang 1994;67:160-5.
26. Gotschall JL, Rzad L, Aster RH. Studies of the minimum temperature at which human platelets can be stored with full maintenance of viability. Transfusion 1986;26:460-2.
27. Rock G, White J, Labow R. Storage of platelets in balanced salt solutions: A simple platelet storage medium. Transfusion 1991;31:21-5.
28. Murphy S, Grode G, Davisson W, Buchholz DFH. Platelet storage in a synthetic medium (PSM) (abstract). Transfusion 1986;26:568.
29. Heddle NM, Klama LN, Griffith R, et al. A prospective study to identify the risk factors associated with acute reactions to platelet and red cell transfusion. Transfusion 1993;33:794-7.
30. Chambers LA, Kruskall MS, Pacini DG, Donovan LM. Febrile reactions after platelet transfusion: The effect of single versus multiple donors. Transfusion 1990;30:219-21.
31. Muylle L, Wouters E, DeBock R, et al. Reactions to platelet transfusions, the effect of the storage time of the concentrates. Transfus Med 1992;2:289-93.
32. Stack G, Snyder E. Generation of cytokines in stored platelet concentrates. Transfusion 1993;34:20-5.
33. Morrow JF, Braine HG, Kickler TS, Ness PM, et al. Septic reactions to platelet transfusion, a persistent problem. JAMA 1991;266:555-8.
34. Lin L, Cook DN, Wiesehahn GP, et al. Photochemical inactivation of viruses and bacteria in platelet concentrates by use of a novel psoralen and long wavelength ultraviolet light. Transfusion 1997;37:423-43.

In: Kickler TS, and Herman JH, eds.
Current Issues in Platelet Transfusion Therapy and Platelet Alloimmunity
Bethesda, MD: AABB Press, 1999

4

The Basic Immunology of Platelet-Induced Alloimmunization

JOHN W. SEMPLE, PhD, AND JOHN FREEDMAN, MD

IT HAS BECOME APPARENT THAT LEUKOCYTES CONtained in transfused platelet components are a major stimulus for the production of HLA antibodies. Hence, considerable effort has been committed to developing methods that reduce or modify leukocytes in platelet transfusion components. Two of the most common strategies, ultraviolet-B (UVB) irradiation and leukocyte reduction of platelets, are aimed at directly affecting the function and quantity, respectively, of leukocytes in the transfusion components. Recently, it

John W. Semple, PhD, Staff Scientist, Division of Hematology, St. Michael's Hospital, Associate Professor, Departments of Pharmacology and Medicine, University of Toronto; and The Toronto Platelet Immunobiology Group, Toronto, Canada; and John Freedman, MD, Director of Transfusion Services, St. Michael's Hospital, Professor, Department of Medicine, University of Toronto; and The Toronto Platelet Immunobiology Group, Toronto, Canada

has been confirmed that both of these approaches significantly reduce the incidence of alloimmunization and immune refractoriness in multitransfused patients with acute leukemia, although a number of patients still become alloimmunized. This chapter focuses on the immune mechanisms responsible for alloimmunization in platelet transfusions and on the role that leukocytes play in affecting these mechanisms. Where possible, the experimental findings are correlated with the clinical observations.

Alloimmunization is generally defined as a recipient's immune response against foreign cells from a donor of the same species. The alloimmune response can be measured by several soluble and cellular factors, but it is primarily confirmed by the identification of donor antibodies and/or cytotoxic T lymphocytes. From the early days of transfusion therapy, it was recognized that whole blood (WB) transfusions are immunogenic, and with the development of component therapy, it became evident that platelets, red blood cells, and even plasma can stimulate the production of donor alloantibodies. The immune mechanisms that result in alloimmunization to blood components are still incompletely understood but are largely related to both the cellular composition of the component transfused (the antigen) and the immune status of the recipient. The complexities of the patient and transfused component can be confounding factors that make it difficult to interpret many of the immunologic changes described in transfusion recipients. For example, experimental immunology often defines immune responses in relation to well-characterized "pure" antigens and then examines how manipulations of the antigen can affect the immune response. Platelet transfusions, however, deliver a complex mixture of primarily major histocompatibility complex (MHC) Class I-positive cells (platelets) and MHC Class II-positive antigen-presenting cells (APCs) included among the leukocytes. Recipient immunity against these cell mixtures can be quite different, depending on the proportion of specific cells in the transfusate. Additionally, with regard to recipient immune responses against transfused components, it is important to recall that most transfusion patients may be immunocompromised because of disease and/or therapy. Animal models help eliminate some of these confounding factors, leading to a clearer understanding of the factors that underlie the immune responses.

The Immune Response

It is beyond the scope of this chapter to review all aspects of the immune response, so only a summary of CD4+ T helper (Th) cell activation and its relationship to B-cell stimulation and IgG antibody production is provided.

The initiation of IgG humoral immune responses against exogenous foreign antigens (eg, soluble proteins, bacteria, or transfused allogeneic cells), involves the interaction and cooperation of several cell types and soluble factors. Secondary IgG immune responses are primarily mediated against protein antigens, such as cell surface glycoproteins, and are initiated when these antigens interact with APCs of the immune system (ie, MHC Class II-positive dendritic cells or macrophages).[1,2] The APCs internalize the antigens into endocytic compartments and, through a number of pH-dependent enzymatic steps and proteolytic (processing) reactions, metabolize them into peptides while they are being transported to intracellular compartments rich in MHC Class II molecules.[3] Through a series of molecular interactions involving, for example, the MHC Class II invariant chain and Class II-associated invariant peptide, the processed antigenic peptides are then loaded into the antigen-binding groove of MHC Class II molecules.[4] Subsequently, the MHC/peptide complexes are reexpressed on the surface of the APCs and presented for interaction with the T-cell receptors (TCRs) of CD4+ Th cells. Th cells, which have sufficient TCR:MHC/peptide affinity together with appropriate APC-dependent costimulatory events (eg, CD28-CD80/86 interaction and cytokine production), become activated.[5-8] For any given protein antigen, only a very small proportion of the recipient's entire Th cell repertoire (1 in 10^4-10^6) is stimulated.[9,10] Once Th cells are activated, however, the processes of Th cell clonal expansion and differentiation can eventually mediate a number of intense immune reactions, such as stimulating antigen-primed B lymphocytes to differentiate into plasma cells and secrete antigen-specific IgG antibodies.[11]

The Alloimmune Response

The advent of transfusion and transplantation medicine provided much of the impetus for the recognition and subsequent study of alloimmune responses. The extraordinary strength of allogeneic responses is intriguing when one considers that alloimmunity has no obvious physiologic function or survival value.[12] It now appears that the immune mechanisms responsible for alloimmune responses depend on the recipient's T-cell responses and on the APC composition of the allogeneic tissue.[12-14] With respect to MHC antibodies (primarily directed to MHC Class I antigens), alloimmunity can occur when donor or allogeneic MHC Class II-positive APCs are present in the blood component; in this case, the requirement for recipient APC function (eg, processing) is overcome and the donor APCs can directly interact with and activate recipient Th cells. Underlying this mechanism of alloimmunity, however, is the normal pathway of immunity, which can generate alloantibodies independently of the APCs in the transfused component.

Two recipient immune recognition mechanisms have been shown to initiate the alloimmune response. The first, the direct pathway, occurs when recipient Th cells directly interact with MHC Class II molecules on donor APCs.[15] This abnormally strong immune mechanism is the result of cross-reactivity of recipient TCRs with polymorphic residues of allogeneic MHC Class I and Class II molecules.[15] It has been estimated that between 1 and 5% of the recipient's entire TCR repertoire can be activated by this mechanism.[9,10] The second mechanism leading to alloimmunization, the indirect pathway, is analogous to the normal immune response[16-19] and occurs when allogeneic non-APCs are administered to the recipient. This mechanism involves the processing and presentation of allelic donor antigens (eg, MHC Class I molecules) by recipient APCs to recipient Th cells.[16-19] The frequency of recipient self-restricted T cells that can recognize processed allo-MHC (indirect recognition) is approximately 100 times lower than that of T cells recognizing intact allo-MHC (direct recognition).[20] Nonetheless, in healthy recipients, indirect allorecognition can generate MHC antibodies with virtually identical titers to those induced by the direct pathway.[21,22] The indirect mechanism is probably responsible for most of the IgG alloimmune responses against antigens derived from platelets, red blood cells, or plasma proteins. A major question still to be answered regarding the indirect pathway is whether it is active in human transfusion recipients in an immunocompromised state. However, since most clinical studies have shown that a proportion of leukemic patients receiving leukocyte-reduced platelets still become alloimmunized, it may be that indirect allorecognition is indeed competent in these patients. Hence, therapeutic manipulations other than leukocyte reduction may be needed. Figure 4-1 summarizes the basic principles of the two allorecognition mechanisms.

Molecular analyses of direct MHC alloreactivity have established that most of the potential antigenic determinants for alloreactive recipient T cells can be identified and mapped to polymorphic amino acid residues surrounding the antigen-binding groove of the Class II MHC molecules. Most Class II MHC molecules contain peptides within their groove, and the contribution of these peptides to direct alloreactive recognition is still under investigation.[23,24] Most alloreactive recognition by T cells probably results from recognition of a variety of different peptides bound to allogeneic MHC molecules; this, together with the many T cells normally specific for peptide plus self MHC, which cross-react with allogeneic MHC, is primar-

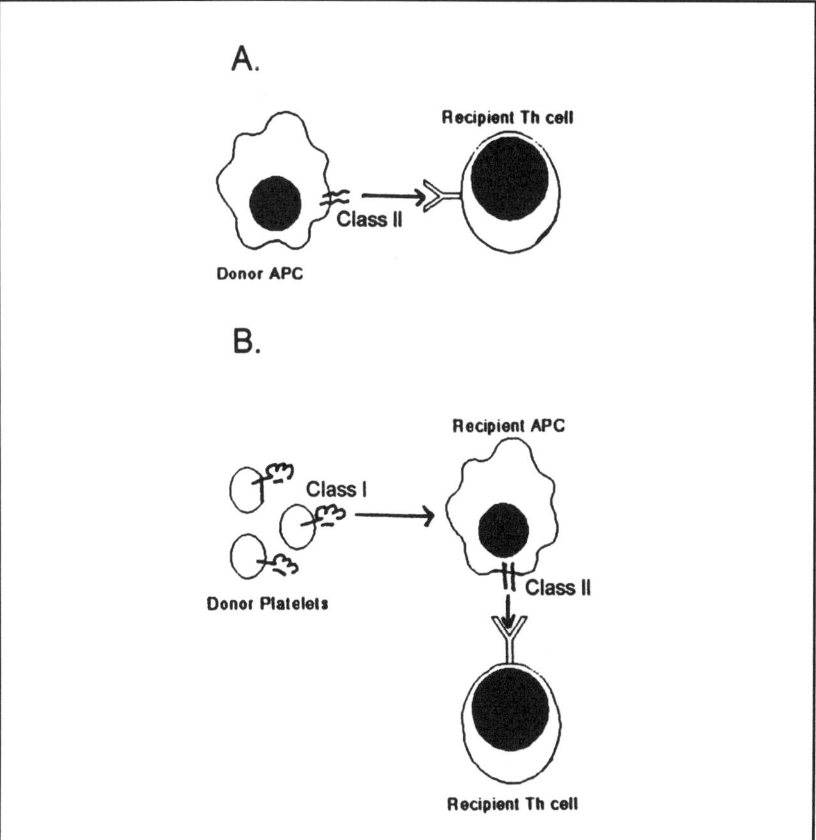

Figure 4-1. Direct and indirect allorecognition. A. Direct allorecognition occurs when the T-cell receptor of recipient T helper (Th) cells directly interacts with the major histocompatibility complex (MHC) Class II molecules on donor antigen-presenting cells (APCs). B. Indirect allorecognition takes place when donor platelet-derived MHC Class I alloantigens are processed and presented by MHC Class II molecules on recipient APCs.

ily responsible for the unusual magnitude of the direct alloreactive response.[23,24] Analogous studies have been performed for peptides involved in indirect MHC allorecognition and have revealed that the majority of peptides recognized by recipient Th cells are derived from the polymorphic residues of donor MHC Class I molecules.[25]

Considerable evidence supports the tenet that functional donor APCs present in blood components induce the majority of recipient humoral responses as a result of direct allorecognition.[26] The hypothesis that removal or modification of leukocytes would prevent or retard transfusion-induced alloimmunization[27] has been shown to be generally correct—at least in patients with leukemia.[28] On the other hand, paradoxically, donor APCs are also responsible for immunosuppressive-like reactions in the transfusion recipients.[29-36] If both alloimmunization and immunosuppression depend on the transfused donor APCs in blood components, it might be envisaged that an optimal number of APCs must be present for maximally reducing alloimmunization.

Transfusion-Induced Immunomodulation

Most of the scientific literature pertaining to animal models of transfusion has dealt with the recipient immunomodulatory effects of transfusion—the so-called transfusion effect. This effect has primarily been associated with an apparent immunosuppression and occurs when allogeneic WB or leukocytes are transfused into a recipient. The effect is subsequently measured by observing, for example, the survival of a donor transfusion-specific allograft. Clinically, the immunosuppressive effect was first identified as an enhancement of renal graft survival following transfusion,[37] and many experimental and clinical studies subsequently confirmed that transfusions containing viable APCs can induce significant recipient immunomodulation.[29-42] These immunomodulatory effects have now also been shown to affect a number of other pathophysiologic processes, such as increased tumor growth[43-45] and increased infections,[46-48] although the evidence supporting these effects remains controversial.[45,48]

The immune mechanisms mediating the transfusion effect are not completely known. However, early studies by Quigley et al[33] identified a recipient splenic T-suppressor activity during blood transfusions. Subsequently, Dallman et al[49] demonstrated a reduced production of interleukin (IL)-2 and a reduced expression of the IL-2 receptor in recipients of WB transfusion, suggesting an IL-2 defect, whereas Babcock and Alexander[50] showed that WB transfusions induce elevated IL-4 and IL-10 cytokine profiles in mice. Similar results have been reported in human recipients of WB.[51] More recently, using transgenic mice expressing a transgenic TCR recognizing the murine MHC Class I molecule L^d, Yang et al[52] demonstrated that a donor-specific transfusion of L^d-positive leukocytes induced tolerance to skin grafts and deleted a majority of donor-reactive T cells. They found that the remaining T cells in the presence of IL-4 were responsible for tolerance induction. These results suggest that WB or leukocyte transfusions tend to shift the recipient's antidonor T-cell immune response toward what is termed a "Th2 response."

For the last decade there has been a trend in immunology to divide Th responses into categories termed "Th1," "Th2," and "Th0."[53-56] These categories are based on the identification of cytokines elaborated. Th1-like responses produce IL-2 and interferon gamma; they primarily mediate cell-mediated immunity and the synthesis of complement-fixing IgG antibodies.[53-56] Th2-like responses, on the other hand, generally produce IL-4, IL-5, IL-6, IL-10, and IL-13 and are superior at inducing noncomplement-fixing IgG and IgE humoral immunity.[53-56] Th0-like responses are thought to be less differentiated than Th1- and Th2-like responses because cytokines characteristic of both (eg, IL-4, interferon gamma, and IL-10) can be identified. What makes these patterns of cytokines so intriguing is that they appear to correlate with different immune functions. With respect to transplantation, for example, there is compelling evidence that Th1 responses are associated with graft rejection,[57-61] whereas Th2 responses may be correlated with immune tolerance toward the graft,[62-65] although several studies have not been consistent with this.[66-68] These cytokine patterns may have relevance to understanding the role that blood transfusions play in nonresponsiveness to alloantigens.

Alloimmunization may be considered an aspect of recipient immunomodulation but may perhaps be better considered as the primary underlying immune response of the host. When a host is exposed to foreign tissue, its main "immunologic concern" is to maintain self-preservation and rid itself of the foreign tissue. With transfusion, depending on the component transfused, the recipient's immune response may be challenged in such a way as to become either deleted, anergic (nonresponsive), and/or altered so that it can no longer maintain immune dominance over the donor tissue and therefore allows graft survival. Related to the latter, Semple et al[22] have shown that recipient mice mount isotypically different IgG antidonor immune responses, depending on the type of blood component transfused. When mice are challenged with WB or leukocytes (containing APCs), they primarily mount a high-titered antidonor IgG1 response, whereas when they are transfused with extremely leukocyte-reduced MHC Class I-positive, Class II-negative platelets, they primarily produce IgG2a antibodies.[22] In mice, the fact that these IgG isotype responses are closely associated with Th1 (IgG2a) and Th2 (IgG1) cytokine responses[53,54] supports the contention that when leukocytes are present in a transfused blood component, Th2 responses can predominate. If the Th1/Th2 paradigm of rejection/tolerance, respectively, is correct, it would appear that leukocyte-containing blood components may drive the recipient's immune system toward Th2-

like responses that may be ineffective in mediating allograft rejection. However, as leukocytes are reduced, such as in platelets, Th1 responses are stimulated, which may significantly change the recipient's response to a graft.[22] A clinical correlate of this murine observation may be seen from evidence that, compared with WB transfusions, platelet transfusions are generally poorer inducers of the transfusion effect.[69,70] Indeed, it is possible that leukocyte-containing blood components do not necessarily cause active immunosuppression but simply generate an alloimmune response (Th2) of a nature that cannot effectively remove donor cells.

Platelet-Induced Alloimmunization

With respect to enriched blood components commonly transfused in clinical medicine, such as leukocyte-reduced platelets, fewer experimental studies have been performed to analyze recipient immune responses. Perhaps the earliest animal study to address platelet immunity was performed by Welsh et al,[71] who found that intraperitoneal injections of allogeneic MHC Class I-positive, Class II-negative rat platelets could not induce an antibody response. A later study in rhesus monkeys also showed that allogeneic platelets could not mount an antibody response.[72] In 1981, Claas et al,[73] using a murine model, demonstrated that allogeneic platelets required at least 10^3 leukocytes to elicit an anti-MHC response. Based on comparative blood volumes, this white blood cell (WBC) dose translates into a human transfusion of 2.5×10^6 WBCs. Subsequent clinical studies have similarly suggested that the threshold of residual leukocytes in human platelet concentrates to prevent alloimmunization should be less than 1-5 $\times 10^6$ WBCs.[74] Although the threshold numbers in the mice and human studies appear to correlate, no clear experimental evidence to date defines the actual leukocyte-reduction level that is required for the maximal reduction of alloimmunization to platelets.

In contrast to the above, several studies in animals and humans have shown that platelet components, including leukocyte-reduced platelets, can mount antibody responses. Platelet immunogenicity was first shown by Nagasawa et al[75] using a rabbit model, and Slichter et al[76] subsequently reported that 18 of 21 dogs became immunologically refractory to subsequent platelet transfusions when given eight weekly transfusions of allogeneic platelets. Blajchman et al[77] used a rabbit model to show that while there was a 91% refractory rate to subsequent platelet transfusions in animals transfused with nonleukocyte-reduced allogeneic blood, the incidence of refractoriness fell to 67% in those transfused with poststorage leukocyte-reduced blood and to 33% in rabbits receiving prestorage leukocyte-reduced blood. Furthermore, Pocsik et al[78] originally reported in 1990 that allogeneic leukocyte-reduced platelet transfusions in healthy human volunteers induced T-lymphocyte activation, particularly with respect to increased levels of IL-2 receptor expression. Thus, transfusions of leukocyte-reduced allogeneic platelets have been shown to stimulate recipient immunity in a variety of species, including humans.

In 1992, Kao[79] demonstrated that leukocyte-reduced (<3 WBC/μL) murine platelets were immunogenic when transfused weekly into allogeneic recipients; MHC antibodies could be detected in the sera of recipient mice by the fourth week of transfusion. Semple et al subsequently confirmed this finding in a different strain combination of mice[80] and also found that leukocyte-reduced platelet transfusions induced CD8+ cytotoxic T lymphocyte and CD4+ T-cell antidonor platelet reactivity. These results were the first to suggest that leukocyte-reduced platelets could elicit their immunogenicity via indirect allorecognition.[80] Concomitantly, Oh et al confirmed these results in a rat model of platelet transfusion.[81] The rat immune response against allogeneic leukocyte-reduced platelets shows several similar characteristics to murine immunity (J. Oh, personal communication).

Surprisingly, investigators found that the platelet-induced IgG antidonor response was preceded by an early (72-hours posttransfusion) stimulation of splenic cytotoxicity against natural killer cell-insensitive target cells. This simulation could be inhibited by N^G-monomethyl-L-arginine (NMMA), but not by depletion of CD8-positive T cells.[80] NMMA is a relatively nonselective inhibitor of a family of enzymes known as the nitric oxide synthases (NOSs).[82] The NOS enzymes catalyze the conversion of L-arginine to L-citrulline, which releases the diffusible gas, nitric oxide.[82] This reaction is responsible for a number of fundamental physiologic homeostatic mechanisms such as blood pressure control, and during inflammatory responses, activated macrophages can use the inducible form of NOS for host defense.[82,83] To characterize this platelet-induced cytotoxicity further, aminoguanidine, a more selective inhibitor of inducible NOS (iNOS),[82,83] was used and both the platelet-induced cytotoxicity and the IgG donor antibody production were selectively inhibited.[84] These results suggest that iNOS may be a recipient enzyme required for the processing and/or presentation of platelet-derived alloantigens to Th cells and for the subsequent stimulation of alloantibody production.[84] Using other metabolic inhibitors of antigen-processing pathways, the authors have obtained preliminary evidence indicating that iNOS activation may be associated with intracellular platelet antigen trafficking (JW Semple, unpublished observations).[85] Of interest, nitric oxide has been shown to be involved with f-actin rearrangements within endothelial cells and macrophage-like cells, which could affect antigen-processing membrane movements.[86,87] Altogether when one considers the literature regarding antigen processing and presentation (reviewed in Watts[3]), allogeneic platelets appear to have rather unique antigen processing and presentation requirements in order to activate Th cells. These observations may help elucidate the basic antigen-processing pathways of allogeneic platelet antigens and may allow for the development of more specific immunotherapies to prevent platelet-induced alloimmunization.

Murine allogeneic platelet transfusion models have shown two other interesting immune reactivities, which still have unknown clinical relevance. First, those murine strains (eg, C57BL/6, ASW, SJL) that lack I-E MHC Class II molecules are immune nonresponders against allogeneic platelet transfusions.[88] Using a series of transgenic and knockout mice, the authors' laboratory determined that the I-E MHC Class II molecule is the permissive restriction element for alloimmunity against platelets; this molecule presents platelet-derived MHC peptides, which positively stimulates alloimmunization. Nonetheless, it suggests that immune responsiveness against allogeneic platelets depends solely on the recipient's MHC Class II phenotype. Second, allogeneic platelet transfusions stimulate CD8+ cytotoxic T-lymphocytes concomitantly with IgG alloantibody production.[80] Intact platelet MHC Class I molecules could potentially engage the TCR of CD8+ T cells but would be expected to anergize the recipient's T cells because of their lack of costimulatory ability.[80,84] The observed cytotoxic T-lymphocyte reactivity, however, suggests that the CD4+ Th cells activated by indirect allorecognition may influence bystander CD8+ T cells, which could ultimately modulate the humoral alloimmune response. Figure 4-2 summarizes the potential T-cell activation pathways induced by allogeneic platelets.

A human model system that is amenable to experimental manipulation would be desirable. The authors have used mice with severe combined immunodeficiency (SCID) reconstituted with human lymphocytes and have successfully employed this model in studies of human platelet alloimmunization. CB.17 SCID mice were derived from BALB/c mice and have a point mutation on chromosome 16, which inhibits their ability to repair double-stranded DNA breaks.[89] Since the proper gene rearrangements for T-cell and B-cell receptors are critically dependent on this DNA repair process, these cells are deleted early in ontogeny. SCID mice are incapable of mounting T-lymphocyte-dependent or -independent immune responses.[90] These mice have been successfully reconstituted with human peripheral blood mononuclear cells (PBMCs) and have served as an in-vivo model of

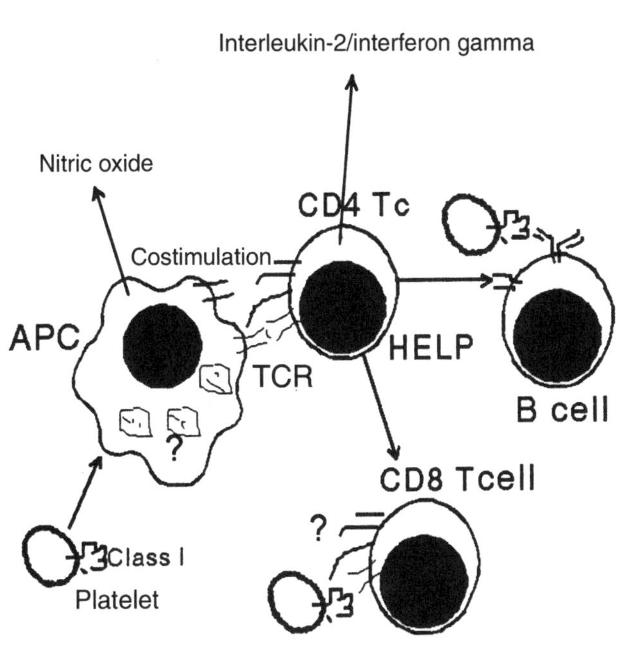

Figure 4-2. Pathways of T-cell activation induced by allogeneic platelets. Donor platelets are phagocytosed by recipient antigen-presenting cells (APCs). This event is associated with the production of nitric oxide, which may have a role in directing platelet-derived major histocompatibility complex (MHC) antigens to intracellular sites rich in recipient MHC Class II molecules. The platelet-derived MHC antigens are processed and presented by recipient MHC Class II molecules to the T-cell receptors (TCRs) of CD4+ T cells. With sufficient costimulation, the CD4+ T cells become activated and secrete cytokines such as interleukin-2 and interferon gamma, which can stimulate (help) either antigen-primed B cells or CD8+ T cells to differentiate into plasma cells or effector cells, respectively. The question marks point out the areas of still unknown potential (eg, exact platelet-processing mechanisms and whether intact platelet MHC Class I molecules can directly interact with CD8+ TCRs).

several human diseases involving the immune system,[90] including D antigen alloimmunization.[91] The immune response of SCID mice reconstituted with human PBMCs (hu-PBMC-SCID mice) to foreign antigens has generally been observed as a secondary immune response[92]; a primary immune response in these mice appears to be more difficult to establish.[92]

The authors developed a SCID mouse model of human alloimmunization and demonstrated that a secondary alloimmune response to platelet transfusions can be achieved in this system.[93] Hu-PBMC-SCID mice receiving weekly HLA-mismatched leukocytes produced IgG anti-human HLA when rechallenged with donor platelets. The use of hu-PBMC-SCID mice has potential for evaluating and manipulating human platelet alloimmunization; for example, the model can be used to study novel immunospecific therapies (eg, competitive antigenic peptides, anti-idiotypic antibodies, CD40L/CD40 interactions) to downregulate alloimmunity.

Testing the Role of Donor Antigen-Presenting Cells in Modulating Platelet Alloimmunization

Several studies, including the recently reported large multicenter Trial to Reduce Alloimmunization to Platelets (TRAP),[28] have indicated that leukocyte reduction is an effective strategy to reduce alloimmunization to platelets. However, it is evident that not all patients benefit from this approach. It remains unknown to what extent of leukocyte reduction is necessary to achieve maximal or optimal benefit. The authors have employed an animal model to address this, using platelets derived from SCID mice.

SCID mouse platelets prepared from platelet-rich plasma can be consistently and reproducibly rendered extremely leukocyte reduced (<0.05 WBC/μL).[94] These platelets, despite having fewer leukocytes, are significantly more immunogenic than BALB/c platelets in allogeneic CBA mouse recipients.[94] The increased immunity to the SCID mouse platelets was found to be due to the absence of leukocytes, since BALB/c WBCs added at levels of 1/μL could significantly inhibit the immune response to SCID mouse platelets.[94] The recipient immune mechanisms responsible for this WBC-induced reduction of platelet immunity are unknown, but several possibilities exist. These include the long-term engraftment of donor-derived hematopoietic cells (microchimerism),[95,96] or the transfer of potentially tolerogenic, costimulatory, molecule-deficient APCs resulting in operational tolerance via clonal anergy.[97] Alternatively, host immunity against purely MHC Class I-positive platelets vs platelets that contain MHC Class II-positive APCs could be unregulated and proceeds at an enhanced rate. In other models of transplantation, particularly liver transplantation, the concept that the amount of donor APCs in the graft plays a key role in either graft acceptance or rejection has found acceptance.[98-100] Whether the findings in this murine model are applicable to human transfusions remains unknown; they suggest that in immunocompetent recipients, excessive leukocyte reduction may be undesirable. Thus, while confirming that leukocyte reduction to levels approaching 1/μL is effective in reducing alloimmunization in a healthy recipient, the murine studies additionally have important implications suggesting that a defined number of selected leukocytes in platelet concentrates may be beneficial to the recipient. This may have relevance to selective leukocyte-reduction strategies. Figure 4-3 summarizes the relationship between platelet leukocyte levels and the magnitude of the donor antibody response.

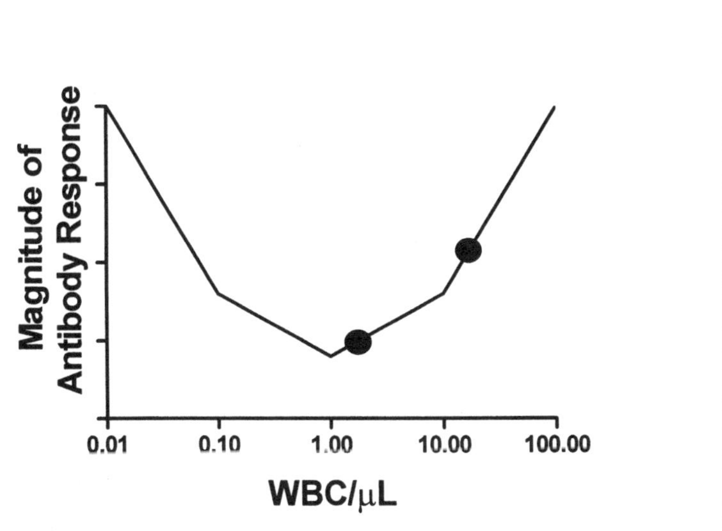

Figure 4-3. Plot showing the relationship between the leukocyte levels within platelets and recipient antidonor major histocompatibility complex (MHC) immunity. A murine model of platelet alloimmunization suggests that as leukocytes within allogeneic platelets are reduced to near zero (<0.05/μL) levels, the platelet-induced antidonor MHC immunity actually increases. The y axis is expressed as the magnitude of response and relates to the IgG antidonor titer. White blood cell (WBC) levels are enumerated by flow cytometry as previously described.[80] For comparison, the solid circles represent where levels of 1 and 5×10^6 WBCs in a 300-mL platelet concentrate would fall on the curve.

Manipulations of Donor Antigen-Presenting Cells in Leukocyte-Containing Platelets

T cells require two signals to become activated. The first is the TCR engagement of the MHC Class II molecule/peptide complex on the surface of APCs; the second includes APC-derived cytokines and the interaction of costimulatory molecules such as CD28-CD80/86.[5-8] Alloreactive T-cell activation by direct recognition of donor APCs also follows this two-signal scheme. If recipient T cells receive donor signal 1 without the donor APC-derived signal 2, anergy or death due to apoptosis ensues, which can lead to recipient unresponsiveness.[101] This reasoning is the basis of UVB irradiation strategies designed to inactivate APC costimulatory function.

UVB irradiation causes protein denaturation, which impairs donor APC processes such as antigen presentation and costimulation (signal 2). It was originally found that UVB-irradiated lymphocytes could no longer stimulate the mixed lymphocyte reaction (MLR).[102] Subsequently, Kahn et al[103] observed that a platelet suspension irradiated with a dose of UVB sufficient to abrogate the ability of its leukocytes to stimulate an MLR had no evident effect on platelet function. Slichter et al[104] reported that only 1 of 12 dogs were alloimmunized after receiving a series of eight weekly transfusions of irradiated platelets compared with 18 of 21 dogs alloimmunized by untreated platelets. Deeg et al[105] reported that donor-specific blood transfusions prior to marrow transplantation led to marrow rejection by littermate dogs, whereas dogs receiving UVB-irradiated blood had successful engraftment. Furthermore, Grijzenhout et al[106] found that the dose of UVB-irradiated leukocytes per transfusion determined the efficacy of alloimmunization reduction. Of interest, they found that lower numbers of transfused UVB-irradiated leukocytes were preferential whereas higher numbers were not effective in the prevention of alloimmunization. Similarly, Kao[107] found that tolerance induction by UVB-irradiated leukocytes was dose-dependent and stimulated the development of splenic regulatory cells, which may be responsible for alloimmunization reduction. In addition, Li et al[108] found that a UVB-irradiated leukocyte transfusion in combination with cyclosporin A induced significant rat renal allograft survival. The TRAP study has now confirmed that UVB irradiation of platelet concentrates can reduce the incidence of alloimmunization.[28] One drawback of this strategy, however, is that UV irradiation cannot be readily applied to red blood cell concentrates, and WBCs in such concentrates are likely to contribute to alloimmunization in at-risk subjects. Nonetheless, UVB irradiation may be a cost-effective alternative to leukocyte-reduction strategies.

Theoretically, any treatment that can cause APC inactivation while maintaining the viability of the platelets has the potential to reduce alloimmunization. For example, photoactivatible compounds such as the psoralens are aromatic compounds that bind reversibly to nucleic acids via intercalation.[109] Upon illumination with long-wavelength UVA light (320-400 nM), the intercalated psoralens form monoadducts and cause interstrand crosslinking.[109] These compounds have been used almost exclusively to inactivate viruses and bacteria in blood components, but their efficacy in preventing alloimmunization has received limited attention. Grana[110] demonstrated that when 8-methoxypsoralen, a psoralen derivative, was used to treat murine platelets, production of donor antibodies was significantly inhibited. More recently, Grass et al[111] have shown that psoralen compounds can reduce in-vitro cytokine production and inhibit the function of APCs. Additionally, others have shown that psoralen compounds can also affect CD69-positive T cells within platelet concentrates.[112] It may be that these types of compounds could be developed to be effective in inactivating donor APCs in blood components for transfusion and in reducing alloimmunization.

Future Considerations

The use of technologies such as leukocyte filtration is significantly increasing and is evolving to produce relatively pure platelet concentrates. One of the major questions still open is, how far one should reduce the levels of APCs in platelet concentrates to achieve maximum benefit to the recipient? Furthermore, does the type of residual leukocyte (eg, MHC Class II APC vs non-APC) within platelets affect recipient immunity?

At present, leukocyte reduction appears to be a relatively efficient means to reduce alloimmunization. However, a number of patients still become alloimmunized to HLA antigens. Furthermore, leukocyte reduction does not appear to reduce the production of platelet-specific alloantibodies.[28] More efficient means of immunotherapy need to be developed to manage patients at risk. With respect to platelet-specific antibodies (including MHC antibodies induced by the platelets themselves), one strategy may be to identify those platelet-derived antigens that are eliciting T-cell activation and modify them to make them nonimmunogenic when they are presented by APCs. Animal models may be useful for addressing this type of strategy.

Platelets are critically involved in many inflammatory reactions. Activated platelets express IL-1β on their surface and can induce endothelial cells to secrete chemokines and express adhesion molecules to initiate such reactions.[113,114] The role of platelet-derived IL-1β in alloimmune responses is unknown, but IL-1 is recognized to play an important role in the generation of immune responsiveness. In addition, the recent exciting observation that activated platelets express the CD40 ligand (CD40L, CD154) suggests that these platelets may directly initiate an inflammatory response of the vessel wall.[115] CD40L is structurally related to tumor necrosis factor-α and was originally identified on stimulated CD4+ T cells; its interaction with CD40 on B cells is critical to the development and function of the humoral immune system.[116] The role of CD40L on activated platelets in the development of recipient inflammatory reactions and alloimmune responses merits further study. Additionally, these proinflammatory molecules expressed by activated platelets may possibly play a role in other recipient reactions, such as febrile nonhemolytic transfusion reactions.

Although no animal model of transfusion can completely mimic the human situation, much of what we do know of the human alloimmune response has come from studying the murine immune system. As presented in this chapter, the animal data suggest that in mammalian species with a functioning immune system, although donor leukocytes play an important role in the recipient's immune response, allogeneic platelets are in themselves immunogenic with respect to MHC antigens. Furthermore, recent studies support the concept that a residual number of defined APCs within an allogeneic platelet transfusion component are required for maximal suppression of antidonor immunity. Leukocyte-reduction strategies may therefore need to take into account both the quantitative and the qualitative nature of residual leukocytes in the platelet transfusion component.

References

1. Unanue ER. Antigen-presenting function of the macrophage. Ann Rev Immunol 1984;2:395-429.
2. Lanzavecchia A. Receptor-mediated antigen uptake and its effect on antigen presentation to Class II-restricted T lymphocytes. Ann Rev Immunol 1990;8:773-93.
3. Watts C. Capture and processing of exogenous antigens for presentation on MHC molecules. Ann Rev Immunol 1997;15:821-50.
4. Cresswell P. Invariant chain structure and MHC Class II function. Cell 1996;84:505-7.
5. Bretscher P, Cohn M. A theory of self-nonself discrimination. Science 1970;169:1042-9.

6. Linsley PS, Clark EA, Ledbetter JA. T-cell antigen CD28 mediates adhesion with B cells by interacting with activation antigen B7/BB-1. Proc Natl Acad Sci U S A 1990;87:5031-6.
7. Liu Y, Linsley PS. Costimulation of T cell growth. Curr Opin Immunol 1992;4:265-70.
8. Lenschow DJ, Walunas TL, Bluestone JA. CD28/B7 system of T cell costimulation. Ann Rev Immunol 1996;14:233-58.
9. Lindahl KF, Wilson DB. Histocompatibility antigen-activated cytotoxic T lymphocytes, II: Estimates of frequency and specificity of precursors. J Exp Med 1977;145:508-22.
10. The HS, Harley E, Phillips RA, Miller RG. Quantitative studies on the precursors of cytotoxic lymphocytes, I: Characteristics of a clonal assay and determination of the size of clones derived from single precursors. J Immunol 1977;118:1049-56.
11. Parker DC. T cell-dependent B cell activation. Ann Rev Immunol 1993;11:331-60.
12. Auchincloss H Jr, Sachs DH. Transplantation and graft rejection. In: Paul WE, ed. Fundamental immunology. New York: Raven, 1993: 1099-141.
13. Rosenberg AS, Mizuochi T, Singer A. Evidence for involvement of dual-function T cells in rejection of MHC Class I disparate skin grafts. Assessment of MHC Class I alloantigens as in vivo helper determinants. J Exp Med 1988;168:33-45.
14. Rosenberg AS, Singer A. Cellular basis of skin allograft rejection: An in vivo model of immune-mediated tissue destruction. Ann Rev Immunol 1992;10:333-58.
15. Sayegh MH, Watschinger B, Carpenter CB. Mechanisms of T cell recognition of alloantigen. The role of peptides. Transplantation 1994;57:1295-302.
16. Adams PW, Lee HS, Waldman WJ, et al. Alloantigenicity of human endothelial cells, III: Quantitated indirect presentation of endothelial alloantigens to human helper T lymphocytes. Transplantation 1994;58:476-83.
17. Steele DJR, Laufer TM, Smiley ST, et al. Two levels of help for B cell alloantibody production. J Exp Med 1996;183:699-703.
18. Chen W, Murphy B, Waaga AM, et al. Mechanisms of indirect allorecognition in graft rejection. Class II allopeptide-specific T cell clones transfer delayed-type hypersensitivity responses in vivo. Transplantation 1996;62:705-10.

19. Clement JD, Chan SY, Bishop DK. Allogeneic Class I MHC requirement for alloantigen-reactive helper T-lymphocyte responses in vivo. Evidence for indirect presentation of alloantigens. Transplantation 1996;62:388-96.
20. Liu Z, Sun Y-K, Xi Y-P, et al. Contribution of direct and indirect recognition pathways to T cell alloreactivity. J Exp Med 1993;177:1643-54.
21. Morton AL, Bell EB, Bolton EM, et al. CD4+ T cell-mediated rejection of major histocompatibility complex Class I-disparate grafts: A role for alloantibody. Eur J Immunol 1993;23:2078-84.
22. Semple JW, Cosgrave D, Speck ER, et al. Recipient immune responses induced by allogeneic whole blood or platelet transfusions: Implications for immunomodulation. In: Smit Sibinga C. Th, Das PC, Löwenberg B, eds. Cytokines and growth factors in blood transfusion. Boston, MA: Kluwer, 1997:29-45.
23. Cuturi MC, Josien R, Douillard P, et al. Prolongation of allogeneic heart graft survival in rats by administration of a peptide (a.a. 75-84) from the $\alpha 1$ helix of the first domain of HLA-B7 01. Transplantation 1995;59:661-8.
24. Shirwan H, Leamer M, Wang HK, et al. Peptides from α-helices of allogeneic Class I major histocompatibility complex antigens are potent inducers of CD4+ and CD8+ T cell and B cell responses after cardiac allograft rejection. Transplantation 1995;59:401-9.
25. Gallon L, Watschinger B, Murphy B, et al. Indirect pathway of allorecognition: The occurrence of self-restricted T cell recognition of allo-MHC peptides early in acute allograft rejection and its inhibition by conventional immunosuppression. Transplantation 1995;59:612-6.
26. Freedman J, Semple JW. Transfusion-induced alloimmunization. In: Singal DP, ed. Immunological effects of blood transfusion. Boca Raton, FL: CRC Press, 1995:19-42.
27. Merryman HT. Transfusion-induced alloimmunization and immunosuppression and the effects of leukocyte depletion. Transfus Med Rev 1989;3:180-93.
28. Trial to Reduce Alloimmunization to Platelets (TRAP) Study Group. Leukocyte reduction and ultraviolet B irradiation of platelets to prevent alloimmunization and refractoriness to platelet transfusions. N Engl J Med 1997;337:1861-915.
29. Lenhard V, Mytilineos J, Hansen B, et al. Immunoregulation after blood transfusions in the rat model—anti-idiotypic antibodies or suppressor cells? Transplant Proc 1985;17:2393-6.

30. Ludwin D, Stary S, Singal DP. Suppressor cell generation in mice after blood transfusions from different H-2 donors. Transplant Proc 1987;21:3402-5.
31. Wood ML, Gottschalk R, Monaco AP. Immune reactivity of congenic mice after allogeneic or isogeneic transfusion. Transplantation 1986; 41:489-97.
32. Bektas H, Jorns Klempnauer J. Differential effect of donor-specific blood transfusion after kidney, heart, pancreas, and skin transplantation in major histocompatibility complex-incompatible rats. Transfusion 1997;37:226-30.
33. Quigley RL, Wood KJ, Morris PJ. Transfusion induces blood donor-specific suppressor cells. J Immunol 1989;142:463-70.
34. Blajchman MA, Bardossy L, Carmen RA, et al. An animal model of allogenic donor platelet refractoriness: The effect of the time of leukodepletion. Blood 1992;79:1371-5.
35. Bordin JO, Bardossy L, Blajchman MA. Experimental animal model of refractoriness to donor platelets: The effect of plasma removal and the extent of white cell reduction on allogeneic alloimmunization. Transfusion 1993;33:798-801.
36. Donnelly PK, Proud G, Shenton BK, et al. Transfusion-induced immunosuppression and red cells clearance. Transfusion Med 1991;1: 217-21.
37. Opelz G, Sengar DPS, Mickey MR, et al. Effect of blood transfusions on subsequent kidney transplants. Transplant Proc 1973;5:253-9.
38. Fabre JW, Bishop M, Sen T, et al. A study of three protocols of blood transfusion before renal transplantation in the dog. Transplantation 1978;26:94-8.
39. Quigley RL, Wood KJ, Morris PJ. Investigation of the mechanism of active enhancement of renal allograft survival by blood transfusion. Immunology 1988;163:373-81.
40. Soulillou J-P, Bignon JD, Peyrat MA. Genetics of the blood transfusion effect on heart allografts in rats. Transplantation 1994;38:63-7.
41. Shirwan H, Wang HK, Barwari L, et al. Pretransplant injection of allograft recipients with donor blood or lymphocytes permits allograft tolerance without the presence of persistent donor chimerism. Transplantation 1996;61:1382-6.
42. Wood PJ, Roberts IS, Yang C-P, et al. Prevention of chronic rejection by donor-specific blood transfusion in a new model of chronic cardiac allograft rejection. Transplantation 1996;61:1440-3.

43. Waymack JP, Fernandez G, Yurt RW, et al. Effect of blood transfusions on immune function, VI: Effect on immunologic response to tumour. Surgery 1990;108:172-8.
44. Bordin JO, Bardossy L, Blajchman MA. Growth enhancement of established tumors by allogeneic blood transfusion in experimental animals and its amelioration by leukodepletion: The importance of the timing of the leukodepletion. Blood 1994;84:344-8.
45. Rustoven JJ. Blood transfusion and cancer: Clinical studies. In: Singal DP, ed. Immunological effects of blood transfusion. Boca Raton, FL: CRC Press, 1995:85-110.
46. Tartter PI. Blood transfusion and bacterial infections: Clinical studies. In: Singal DP, ed. Immunological effects of blood transfusion. Boca Raton, FL: CRC Press, 1995:111-26.
47. Jensen LS, Anderson AJ, Christiansen PM, et al. Postoperative infection and natural killer cell function following blood transfusion in patients undergoing elective colorectal surgery. Br J Surg 1992;79: 513-6.
48. Vamvakas EC, Moore SB. Blood transfusion and postoperative septic complications. Transfusion 1994;34:714-27.
49. Dallman MJ, Wood KJ, Morris PJ. Recombinant interleukin-2 (IL-2) can reverse the blood transfusion effect. Transplant Proc 1989;21: 1165-7.
50. Babcock GF, Alexander JW. The effects of blood transfusion on cytokine production by Th1 and Th2 lymphocytes in the mouse. Transplantation 1996;61:465-70.
51. Kalechman Y, Gafter U, Sobelman D, Sredni B. The effect of a single whole-blood transfusion on cytokine secretion. J Clin Immunol 1990;10:99-105.
52. Yang L, DuTemple B, Khan Q, Zhang L. Mechanisms of long-term donor-specific allograft survival induced by pretransplant infusion of lymphocytes. Blood 1998;91:324-30.
53. Mosmann TR, Coffman RL. Th1 and Th2 cells: Different patterns of lymphokine secretion lead to different functional properties. Ann Rev Immunol 1989;7:145-73.
54. Romagnani S. Th1 and Th2 in human diseases. Clin Exp Immunol 1996;80:225-35.
55. Snapper CM, Paul WE. Interferon-γ and B cell stimulatory Factor-1 reciprocally regulate Ig isotype production. Science 1986;236:944-7.

56. Cher D, Mosman TR. Two types of mouse helper T cell clones, II: Delayed-type hypersensitivity is mediated by Th1 clones. J Immunol 1987;138:3688-95.
57. O'Connell P, Pacheco-Silva A, Nickerson P. Unmodified pancreatic islet allograft rejection results in the preferential expression of certain T cell activation transcripts. J Immunol 1993;150:1093-104.
58. Thai NL, Fu F, Qian S, et al. Cytokine mRNA profiles in mouse orthotopic liver transplantation. Graft rejection is associated with augmented Th1 function. Transplantation 1995;59:274-81.
59. Egawa H, Martinez OM, Quinn MB, et al. Acute liver allograft rejection in the rat. An analysis of the immune response. Transplantation 1995;59:97-104.
60. Takeuchi T, Lowry RP, Konieczny B. Heart allografts in mouse systems: The differential activation of Th2-like effector cells in peripheral tolerance. Transplantation 1992;53:1281-9.
61. Hayashi M, Martinez OM, Garcia-Kennedy R, et al. Expression of cytokines and immune mediators during chronic liver allograft rejection. Transplantation 1995;60:1533-41.
62. Landorfo S, Cofano F, Giovarelli P, et al. Inhibition of interferon-gamma may suppress allograft reactivity by T lymphocytes in vitro and in vivo. Science 1985;229:176-9.
63. Chen N, Field EH. Enhanced type 2 and diminished type 1 cytokines in neonatal tolerance. Transplantation 1995;59:933-41.
64. Mottra PL, Han W-R, Purcell LJ, et al. Increased expression of IL-4 and IL-10 and decreased expression of IL-2 and interferon-γ in long-surviving mouse heart allografts after brief CD4-monoclonal antibody therapy. Transplantation 1995;59:559-65.
65. Donckier V, Wissing M, Bruyns C, et al. Critical role of interleukin 4 in the induction of neonatal transplantation tolerance. Transplantation 1995;59:1571-6.
66. Piccotti JR, Chan SY, VanBuskirk AM, et al. Are Th2 helper T lymphocytes beneficial, deleterious, or irrelevant in promoting allograft survival? Transplantation 1997;63:619-24.
67. Martinez OM, Vilanueva JC, Lake J, et al. IL-2 and IL-5 gene expression in response to alloantigen in liver allograft recipients and in vitro. Transplantation 1993;55:1159-67.
68. Chan SY, DeBruyne LA, Goodman RE, et al. In vivo depletion of CD8+ T cells results in Th2 cytokine production and alternative mechanisms of allograft rejection. Transplantation 1995;59:1155-61.

69. Bijnen AB, Heineman E, Marquet RL, et al. Lack of beneficial effect of thrombocyte transfusions on the kidney graft survival in dogs. Transplantation 1984;37:213-4.
70. Chapman JR, Ting A, Fisher M, et al. Failure of platelet transfusion to improve human renal allograft survival. Transplantation 1986;41:468-73.
71. Welsh KI, Burgos H, Batchelor JR. The immune response to allogeneic rat platelets; Ag-B antigens in matrix form lacking Ia. Eur J Immunol 1977;7:267-72.
72. Oh JH, McClure HM, Tuttle EP. Immunological unresponsiveness induced by platelet transfusions in rhesus monkeys. Transplantation 1983;36:727-32.
73. Claas FHJ, Smeenk RJT, Schmidt R, et al. Alloimmunization against the MHC antigens after platelet transfusions is due to contaminating leukocytes in the platelet suspension. Exp Hematol 1981;9:84-9.
74. Freedman JJ, Blajchman MA, McCombie N. Canadian Red Cross Society symposium on leukocyte-reduction: Report of proceedings. Transfus Med Rev 1994;8:1-14.
75. Nagasawa T, Kim BK, Baldini MG. Temporary suppression of circulating anti-platelets allo-antibodies by the massive infusion of fresh stored and lyophilized platelets. Transfusion 1978;18:429-35.
76. Slichter SJ, O'Donnell MR, Weiden PL, et al. Canine platelet alloimmunization: The role of donor selection. Br J Haematol 1986;63:713-27.
77. Blajchman MA, Bardossy L, Carmen RA, et al. An animal model of allogeneic platelet refractoriness: The effect of the time of leukodepletion. Blood 1992;79:1371-5.
78. Pocsik E, Mihalik R, Gyodi E, et al. Activation of lymphocytes after platelet allotransfusion possessing only Class I MHC product. Clin Exp Immunol 1990;82:102-8.
79. Kao KJ. Effects of leukocyte depletion and UVB irradiation on alloantigenicity of major histocompatibility complex antigens in platelet concentrates: A comparative study. Blood 1992;80:2931-7.
80. Semple JW, Speck ER, Milev YP, et al. Indirect allorecognition of platelets by T helper cells during platelet transfusions correlates with anti-MHC antibody and cytotoxic T lymphocyte formation. Blood 1995;86:805-12.
81. Oh JH, Taysavong P, Whelchel JD. Conferring immunogenicity to platelets by preincubation with recipients' adherent cells (abstract).

In: Proceedings IX International Congress of Immunology. San Francisco, CA, 1995:69.
82. Fukuto JM, Chaudhuri G. Inhibition of constitutive and inducible nitric oxide synthase: Potential selective inhibition. Annu Rev Pharmacol Toxicol 1995;35:165-93.
83. Misko TP, Moore WM, Kasten TP, et al. Selective inhibition of the inducible nitric oxide synthase by aminoguanidine. Eur J Pharmacol 1993;233:119-27.
84. Bang A, Speck ER, Blanchette VS, et al. Recipient humoral immunity against leukoreduced allogeneic platelets is suppressed by aminoguanidine, a selective inhibitor of inducible nitric oxide synthase (iNOS). Blood 1996;88:2959-66.
85. Bang A, Hicks KJ, Speck ER, et al. Allogeneic platelets require unique antigen processing mechanisms within recipient antigen presenting cells (APC) in order to stimulate alloantibody production (abstract). Blood 1996;88:162a.
86. Clancy RJ, Leszcynska J, Amin A, et al. Nitric oxide stimulates ADP ribosylation of actin in association with the inhibition of actin polymerization in human neutrophils. J Leukoc Biol 1995;58:196-203.
87. Liu SM, Sundqvist T. Involvement of nitric oxide in permeability alteration and F-actin redistribution induced by phorbol myristate acetate in endothelial cells. Exp Cell Res 1995;221:289-98.
88. Semple JW, Speck ER, Blanchette V, Freedman J. Immune nonresponsiveness to allogeneic platelets in murine strains which lack MHC Class II I-E molecules is due to the presence of CD8+ T cells (abstract). Blood 1996;88:162a.
89. Fischer A, Cavazzana-Calvo M, De Saint Basile G, et al. Naturally occurring primary deficiencies of the immune system. Annu Rev Immunol 1997;15:93-124.
90. Barry TS, Haynes BF. In vivo models of human lymphopoiesis and autoimmunity in severe combined immune deficient mice. J Clin Immunol 1992;12:311-24.
91. Leader KA, Macht LM, Steers JH Jr. Antibody responses to the blood group antigen D in SCID mice reconstituted with human blood mononuclear cells. Immunology 1992;76:229-34.
92. Tary-Lehmann M, Saxon A, Lehmann PV. The human immune system in hu-PBL-SCID mice. Immunol Today 1995;16:529-33.
93. Lazarus AH, Crow AR, Semple JW, et al. Induction of a secondary human anti-HLA alloimmune response in severe combined immu-

nodeficient mice engrafted with human lymphocytes. Transfusion 1997;37:1192-9.

94. Semple JW, Speck ER, Cosgrave D, et al. Extreme leukoreduction of major histocompatibility complex class II positive B cells enhances allogeneic platelet immunity. Blood 1999;93.
95. Starzl TE, Demetris AJ, Murase N, et al. Cell migration, chimerism and graft acceptance. Lancet 1992;339:1579-82.
96. Starzl TE, Demetris AJ, Trucco M, et al. Cell migration and chimerism after whole organ transplantation: The basis of graft acceptance. Hepatology 1993;17:1127-52.
97. Schwartz RH. Immunological tolerance. In: Paul WE, ed. Fundamental immunology. New York: Raven, 1993:677-732.
98. Sun J, McCaughan GW, Gallager N, et al. Deletion of spontaneous rat liver allograft acceptance by donor irradiation. Transplantation 1995;60:233-6.
99. Tu Y, Arima T, Flye MW. Rejection of spontaneously accepted rat liver allografts with recipient interleukin-2 treatment or donor irradiation. Transplantation 1997;63:177-81.
100. Steptoe RJ, Fu F, Li W, et al. Augmentation of dendritic cells in murine organ grafts by Flt3 ligand alters the balance between transplant tolerance and immunity. J Immunol 1997;159:5483-91.
101. Jenkins MK, Schwartz RH. Antigen presentation by chemically modified splenocytes induces antigen-specific T cell unresponsiveness in vitro and in vivo. J Exp Med 1987;165:302-9.
102. Lindahl-Kiessling K, Safwenberg J. Inability of UV-irradiated lymphocytes to stimulate allogeneic cells in mixed lymphocyte culture. Int Arch Allergy Immunol 1971;41:670-80.
103. Kahn RA, Duffy BF, Rodey GG. Ultraviolet irradiation of platelet concentrates abrogates lymphocyte activation without affecting platelet function in vitro. Transfusion 1985;25:547-50.
104. Slichter SJ, Deeg HJ, Kennedy MS. Prevention of platelet alloimmunization in dogs with systemic cyclosporin and by UV-irradiation or cyclosporin-loading of donor platelets. Blood 1987;69:414-8.
105. Deeg HJ, Aprile J, Graham TC, et al. Ultraviolet irradiation of blood prevents transfusion-induced sensitization and marrow graft rejection in dogs. Blood 1996;87:537-9.
106. Grijzenhout MA, Aarts-Riemens MI, Claas FHJ, et al. Prevention of MHC-alloimmunization by UVB-irradiation in a murine model: Ef-

fects of UV dose and number of transfused cells. Br J Haematol 1994;87:598-604.

107. Kao KJ. Induction of humoral immune tolerance to major histocompatibility complex antigens by transfusions of UVB-irradiated leukocytes. Blood 1996;88:4375-82.

108. Li S, Hart ME, Bloom A, Miller J. The impact of ultraviolet B-irradiated leukocyte transfusion and cyclosporin in rat kidney transplantation. Transplantation 1996;61:320-39.

109. Cimino G, Gamper H, Isaacs S, Hearst J. Psoralens as photoactive probes of nucleic acid structure and function: Organic chemistry, photochemistry, and biochemistry. Ann Rev Biochem 1985;54:1151-78.

110. Grana NH. Use of 8-methoxypsoralen and ultraviolet-A pretreated platelet concentrates to prevent alloimmunization against Class I major histocompatibility antigens. Blood 1991;77:2530-7.

111. Grass JA, Hei DJ, Metchette K, et al. Inactivation of leukocytes in platelet concentrates by photochemical treatment with psoralen plus UVA. Blood 1998;91:2180-8.

112. Fiebig E, Hirschkorn D, Busch M, et al. Loss of inducible CD69 expression on donor T cells (CD3+69+ind) in platelet concentrates (PCS) by storage, irradiation and photochemical treatment (abstract). Transfusion 1997;37(suppl):92S.

113. Hawrylowicz CM, Santoro SA, Platt FM, Unanue ER. Activated platelets express IL-1 activity. J Immunol 1989;143:4015-21.

114. Hawrylowicz CM, Howels GL, Feldman M. Platelet-derived interleukin 1 induced human endothelial adhesion molecule expression and cytokine production. J Exp Med 1991;174:785-90.

115. Henn V, Slupsky JR, Grafe M, et al. CD40 ligand on activated platelets triggers an inflammatory reaction of endothelial cells. Nature 1998;391:591-4.

116. Foy TM, Aruffo A, Bajorath A, et al. Immune regulation by CD40 and its ligand GP39. Ann Rev Immunol 1996;14:591-617.

In: Kickler TS, and Herman JH, eds.
Current Issues in Platelet Transfusion Therapy and Platelet Alloimmunity
Bethesda, MD: AABB Press, 1998

5

A Critical Analysis of Clinical Trials to Prevent Platelet Alloimmunization

K. J. KAO, MD, PhD

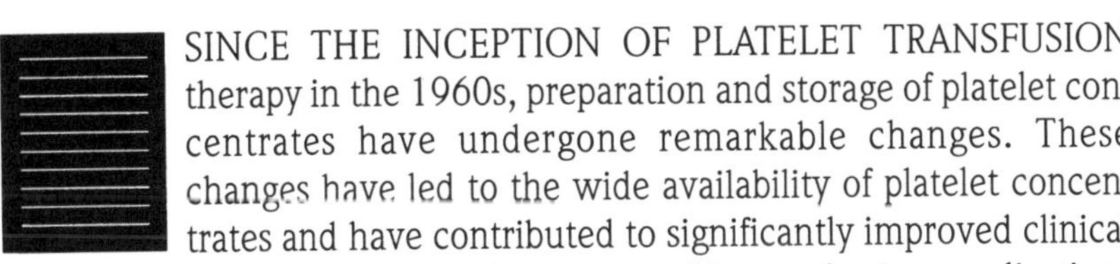

SINCE THE INCEPTION OF PLATELET TRANSFUSION therapy in the 1960s, preparation and storage of platelet concentrates have undergone remarkable changes. These changes have led to the wide availability of platelet concentrates and have contributed to significantly improved clinical outcomes in the prevention and treatment of hemorrhagic complications associated with thrombocytopenia. Today, more than 4 million units of platelets are transfused annually.[1] Unfortunately, because platelet concentrates, like other blood products, are immunogenic, the increased platelet usage has been accompanied by a concomitant increase in immunologic

K. J. Kao, MD, PhD, Professor, Department of Pathology, Immunology and Laboratory Medicine, and Medical Director, Shands Hospital Blood Bank, University of Florida, Gainesville, Florida

complications, the most common of which is antibody development to donor Class I HLA antigens.[2,3] Because high concentrations of HLA antigens are present on platelets,[4] donor platelets are highly susceptible to HLA antibodies. Many immunized patients therefore become unresponsive to pooled random-donor platelets and require HLA-matched apheresis platelets.

Because of the highly polymorphic nature of HLA antigens,[5,6] a pool of several thousand HLA-typed individuals is needed to find a few HLA-matched platelet donors. HLA alloimmunization therefore has emerged as one of the most challenging issues in platelet transfusion therapy. For this reason, considerable research has been conducted to understand the mechanisms by which HLA alloimmunization is induced through transfusions of blood components. Results generated from these works indicate that donor leukocytes play a dominant role in causing HLA alloimmunization. This finding has led to numerous clinical trials using leukocyte-reduced blood components to prevent HLA alloimmunization. This chapter reviews what has been learned from these trials, how the generated information should be applied for routine patient care, and what issues remain to be addressed to prevent platelet alloimmunization.

Platelet Alloimmunization

Three different groups of alloantigens are present on platelets: 1) blood group antigens, 2) platelet-specific antigens, and 3) HLA antigens. Although blood group antigens and HLA antigens are not platelet-specific, they are intrinsic components of the platelet membrane. Alloimmunizations to these three groups of alloantigens after platelet transfusion are expected and have different clinical implications.

Alloimmunization to Blood Group Antigens

Blood group antigens on platelets include ABH, Lewis, Ii, and P antigens.[7-12] These antigens are part of platelet membrane glycoproteins.[9] Portions of ABH and Lewis antigens are acquired from plasma by adsorption.[10-12] Antibodies to ABH, Lewis, and P antigens often develop spontaneously in antigen-negative individuals, and antibodies to I antigens often occur as cold-reacting autoantibodies.[32] Antibodies to Lewis and P antigens usually do not adversely affect recovery of donor platelets carrying these antigens, so transfusion-induced alloimmunization to these antigens is not clinically significant. While some investigators have shown that ABO incompatibility could have some negative impact on posttransfusion platelet recovery,[14-17] others have not found a similar negative effect.[18-20] These discrepant findings indicate that the effect of ABO incompatibility on platelet transfusion is subtle. This subtle effect is likely due to the highly variable expression of ABH antigens on platelets between individuals[21] and the varying titers of ABO isoagglutinin in transfusion recipients.[15,17]

Platelet units contain small but significant quantities of donor red cells.[22,23] Platelet transfusions can cause alloimmunization to red cell antigens that are absent in transfusion recipients.[24-26] Since these blood group antigens are not present on platelets, antibody development to these antigens does not have a direct impact on platelet transfusion response.

Alloimmunization to Platelet-Specific Alloantigens

In addition to blood group antigens, platelets contain antigenic epitopes that are not found on other types of blood cells. More than 20 such platelet-specific alloantigens have been identified.[27-29] These antigens are part of platelet membrane glycoproteins and have been well-characterized at the molecular level.[28,29] Platelet transfusions or pregnancy could result in alloimmunization to these antigens. The antibodies to these antigens could lead to one of the following clinical conditions: 1) neonatal alloimmune thrombocytopenia among mothers who become immunized to platelet alloantigen of infants and give birth to thrombocytopenic infants; 2) posttransfusion purpura among patients who become immunized to platelet-specific alloantigens after blood transfusion and develop thrombocytopenia; and 3) alloimmune platelet transfusion refractoriness among patients who receive multiple platelet transfusions, develop the antibodies, and become refractory to random-donor platelets.[27,30]

According to the recent multicenter Trial to Reduce Alloimmunization to Platelets (TRAP),[3] the development of antibodies to platelet-specific alloantigens was detected in 8% of recipients after multiple platelet transfusions. This finding is consistent with results of earlier studies.[31-34] Despite their detection by in-vitro assays, these antibodies often do not have significant impact on platelet transfusion response.[33,35-36] Only a few cases of platelet transfusion failures can be attributed to their presence,[38-40] although the exact reason for this finding is not clear. Since platelet-specific antigens are present in dimorphic forms and are unequally distributed in a high-incidence public form and a low-incidence private form,[27,29,40] antibodies to them are often against platelets from a fraction of blood donors and are clinically inconsequential. Although refractoriness due to alloimmunization to high-incidence platelet-specific antigens potentially does pose a major challenge in finding compatible donors, these cases are fortunately rare.[38,41]

Alloimmunization to HLA Antigens

HLA Class I molecules make up the third group of platelet alloantigens. These antigens are heterodimeric membrane glycoproteins that consist of a 44-kD highly polymorphic heavy chain and a 12-kD invariant β2 microglobulin.[42] These two polypeptides are noncovalently associated with each other and are present in varying quantities on almost all cells in an individual. The genes encoding HLA heavy chains are found at three different loci (A, B, and C) of chromosome 6. Functionally, HLA antigens play a major role in presenting antigenic peptides to cytotoxic T lymphocytes[43] and are essential for ontogenetic development of CD8+ cytotoxic T cells in the thymus.[44,45] Clinically, it is the HLA antigenic system that primarily determines the survival of transplanted allografts.

The number of HLA antigens per platelet varies widely between individuals ranging from 50,000 to 180,000 molecules.[4,46] On the average, there are 100,000 HLA molecules per platelet.[4] Considering the small size of platelets, the density of HLA antigens on platelets is highest among all types of blood cells. HLA antigens on platelets are integral membrane proteins and are not derived from plasma.[4,47-49] This high density renders the HLA antigens susceptible to HLA antibodies. Thus, HLA antibodies are responsible for more than 90% of immune-mediated platelet transfusion refractoriness.[3,31] According to earlier studies,[50-57] HLA alloimmunization occurred in 30-70% of patients with various hematologic and nonhematologic malignancies after they received multiple platelet and red cell transfusions. In immunocompetent patients who had one-time exposure to platelets and red cells during open-heart surgery, 74% of patients became immunized to HLA antigens.[55]

Mechanism of Transfusion-Induced HLA Alloimmunization

In 1978, Batchelor et al[56] used rat and mouse models to demonstrate that Class I major histocompatibility complex (MHC) antigens are poor immunogens. To induce antibodies to non-self MHC antigens, viable and functioning donor leukocytes are necessary. The importance of viable donor leukocytes for HLA alloimmunization is further supported by the finding that stored blood has reduced HLA immunogenicity.[57] These findings suggest that direct interaction between functional donor leukocytes and the immune system of transfusion recipients is critical for the induction of antibody responses to non-self MHC antigens within the same species. This conclusion was further corroborated by showing that removal of leukocytes from platelet concentrates can prevent platelet transfusion-induced alloimmunization to donor MHC antigens in a mouse model.[58] The importance of leukocytes in immunizing recipients to donor MHC antigens is also supported by the findings that passenger leukocytes in renal allografts are the primary immunogenic elements causing graft rejection,[59] and that the synthesis and expression of costimulatory signals by viable Class II MHC antigen-positive donor leukocytes are critical for transfusion-induced alloimmunization to donor MHC antigens.[60,61]

On the basis of results from the aforementioned studies, the sequence of events responsible for transfusion-induced HLA alloimmunization is most likely as follows: After Class II-positive donor leukocytes, including dendritic cells, monocytes, and B cells, are infused into a recipient, these cells are recognized by alloreactive helper T cells in the recipient. The initial interaction between Class II MHC molecules on donor antigen-presenting leukocytes and T-cell receptors on recipient helper T cells activates the donor leukocytes,[62-64] which then begin to produce interleukin-1 (IL-1), IL-12, and other cytokines and to express CD80 and CD86 costimulatory signals on their cell surface.[65,66] The CD80 and CD86 costimulatory signals then further activate recipient helper T cells by binding to CD28 receptors.[67,68] Activation of helper T cells by costimulatory signals leads to the increased expression of CD40 ligand (CD40L) and IL-2 receptors and to the secretion of IL-2, IL-3, IL-4, IL-5, IL-6, IL-10, IL-13, tumor necrosis factor-beta, and/or gamma interferon. CD40L, IL-4, IL-5, IL-10, and IL-13 provide critical T-cell help to recipient B lymphocytes for their proliferation, maturation, and antibody production.[62,69,70] The secreted IL-2 stimulates T cells to proliferate and amplifies T-cell help to B cells. At the same time, the Class II MHC molecules on recipient B cells allow their intimate interaction with activated helper T cells in an antigen-specific manner. These intricate interactions finally culminate in the production of antibodies to donor Class I MHC antigens.

Therefore, any removal or inactivation of donor antigen-presenting leukocytes should prevent HLA alloimmunization and consequent immune refractoriness. On this basis and that of previous transfusion studies in animals, many clinical trials have been launched to assess the efficacy of using leukocyte reduction and inactivation to reduce alloantigenicity of platelet concentrates.

Strategies and Trials for Prevention of HLA Alloimmunization and Platelet Refractoriness

To prevent transfusion-induced HLA alloimmunization and/or alloimmune platelet refractoriness, two general strategies can be applied: 1) to reduce the immunogenicity of platelet concentrates and red cells, and 2) to modify the immune response in transfusion recipients. These two strategies are not mutually exclusive; however, using a single approach to modify the immunoregulatory mechanism in transfusion recipients and to reduce the immunogenicity of the transfused platelet concentrates simultaneously has yet to be established. In the past 2 decades, however, most clinical trials for the prevention of alloimmune platelet refractoriness have been confined to the first strategy. The reported results, albeit encouraging, were inconclusive for reasons that are discussed below.

Reduction of Immunogenicity of Platelet Concentrates

Prospective Use of Single-Donor Apheresis Platelets

Since HLA alloimmunization is responsible for most alloimmune platelet transfusion refractoriness and the severity of refractoriness is proportional to the immune responses against different HLA antigens,[71] one approach to limit the extent of HLA alloimmunization is to reduce donor exposure. This can be accomplished by giving thrombocytopenic patients single-donor apheresis platelets (SDPs). In a small-scale, randomized trial involving 34 patients with various hematologic malignancies, lymphoma, Hodgkin's disease, or breast carcinoma, Sintnicolaas et al[72] reported in 1981 that the use of SDP transfusion delayed HLA alloimmunization longer than the use of pooled random-donor platelets (PDPs). However, the difference was not statistically significant, and only three patients—one in the SDP treatment arm and two in the PDP treatment arm—became alloimmunized to HLA antigens. The low incidences of HLA alloimmunization in this study likely resulted from relatively low degrees of leukocyte content in platelet components ($0.2\text{-}13.8 \times 10^7$ leukocytes per transfusion) and the heterogeneity of patients' diagnoses.

Two years later, a better-designed trial to evaluate use of SDPs in this regard was reported.[73] A total of 54 newly diagnosed adult patients with acute leukemia were studied in this randomized trial. Eligibility criteria, platelet and red cell transfusion triggers, criteria for HLA alloimmunization and platelet transfusion refractoriness, study period, and endpoints were clearly defined. All red cell components were leukocyte-reduced, and only ABO-identical platelets were used. The mean leukocyte contents per 1.0×10^{11} platelets were 8.9×10^8 and 2.0×10^8 for SDPs and PDPs, respectively. The results of this study show that HLA alloimmunization (56% vs 15%, $p<0.001$) and platelet transfusion refractoriness (52% vs 15%, $p<0.01$) were effectively forestalled by transfusions of random SDPs, compared with PDPs.

However, results of a large multicenter trial (TRAP) to prevent HLA alloimmunization showed no benefit from using SDPs instead of PDPs after leukocytes were removed from both products.[3] Since primary HLA alloimmunization is induced mainly by donor leukocytes, it is not surprising that the removal of immunogenic leukocytes from PDPs or SDPs is equally effective in preventing it from occurring. Consequently, the benefit of transfusing patients with SDPs to prevent HLA alloimmunization is no longer discernible after leukocytes are removed. The only advantage of using leukocyte-reduced SDPs is to limit the risk of contracting transfusion-transmitted infectious diseases.

Prospective Use of Leukocyte-Reduced Red Cells and Platelets

As mentioned previously, animal studies have indicated that leukocytes are the primary cellular element responsible for alloimmunization to donor MHC antigens. Prompted by this observation, a series of clinical trials[3,39,74-89] has been conducted using leukocyte-reduced blood components to prevent HLA alloimmunization/platelet transfusion refractoriness. These 18 clinical trials are summarized in Tables 5-1, 5-2, 5-3, and 5-4. Although 14 of the trials showed positive results using leukocyte-reduced blood components to prevent or forestall transfusion-induced HLA alloimmunization and/or platelet transfusion refractoriness, only 5 trials (Trials 6, 9, 11, 14, and 18) showed statistically significant differences between the control and the treatment groups. Negative findings were reported in three trials (Trials 3, 15, and 16).

Although the majority of these trials yielded encouraging findings, many of them suffered from multiple deficiencies. These common deficiencies included 1) small numbers of evaluable patients (≤50 patients in 10 trials; between 51 and100 patients in 5 trials), 2) significant heterogeneity in underlying diseases and treatments that resulted in varying degrees of immunosuppression (12 trials), 3) high numbers of residual leukocytes ($>1 \times 10^7$) after leukocyte reduction, 4) lack of stratification of important confounding factors such as prior pregnancy/transfusion and 5) lack of blinding of components (in all except Trial 18). Other, less frequent problems included a lack of randomization, overly strict definition for HLA alloimmunization (>20% panel reactive lymphocytoxic antibody [PRA]), wide variations in numbers of transfusions among patients, ill-defined study period, use of both pooled and apheresis platelets in the same treatment arm, unknown sensitivity and precision of leukocyte-counting methods for quality control of leukocyte-reduced blood components, and incomparable treatment and control groups. For these reasons, it has been

Table 5-1. Clinical Trials for Prevention of HLA Alloimmunization and Platelet Transfusion Refractoriness—Design and Patient Data

	Investigator Year (reference)	Trial Design				Evaluable Patients	
		Prospective	Randomized	Controlled	Stratification	No. Control/ Treatment	Type
1	Eernisse & Brand 1981[74]	No	No	Historical	No	16/68	ANLL, ALL lymphoma, aplastic anemia
2	Sirchia et al 1982[75]	Yes	No	Yes	No	6/5	Thalassemia major
3	Schiffer et al 1983[76]	Yes	Yes	Yes Sex, prior pregnancy/ transfusion	Yes	31/25	ANLL
4	Fisher et al 1985[77]	Yes	No	Yes	No	12/12	Nontransfused renal patients
5	Sirchia et al 1986[78]	Yes	No	Yes	No	13/11	Thalassemia major
6	Murphy et al 1986[79]	Yes	No	Yes	No	31/19	Acute leukemia
7	Brand et al 1988[80]	Yes	No	No	No	0/335	ANLL, ALL lymphoma, aplastic anemia, BMT
8	Sniecinski et al 1988[81]	Yes	Yes	Yes Age, prior pregnancy/ transfusion	Yes	20/20	Hematologic malignancy, aplastic anemia

Table 5-1. Clinical Trials for Prevention of HLA Alloimmunization and Platelet Transfusion Refractoriness—Design and Patient Data (continued)

		Trial Design				Evaluable Patients	
	Investigator Year (reference)	Pros-pective	Ran-domized	Con-trolled	Stratifi-cation	No. Control/ Treatment	Type
9	Andreu et al 1988[82]	Yes	Yes	Yes	No	35/34	Leukemia, lymphoma, refractory anemia
10	Saarinen et al 1990[83]	No	No	Historical	No	21/26	Pediatric patients leukemia, aplastic anemia, solid tumors, BMT
11	van Marwijk Kooij et al 1991[84]	Yes	Yes	Yes	No	26/27	ANLL, ALL
12	Oksanen et al 1991[85]	Yes	Yes	Yes	No	15/16	ANLL, ALL
13	Ten Haaft et al 1992[86]	Yes	No	No	No	0/25	ANLL, ALL lymphoma, autologous BMT
14	Bedford Russell et al 1993[87]	Yes	Yes	Yes	No	23/19	Premature newborns
15	Williamson et al 1994[88]	Yes	Yes	Yes	No	56/67	ANLL, ALL, CLL lymphoma, myeloma, Hodgkin's disease

(continued)

Table 5-1. Clinical Trials for Prevention of HLA Alloimmunization and Platelet Transfusion Refractoriness—Design and Patient Data (continued)

		Trial Design				Evaluable Patients	
	Investigator Year (reference)	Prospective	Randomized	Controlled	Stratification	No. Control/ Treatment	Type
16	Sintnicolaas et al 1995[89]	Yes	Yes	Yes Hospital sites	Yes	25/21	Female patients with hematologic malignancies and prior pregnancy
17	Novotny et al 1995[38]	Yes	No	No	No	0/164	ANLL, ALL, non-Hodgkin's lymphoma, Hodgkin's disease, aplastic anemia, MDS, and others
18	TRAP Study Group 1997[3]	Yes	Yes	Yes Trial sites, prior pregnancy/ transfusion	Yes	131/130, 137,132	ANLL

BMT = Bone marrow transplantation; ALL = acute lymphocytic leukemia; ANLL = Acute nonlymphocytic leukemia; MDS = myelodysplastic syndrome; CLL = chronic lymphocytic leukemia; TRL = total residual leukocytes

Table 5-2. Clinical Trials for Prevention of HLA Alloimmunization and Platelet Transfusion Refractoriness—Blood Components and Treatment

	Investigator Year (reference)	Blood Components	
		Control	Treatment
1	Eernisse & Brand 1981[74]	Standard pooled platelets and leukocyte-reduced (TRL >5×10^6) red cells	Leukocyte-reduced (TRL <5×10^6) pooled platelets and red cells
2	Sirchia et al 1982[75]	Leukocyte-reduced (TRL >5×10^6) red cells	Leukocyte-reduced (TRL <5×10^6) red cells
3	Schiffer et al 1983[76]	Standard pooled platelets and leukocyte-reduced (TRL >5×10^6) red cells	Leukocyte-reduced (TRL >5×10^6) pooled platelets and red cells
4	Fisher et al 1985[77]	Standard apheresis platelets; no red cell transfusions	Leukocyte-reduced apheresis platelets (TRL <5×10^6); no red cell transfusions
5	Sirchia et al 1986[78]	Standard or leukocyte-reduced (TRL >5×10^6) red cells	Leukocyte-reduced (TRL <5×10^6) red cells
6	Murphy et al 1986[79]	Standard apheresis platelets and red cells	Leukocyte-reduced apheresis platelets and red cells (TRL >5×10^6)
7	Brand et al 1988[80]	No control group	All patients received leukocyte-reduced (TRL <5×10^6) components
8	Sniecinski et al 1988[81]	Standard pooled platelets and red cells	Leukocyte-reduced (TRL >5×10^6) pooled platelets and red cells

(continued)

Table 5-2. Clinical Trials for Prevention of HLA Alloimmunization and Platelet Transfusion Refractoriness—Blood Components and Treatment (continued)

	Investigator Year (reference)	Blood Components: Control	Blood Components: Treatment
9	Andreu et al 1988[82]	Standard pooled or apheresis platelets and red cells	Leukocyte-reduced (TRL >5×10^6) pooled or apheresis platelets and red cells
10	Saarinen et al 1990[83]	Standard pooled platelets and red cells	Leukocyte-reduced (TRL >5×10^6) pooled platelets and red cells
11	van Marwijk Kooij et al 1991[84]	Standard pooled platelets and leukocyte-reduced (TRL >5×10^6) red cells	Leukocyte-reduced (TRL <5×10^6) pooled platelets and red cells
12	Oksanen et al 1991[85]	Standard pooled platelets and red cells	Leukocyte-reduced (TRL <5×10^6) pooled platelets and red cells
13	Ten Haaft et al 1992[86]	No control group	Leukocyte-reduced (TRL >5×10^6) blood components
14	Bedford Russell et al 1993[87]	Standard red cells	Leukocyte-reduced (TRL <5×10^6) red cells

Table 5-2. Clinical Trials for Prevention of HLA Alloimmunization and Platelet Transfusion Refractoriness—Blood Components and Treatment (continued)

	Investigator Year (reference)	Blood Components	
		Control	Treatment
15	Williamson et al 1994[88]	Standard pooled/apheresis platelets and red cells	Leukocyte-reduced (TRL $<5\times10^6$) pooled/apheresis platelets and red cells
16	Sintnicolaas et al 1995[89]	Standard apheresis platelets and buffy-coat-removed red cells	Leukocyte-reduced (TRL $<5\times10^6$) apheresis platelets and red cells
17	Novotny et al 1995[38]	No control group	Leukocyte-reduced (TRL $>5\times10^6$) blood components
18	TRAP Study Group 1997[3]	Control; standard pooled platelets; all red cell units were leukocyte-reduced for control and treatment arms	Ultraviolet B-irradiated pooled platelets; (F-PC): leukocyte-reduced pooled platelets (TRL $<5\times10^6$); (F-AP): leukocyte-reduced apheresis platelets (TRL $<5\times10^6$)

F-PC = pooled and filtered platelet concentrates; F-AP = filtered apheresis platelet concentrates; TRL = total residual leukocytes

Table 5-3. Clinical Trials for Prevention of HLA Alloimmunization and Platelet Transfusion Refractoriness—Methods

	Methods of WBC Reduction		Residual WBC		Endpoint	
Investigator Year (reference)	RBC	Platelets	RBC	Platelets	LCA	Platelet Refractoriness
1 Eernisse & Brand 1981[74]	Cotton-wool filters	Differential centrifugation	95% reduction	$<5\times10^6$	Yes	Yes
2 Sirchia et al 1982[75]	Erypur or Imugard IG500 filter	No platelets	$<1\times10^6$ (65-96% units) $1\text{-}50\times10^6$ (4-35% units)		Yes	No
3 Schiffer et al 1983[76]	Frozen and washed	Differential centrifugation	3×10^7	1.2×10^7	Yes (≥20% PRA)	No
4 Fisher et al 1985[77]	Imugard IG500 filter		$\leq5\times10^6$		Yes	No
5 Sirchia et al 1986[78]	Erypur filter		Not available		Yes	No
6 Murphy et al 1986[79]	Imugard IG500 filter	Differential centrifugation	$\leq8\times10^6$	$0.9\text{-}2.2\times10^8$	Yes	Yes
7 Brand et al 1988[80]	CellSelect filter after buffy coat removal	Differential centrifugation	$\leq0.5\times10^6$	2×10^7	Yes	Yes

Table 5-3. Clinical Trials for Prevention of HLA Alloimmunization and Platelet Transfusion Refractoriness—Methods (continued)

	Methods of WBC Reduction		Residual WBC		Endpoint	
Investigator Year (reference)	RBC	Platelets	RBC	Platelets	LCA	Platelet Refractoriness
8 Sniecinski et al 1988[81]	Imugard IG500 filter	Imugard IG500 filter	5×10^{7}	6×10^{6}	Yes (≥10%PRA)	Yes
9 Andreu et al 1988[82]	Imugard IG500 filter	Imugard IG500 filter	6.1×10^{7}	Pooled platelets: 4.7×10^{7}; pheresis platelets: 1.5×10^{8}	Yes (≥10%PRA)	No
10 Saarinen et al 1990[83]	Imugard IG500 filter	Imugard IG500 filter	$<1\times10^{6}$	$<0.2\times10^{6}$	Platelet count increment	
11 van Marwijk Kooij et al 1991[84]	CellSelect filter after buffy coat removal	Differential centrifugation or filtration	$<5\times10^{6}$	3.5×10^{7} (centrifuged), $<5\times10^{6}$ (filtered)	Yes (≥10%PRA)	No
12 Oksanen et al 1991[85]	CellSelect filter after buffy coat removal	Imugard IG500 filter	0.1×10^{6}	0.04×10^{6}	Yes	Yes

(continued)

Table 5-3. Clinical Trials for Prevention of HLA Alloimmunization and Platelet Transfusion Refractoriness—Methods (continued)

Investigator Year (reference)	Methods of WBC Reduction		Residual WBC		Endpoint	
	RBC	Platelets	RBC	Platelets	LCA	Platelet Refractoriness
13 Ten Haaft et al 1992[86]	CellSelect filter	Differential centrifugation	8.5×10^6	$7.8\text{x}10^6$	Yes	Yes
14 Bedford Russell et al 1993[87]	Sepacell filter		0.2×10^6/mL		Yes	No
15 Williamson et al 1994[88]	PALL RC filter bedside filtration	Pall PL filter	>99.9% removal	>99.9% removal	Yes (≥10%PRA)	No
16 Sintnicolaas et al 1995[89]	CellSelect filter after buffy coat removal	CellSelect filter	0.4×10^6	2×10^6	Yes (≥10%PRA)	No
17 Novotny et al 1995[38]	CellSelect filter after buffy coat removal	CellSelect filter	$<5\times10^6$	$<1\times10^6$	Yes (≥20%PRA)	No
18 TRAP Study Group 1997[3]	Pall RC-100 or BPF-4 filter	Pall PL-100 filter	$<5\times10^6$	$<5\times10^6$	Yes	Yes

WBC = white blood cell; RBC = red blood cell; PRA = panel reactive lymphocytotoxicity antibody; LCA = lymphocytotoxic antibody

Table 5-4. Clinical Trials for Prevention of HLA Alloimmunization and Platelet Transfusion Refractoriness—Results

	Results				
	% HLA Alloimmunization		% Immune Refractoriness		
Investigator Year (reference)	Control	Treatment	Control	Treatment	Difference
1 Eernisse & Brand 1981[74]	10/16 (63%)	19/68 (28%)	10/16(63%)	12/68(18%)	
	No statistical analysis		No statistical analysis		
2 Sirchia et al 1982[75]	3/6 (50%)	0/5 (0%)			
	No statistical analysis				
3 Schiffer et al 1983[76]	13/31(42%)	5/25(20%)			No
	p=0.07				
4 Fisher et al 1985[77]	4/12 (33%)	0/12 (0%)			
	No statistical analysis				
5 Sirchia et al 1986[78]	8/13 (62%)	0/11 (0%)			
	No statistical analysis				
6 Murphy et al 1986[79]	15/31 (48%)	3/19 (16%)	7/31 (23%)	1/19 (5%)	Yes
	p=0.02				
	7/14 (50%)*	1/11 (9%)*			

(continued)

Table 5-4. Clinical Trials for Prevention of HLA Alloimmunization and Platelet Transfusion Refractoriness—Results (continued)

Investigator Year (reference)	Results				
	% HLA Alloimmunization		% Immune Refractoriness		
	Control	Treatment	Control	Treatment	Difference
7 Brand et al 1988[80]	NA	69/335 (21%)	NA	31/335 (9%)	
8 Sniecinski et al 1988[81]	10/20 (50%)	3/20 (15%)	10/20(50%)†	3/20 (15%)†	
	No statistical analysis				
9 Andreu et al 1988[82]	11/35 (31%)	4/34 (12%)			Yes
	p<0.05				
10 Saarinen et al 1990[83]	NA		NA		
11 van Marwijk Kooij et al 1991[84]	11/26 (42%)	3/27 (11%)	12/26 (46%)†	3/27 (11%)†	Yes
	p<.004		p<0.005		
12 Oksanen et al 1991[85]	3/15 (20%)	2/16 (12.5%)	1/15 (7%)	0/16 (0%)	
	No statistical analysis				
13 Ten Haaft et al 1992[86]	NA	3/25 (12%)	NA	6/25(24%)	

Table 5-4. Clinical Trials for Prevention of HLA Alloimmunization and Platelet Transfusion Refractoriness—Results (continued)

Investigator Year (reference)	Results				Difference
	% HLA Alloimmunization		% Immune Refractoriness		
	Control	Treatment	Control	Treatment	
14 Bedford Russell et al 1993[87]	7/23 (30%) p=0.02	0/19 (0%)			Yes
15 Williamson et al 1994[88]	21/56 (38%) p=0.07	15/67 (22%)	30%	26%	No
16 Sintnicolaas et al 1995[89]	11/25 (44%) p=0.41	9/21 (43%)	14/34 (41%) p=0.52	8/28 (29%)	No
17 Novotny et al 1995[38]	NA NA	19/164 (12%) 3/112 (3%)*			
18 TRAP Study Group 1997[3]	Control UVB F-PC 45% 21% 18% p<0.001	F-AP 17%	Control UVB 13 % 5% p=0.03	F-PC F-AP 3% 4% p=0.004 p=0.01	Yes

*Patients without prior transfusion and pregnancy
†Clinical platelet transfusion refractoriness
NA = Not available; UVB = ultraviolet B; F-PC = pooled and filtered platelet concentrates; F-AP = filtered apheresis platelet concentrates

difficult to draw any definitive conclusions from these studies until TRAP was completed and its findings reported in 1997.[3]

Among the first 17 trials listed in Table 5-1, only those reported by Schiffer et al[76] and Sintnicolaas et al[89] were carefully planned and randomized prospective trials. The eligibility criteria, the study endpoints, and the follow-up period were clearly defined. Both trials also enrolled relatively larger numbers of patients than others. In the study reported by Schiffer et al, randomization was also stratified according to gender and prior exposure to histocompatibility antigens through transfusion and/or pregnancy.[76] More important, to minimize varying degrees of immunologic suppression and responsiveness among subjects, only patients with newly diagnosed acute nonlymphocytic leukemia who received the same chemotherapeutic regimen were included. Unfortunately, a significant number of patients (43%) had to be excluded from the final analysis because of granulocyte transfusions, loss to follow-up, and early death. The study also suffered from not having effective methods for preparing high-quality, leukocyte-reduced platelet concentrates. Consequently, high numbers of residual leukocytes (0.5-1 $\times$ 10^8/transfusion) were present in the treated platelets. The use of at least 20% PRA to define HLA alloimmunization was probably too stringent and could have led to an underestimation of alloimmunized patients in the control arm. For these reasons, Schiffer and his colleagues did not discern any significant benefits from using leukocyte-reduced platelets to prevent HLA alloimmunization and alloimmune platelet transfusion refractoriness.[76]

In the trial reported by Sintnicolaas et al,[89] 62 patients with hematologic malignancies and previous pregnancies were studied and 55 patients were evaluable.[89] This trial was stratified according to hospital sites. All patients were transfused with SDPs, and third-generation, high-efficiency leukocyte-removal filters were used to reduce all red cells of leukocytes. Unlike other studies, this trial aimed to determine whether leukocyte-reduced SDPs could prevent secondary HLA alloimmunization in patients who had prior exposure to HLA antigens through pregnancy. The investigators found that leukocyte-reduced SDPs are not able to prevent secondary HLA alloimmunization or platelet transfusion refractoriness. In contrast, the recently reported TRAP trial[3] showed that the use of leukocyte-reduced SDPs can reduce HLA alloimmunization in women who had prior pregnancy. However, PDPs instead of SDPs were used in the control arm of the TRAP trial. Since the latter are less immunogenic,[72,73] this discrepant finding is likely due to different types of platelet components used in the control groups.

To avoid all the aforementioned shortcomings and to obtain conclusive results regarding the effectiveness of using leukocyte-reduced platelet components and red cells to prevent HLA alloimmunization and platelet transfusion refractoriness, a carefully designed multicenter study known as the TRAP trial was launched in 1991. This randomized and blinded prospective trial studied patients with de novo acute nonlymphocytic leukemia who met the eligibility criteria, which were clearly defined to avoid varying immunologic suppression and responsiveness associated with underlying diseases, chemotherapy, and/or prior alloimmunization. The primary and the secondary endpoints for the study were also clearly defined. Randomization was stratified according to trial sites, prior pregnancy, and prior transfusion. Considerable efforts were made to ensure the high quality of leukocyte reduction by filtration and of leukocyte inactivation by irradiation with medium wavelength ultraviolet (UVB) light. There were three treatment groups in this trial. The control group was treated with unmodified pooled platelet concentrates; the three treatment groups received leukocyte-reduced pooled platelets, UVB-irradiated pooled platelets, or leukocyte-reduced apheresis platelets. Red cell units given to all patients were leukocyte-reduced. There were 530 evaluable patients. The results generated from this study conclusively demonstrate that both leukocyte reduction and UVB irradiation were effective in preventing primary HLA alloimmunization and alloimmune platelet transfusion refractoriness. Additional important findings are that the incidence of platelet transfusion refractoriness during the 8 weeks of chemotherapy was 16%—not as high as reported previously—and that both leukocyte reduction by filtration and inactivation by UVB irradiation are effective in forestalling HLA alloimmunization in women with prior pregnancy. The low incidence of platelet transfusion refractoriness in patients transfused with standard pooled platelets might have resulted from a stricter definition of platelet refractoriness (corrected count increment <5000/µL) and more accurate assessment of pre- and postplatelet transfusion counts for calculation of the corrected count increment.

Prospective Use of UVB-Irradiated Platelet Concentrates

As discussed previously, various experimental studies have indicated that inactivation of antigen-presenting leukocytes in platelet concentrates by irradiation with short (UVC) or medium (UVB) wavelength UV light is an effective approach to reducing the alloantigenicity of platelet concentrates. Since UVB penetrates plastic bags with higher efficiency than UVC, UVB is the preferred UV light for leukocyte inactivation. The first preliminary clinical trial of UVB-irradiated platelet concentrates in healthy volunteers and thrombocytopenic patients was reported in 1992.[90] This trial demonstrated the safety and hemostatic efficacy of UVB-irradiated platelet concentrates. Two years later, Grijzenhout et al[91] studied HLA alloimmunization after a single transfusion of pooled platelets with or without UVB irradiation in 101 male patients undergoing cardiopulmonary bypass procedure and without prior exposure to allogeneic blood components. In this study, leukocytes were removed from all red cell units by third-generation high-efficiency filters. The results of this study showed that UVB irradiation of platelet concentrates failed to reduce the incidence of HLA alloimmunization. The negative finding was probably related to the use of a relatively low dose of UVB (0.5 J/cm^2) for irradiation, which might have led to the incomplete inactivation of donor leukocytes. Two years later, Blundell et al[92] conducted another study in 50 patients with various hematologic malignancies. Again, no significant difference was noted between the control and the treatment groups, probably because of the insufficient number of patients. Conclusive demonstration of the effectiveness of using UVB-irradiated platelet concentrates was not available until the multicenter TRAP trial was completed,[3] the results of which show that UVB irradiation is as effective and safe as leukocyte reduction of platelets for preventing HLA alloimmunization.

Technically, UVB irradiation is not more complicated or time-consuming than leukocyte reduction by filtration. One drawback of UVB irradiation is that the irradiated platelet concentrates may shorten the platelet shelf life and that irradiation should be performed shortly before transfusion.[93,94] But despite this minor inconvenience, UVB irradiation not only can reduce the immunogenicity but also may induce specific immune tolerance to donor HLA antigens, as reported in different animal models.[95,96] This induced tolerance may reduce risks of immune platelet refractoriness from subsequent exposures to untreated blood components and may offer the unique advantage of using less intense conditioning regimens for allogeneic marrow transplantation. All these interesting possibilities remain to be investigated. It is also of interest to learn whether UVB-irradiated platelet concentrates can prevent anamnestic response in patients with prior immunization to HLA antigens. However, results of an experimental transfusion study conducted in a murine model suggest that UVB irradiation is unlikely to accomplish this goal.[96]

Modification of Recipient Immune Response

The second strategy for preventing HLA alloimmunization and immune platelet transfusion refractoriness is to modify the immune response in transfusion recipients. There are two approaches for this strategy: 1) immunosuppressive therapy, and 2) the induction of specific immune tolerance to donor platelets.

Immunosuppressive Therapy

Several investigators have found that patients treated with intensive chemotherapy have a lower rate of alloimmunization.[97,98] The effectiveness of using immunosuppressive drugs such as azathioprine to prevent transfusion-induced alloimmunization has been demonstrated in patients transfused with donor-specific blood before transplantation of renal allografts.[99] The success of using cyclosporin has also been reported in a dog transfusion model.[95] However, since most patients who require multiple platelet transfusions are already receiving intensive chemo- and/or radiotherapy, further immunosuppressive therapy could increase their risk of serious infection and outweigh the potential benefit. For this reason, clinical trials of immunosuppressive agents to prevent platelet alloimmunization and refractoriness have not been conducted.

Induction of Immunologic Tolerance

Recent progress in understanding the basic immunobiology of alloimmunization has led to the study of using leukocytes inactivated with UV light to induce specific tolerance to donor MHC antigens in various animal models.[95,96] The results of these studies indicate that partial immune tolerance can be induced by transfusions of UVB- or UVC-irradiated platelet concentrates, and complete humoral immune tolerance can be induced by transfusions of purified donor leukocytes inactivated with UVB.[96] The tolerance induction likely results from the absence of CD80 and CD86 costimulatory signal expression on donor leukocytes inactivated with UVB.[100] Although the TRAP trial showed that transfusions of UVB-irradiated platelet concentrates were effective in preventing HLA alloimmunization, the trial did not address the possible induction of immune tolerance in the treated patients. Thus, the use of UVB-irradiated platelet concentrates to induce tolerance to donor MHC antigens remains to be determined.

Conclusions

Since the first study using leukocyte-reduced blood components to prevent alloimmune platelet transfusion refractoriness reported by Eernisse and Brand[74] in 1981, many clinical trials have been conducted to answer the same question. For various reasons, the results of these studies remained inconclusive until the findings from the TRAP trial became available in 1997. Then for the first time, leukocyte reduction and UVB irradiation were clearly demonstrated to be equally effective in preventing HLA alloimmunization and alloimmune platelet transfusion refractoriness. But despite this significant accomplishment, many questions remain unanswered. For instance, factors contributing to the failed prevention of HLA alloimmunization by leukocyte-reduced or inactivated platelet concentrates in patients without any prior exposure to non-self HLA antigens still need to be identified. Is this failure due to varying immune responsiveness or to insufficient reduction of leukocytes? What is the upper limit of donor leukocytes that can be allowed in the filtered red cell and platelet units for preventing HLA alloimmunization? Can the combination of UVB irradiation and leukocyte reduction offer any additive or synergistic protection? Is there any induction of immune tolerance after transfusions of UVB-irradiated platelets?

While we await answers to these questions, the following recommendations regarding the use of leukocyte-reduced blood components to prevent HLA alloimmunization and/or alloimmune platelet transfusion refractoriness can be made on the basis of the information generated from the published clinical trials:

1. Transfusions of leukocyte-depleted or leukocyte-inactivated blood components can be considered for patients who require chronic platelet transfusion support and have not had a prior pregnancy or transfusion.
2. Patients who require chronic platelet transfusion support and have history of prior pregnancy or blood transfusion should be tested for the presence of HLA antibodies. If they are negative for these antibodies, the use of leukocyte-reduced or inactivated blood components can be considered to forestall HLA alloimmunization.
3. The use of leukocyte-reduced or inactivated blood components is particularly important for patients with no detectable HLA antibodies who are awaiting allogeneic marrow or solid organ transplantation.
4. It is important to ensure that leukocytes are properly inactivated or reduced in all blood components for all patients mentioned above. The residual leukocyte content in the reduced blood components should be as low as possible and no more than 5×10^6 cells per transfusion.

As new information regarding the cellular and molecular basis of transfusion-induced HLA alloimmunization becomes available, these recommendations will undoubtedly need to be revised. The new information will allow us to develop more effective methods for preventing transfusion-induced HLA sensitization. Knowledge acquired from studies on the immunomodulatory effects of UVB-irradiated leukocytes could lead to the clinical application of UVB leukocytes to induce specific immunologic tolerance and open a new chapter in transfusion medicine.

References

1. Surgenor DM, Wallace EL, Hao SH, Chapman RH. Collection and transfusion of blood components in the United States, 1982–1988. N Engl J Med 1990;322:1646-51.
2. Schiffer CA. Prevention of alloimmunization against platelets. Blood 1991;77:1-4.
3. Trial to Reduce Alloimmunization to Platelets (TRAP) Study Group. Leukocyte reduction and ultraviolet B irradiation of platelets to prevent alloimmunization and refractoriness to platelet transfusions. N Engl J Med 1997;337:1861-915.
4. Kao KJ. Plasma and platelet HLA in normal individuals: Quantitation by competitive enzyme-linked immunoassay. Blood 1987;70:282-6.
5. Opelz G, Mickey MR, Terasaki PI. Unrelated donors for bone marrow transplantation and transfusion support: Pool sizes required. Transplant Proc 1974;6:405-9.
6. Bolgiano DC, Larson EB, Slichter SJ. A model to determine required pool size for HLA-typed community donor apheresis programs. Transfusion 1989;29:306-10.
7. Dunstan RA, Simpson MB. Heterogeneous distribution of antigens on human platelets demonstrated by fluorescence flow cytometry. Br J Haematol 1985;61:603-9.
8. Dunstan RA, Simpson MB, Rosse WF. Presence of P blood group antigens on human platelets. Am J Clin Pathol 1985;83:731-5.
9. Santoso S, Kiefel V, Mueller-Eckhardt C. Blood group A and B determinants are expressed on platelet glycoproteins IIa, IIIa, and Ib. Thromb Haemost 1991;65:196-201.
10. Kelton JG, Hamid C, Aker S, et al. The amount of blood group A substance on platelets is proportional to the amount in plasma. Blood 1982;59:980-5.
11. Dunstan RA, Simpson MB, Knowles RW, et al. The origin of ABH antigens on human platelets. Blood 1985;65:615-9.
12. Mollicone R, Caillard T, Le Pendu J, et al. Expression of ABH and X (Lex) antigens on platelets and lymphocytes. Blood 1988;71:1113-9.

13. Mollison PL, Engelfriet CP, Contreras M. Blood transfusion in clinical medicine. 10th ed. Oxford, England: Blackwell Scientific Publications, 1997:115-50.
14. Lee EJ, Schiffer CA. ABO compatibility can influence the results of platelet transfusion: Results of a randomized trial. Transfusion 1989; 29:384-9.
15. Duquesnoy RJ, Anderson AJ, Tomasulo PA, et al. ABO compatibility and platelet transfusions of alloimmunized thrombocytopenic patients. Blood 1979;54:595-9.
16. Heal JM, Blumberg N, Masel D. An evaluation of crossmatching, HLA, and ABO matching for platelet transfusions to refractory patients. Blood 1987;70:23-30.
17. Brand A, Sintnicolaas K, Claas FHJ, et al. ABH antibodies causing platelet transfusion refractoriness. Transfusion 1986;26:463-6.
18. Freireich EJ, Kliman A, Gaydos LA, et al. Response to repeated platelet transfusion from the same donor. Ann Intern Med 1963;59:277-87.
19. Tosato G, Appelbaum FR, Deisseroth AB. HLA-matched platelet transfusion therapy of severe aplastic anemia. Blood 1978;52:846-54.
20. Shulman NR. Immunological considerations attending platelet transfusion. Transfusion 1966;6:39-49.
21. Ogasawara K, Ueki J, Takenaka M, Furihata K. Study on the expression of ABH antigens on platelets. Blood 1993;82:993-9.
22. Herman JH. Single-donor (apheresis) vs pooled platelet concentrates. In: Kurtz SR, Brubaker DB, eds. Clinical decisions in platelet therapy. Bethesda, MD: American Association of Blood Banks, 1992:19-30.
23. Skinnider L, Wrobel H, McSheffrey B. The nature of the leukocyte "contamination" in platelet concentrates. Vox Sang 1985;49:309-14.
24. Goldfinger D, McGinniss MH. Rh-incompatible platelet transfusions—risks and consequences of sensitizing immunosuppressed patients. N Engl J Med 1971;284:942-4.
25. Lichtiger B, Surgeon J, Rhorer S. Rh-incompatible platelet transfusion therapy in cancer patients. A study of 30 cases. Vox Sang 1983;45:139-43.
26. Baldwin ML, Ness PM, Scott D, et al. Alloimmunization to D antigen and HLA in D-negative immunosuppressed oncology patients. Transfusion 1988;28:330-3.
27. Warkentin TE, Smith JW. The alloimmune thrombocytopenic syndromes. Transfus Med Rev 1997;11:296-307.

28. Kunicki TJ, Newman PJ. The molecular immunology of human platelet proteins. Blood 1992;80:1386-404.
29. Newman PJ, Valentin N. Human platelet alloantigens: Recent findings, new perspectives. Thromb Haemost 1995;74:234-9.
30. McFarland JG. Alloimmunization and platelet transfusion. Semin Hematol 1996;33:315-28.
31. Murphy MF, Metcalfe P, Ord J, et al. Disappearance of HLA and platelet-specific antibodies in acute leukaemia patients alloimmunized by multiple transfusions. Br J Haematol 1987;67:255-60.
32. Pamphilon DH, Farrell DH, Donaldson C, et al. Development of lymphocytotoxic and platelet reactive antibodies: A prospective study in patients with acute leukaemia. Vox Sang 1989;57:177-81.
33. Godeau B, Fromont P, Seror T, et al. Platelet alloimmunization after multiple transfusions: A prospective study of 50 patients. Br J Haematol 1992;81:395-400.
34. Uhrynowska M, Zupanska B. Platelet-specific antibodies in transfused patients. Eur J Haematol 1996;56:248-51.
35. Bishop JF, McGrath K, Wolf MM, et al. Clinical factors influencing the efficacy of pooled platelet transfusions. Blood 1988;71:383-7.
36. Meenaghan M, Judson P, Yousaf K, et al. Antibodies to platelet glycoprotein V in polytransfused patients with hematological disease. Vox Sang 1993;64:167-70.
37. Murata M, Furihata K, Ishida F, et al. Genetic and structural characterization of an amino acid dimorphism in glycoprotein Ib alpha involved in platelet transfusion refractoriness. Blood 1992;79:3086-90.
38. Novotny VMJ, van Doorn R, Witvliet MD, et al. Occurrence of allogeneic HLA and non-HLA antibodies after transfusion of prestorage filtered platelets and red blood cells: A prospective study. Blood 1995;85:1736-41.
39. Saji H, Maruya E, Fujii H, et al. New platelet antigen, Siba, involved in platelet transfusion refractoriness in a Japanese man. Vox Sang 1989;56:283-7.
40. Kim HO, Jin Y, Kickler TS, et al. Gene frequencies of the five major human platelet antigens in African-American, white and Korean populations. Transfusion 1995;35:863-7.
41. Reznikoff-Etievant MF, Muller JY, Julien F, et al. An immune response gene linked to MHC in man. Tissue Antigens 1983;22:312-4.

42. Ploegh HL, Orr HT, Strominger JL. Major histocompatibility antigens: The human (HLA-A,B,C) and murine (H-2K, H2-D) class I molecules. Cell 1981;24:287-99.
43. Zinkernagel RM, Doherty PC. MHC restricted cytotoxic cells: Studies on the biological role of polymorphic major transplantation antigens determine T-cell restriction specificity function and responsiveness. Adv Immunol 1979;27:51-177.
44. Zijlstra M, Bix M, Simister NE, et al. β2-microglobulin deficient mice lack CD4-8+ cytolytic T cells. Nature 1990;344:742-6.
45. Koller BH, Marrack P, Kappler JW. Normal development of mice deficient in β2M, MHC Class I proteins and CD8+ T cells. Science 1990;248:1227-30.
46. Kao KJ, Cook DJ, Scornik JC. Quantitative analysis of platelet surface HLA by W6/32 anti-HLA monoclonal antibody. Blood 1986;68:627-32.
47. Kao KJ. Selective elution of HLA antigens and β_2-microglobulin from human platelets by chloroquine diphosphate. Transfusion 1988;28: 14-7.
48. Santoso S, Mueller-Eckhardt C, Santoso S, et al. HLA antigens on platelet membranes: In vitro and in vivo studies. Vox Sang 1986;51: 327-33.
49. Santoso S, Kalb R, Kiefel V, et al. The presence of messenger RNA for HLA Class I in human platelets and its capability for protein synthesis. Br J Haematol 1993;84:451-6.
50. Schiffer CA, Lichtenfeld JL, Wiernik PH, et al. Antibody response in patients with acute non-lymphocytic leukemia. Cancer 1976;37: 2177-82.
51. Howard JE, Perkins HA. The natural history of alloimmunization to platelets. Transfusion 1978;18:496-503.
52. MacPherson BR. HLA antibody formation within the HLA-A1, cross-reactive group in multitransfused platelet recipients. Am J Hematol 1989;30:228-32.
53. Atlas E, Freedman J, Blanchette V, et al. Downregulation of the anti-HLA alloimmune response by variable region reactive (anti-idiotypic) antibodies in leukemic patients transfused with platelet concentrates. Blood 1993;81:538-42.
54. Hogge DE, McConnell M, Jacobson C, et al. Platelet refractoriness and alloimmunization in pediatric oncology and bone marrow transplant patients. Transfusion 1995;35:645-52.

55. Gleichmann H, Breininger J. Over 95% sensitization against allogeneic leukocytes following single massive blood transfusion. Vox Sang 1975;28:66-73.
56. Batchelor JR, Welsh KI, Burgos H. Transplantation antigens per se are poor immunogens within species. Nature 1978;273:54-6.
57. Galvao MM, Peixinho ZF, Mendes NF, Sabbaga E. Stored blood—an effective immunosuppressive method for transplantation of kidneys from unrelated donors: An 11-year follow-up. Braz J Med Biol Res 1997;30:727-34.
58. Claas FHJ, Smeenk RJT, Schmidt R, et al. Alloimmunization against the MHC antigens after platelet transfusions is due to contaminating leukocytes in the platelet suspension. Exp Hematol 1981;9:84-9.
59. Parthenais MA, Soots A, Nemlander A, et al. Immunogenicity of allograft components. II: Relative immunogenicity of rat kidney parenchymal versus passenger cells. Cell Immunol 1981;57:92-8.
60. Fujihara M, Takahashi TA, Azuma M, et al. Decreased inducible expression of CD80 and CD86 in human monocytes after ultraviolet-B: Its involvement in inactivation of alloantigenicity. Blood 1996;87:2386-93.
61. Kao KJ, del Rosario MLU. Role of Class II major histocompatibility complex (MHC) antigen-positive donor leukocytes in transfusion-induced alloimmunization to donor Class I MHC antigens. Blood 1998;92:690-4.
62. Clark EA, Ledbetter JA. How B and T cells talk to each other. Nature 1994;367:425-8.
63. Dubey C, Croft M, Swain SL. Costimulatory requirements of naive CD4+ T cells: ICAM-1 or B7-1 can costimulate naive CD4 T cell activation but both are required for optimal response. J Immunol 1995;155:45-57.
64. Bachmann MF, McKall-Faienza K, Schmits R, et al. Distinct roles for LFA-1 and CD28 during activation of naive T cells: Adhesion versus costimulation. Immunity 1997;7:549-57.
65. Nabavi N, Freeman GJ, Gault A, et al. Signalling through the MHC Class II cytoplasmic domain is required for antigen presentation and induces B7 expression. Nature 1992;360:266-8.
66. Fleischer J, Soeth E, Reiling N, et al. Differential expression and function of CD80 (B7-1) and CD86 (B7-2) on human peripheral blood monocytes. Immunology 1996;89:592-8.

67. Thompson CB. Distinct roles for the costimulatory ligands B7-1 and B7-2 in T helper cell differentiation? Cell 1995;81:979-82.
68. Reiser H, Stadecker MJ. Costimulatory B7 molecules in the pathogenesis of infectious and autoimmune diseases. N Engl J Med 1996;335:1369-77.
69. Klaus SJ, Pinchuk LM, Ochs HD, et al. Costimulation through CD28 enhances T cell-dependent B cell activation via CD40-CD40L interaction. J Immunol 1994;152:5643-52.
70. Yang Y, Wilson JM. CD40 ligand-dependent T cell activation: Requirement of B7-CD28 signaling through CD40. Science 1996;273:1862-4.
71. Daly PA, Schiffer CA, Aisner J, Wiernik PH. Platelet transfusion therapy—one hour posttransfusion increments are valuable in predicting the need for HLA-matched preparations. JAMA 1980;243:435-8.
72. Sintnicolaas K, Sizoo W, Haije WG, et al. Delayed alloimmunization by random single donor platelet transfusions: A randomised study to compare single donor and multiple donor platelet transfusions in cancer patients with severe thrombocytopenia. Lancet 1981;1:750-4.
73. Gmur J, von Felten A, Osterwalder B, et al. Delayed alloimmunization using random single donor platelet transfusion: A prospective study in thrombocytopenic patients with acute leukemia. Blood 1983;62:473-9.
74. Eernisse JG, Brand A. Prevention of platelet refractoriness due to HLA antibodies by administration of leukocyte-poor blood components. Exp Hematol 1981;9:77-83.
75. Sirchia G, Parravicini A, Rebulla P, et al. Effectiveness of red blood cells filtered through cotton wool to prevent antileukocyte antibody production in multitransfused patients. Vox Sang 1982;42:190-7.
76. Schiffer CA, Dutcher JP, Aisner J, et al. A randomized trial of leukocyte-depleted platelet transfusion to modify alloimmunization in patients with leukemia. Blood 1983;62:815-20.
77. Fisher M, Chapman JR, Ting A, et al. Alloimmunisation to HLA antigens following transfusion with leukocyte-poor and purified platelet suspensions. Vox Sang 1985;49:331-5.
78. Sirchia G, Rebulla P, Mascaretti L, et al. The clinical importance of leukocyte-depletion in regular erythrocyte transfusions. Vox Sang 1986;51:2-8.
79. Murphy MF, Metcalfe P, Thomas H, et al. Use of leukocyte-poor blood components and HLA-matched-platelet donors to prevent HLA alloimmunization. Br J Haematol 1986;62:529-34.

80. Brand A, Claas FHJ, Voogt PJ, et al. Alloimmunization after leukocyte-depleted multiple random donor platelet transfusions. Vox Sang 1988;54:160-6.
81. Sniecinski I, O'Donnell MR, Nowicki B, et al. Prevention of refractoriness and HLA-alloimmunization using filtered blood products. Blood 1988;71:1402-7.
82. Andreu G, Dewailly J, Leberre C, et al. Prevention of HLA alloimmunization with leukocyte-poor packed red cells and platelet concentrates obtained by filtration. Blood 1988;72:964-9.
83. Saarinen UM, Kekomaki R, Siimes MA, et al. Effective prophylaxis against platelet refractoriness in multitransfused patients by use of leukocyte-free blood components. Blood 1990;75:512-7.
84. van Marwijk Kooij M, van Prooijen HC, Moes M, et al. Use of leukocyte-depleted platelet concentrates for the prevention of refractoriness and primary HLA alloimmunization: A prospective randomized trial. Blood 1991;77:201-5.
85. Oksanen K, Kekomaki R, Ruutu T, et al. Prevention of alloimmunization in patients with acute leukemia by use of white cell-reduced blood components—a randomized trial. Transfusion 1991;31:588-94.
86. Ten Haaft MA, van den Berg-Loonen PM, van Rhenen DJ. Prevention of primary HLA class I alloimmunization with leukocyte-poor blood components produced without the use of platelet filters. Vox Sang 1992;63:257.
87. Bedford Russell AR, Rivers RP, Davey N. The development of anti-HLA antibodies in multiply transfused preterm infants. Arch Dis Child 1993;68:49-51.
88. Williamson LM, Wimperis JZ, Williamson P, et al. Bedside filtration of blood products in the prevention of HLA alloimmunization—a prospective randomized study. Blood 1994;83:3028-35.
89. Sintnicolaas K, van Marwijk Kooij M, van Prooijen HC, et al. Leukocyte depletion of random single-donor platelet transfusion does not prevent secondary human leukocyte antigen-alloimmunization and refractoriness: A randomized prospective study. Blood 1995;85: 824-8.
90. Sherman L, Menitove J, Kagen LR, et al. Ultraviolet-B irradiation of platelets: A preliminary trial of efficacy. Transfusion 1992;32:402-7.
91. Grijzenhout MA, Aarts-Riemens MI, de Gruijl FR, et al. UVB irradiation of human platelet concentrates does not prevent HLA alloimmunization in recipients. Blood 1994;84:3524-31.

92. Blundell EL, Pamphilon DH, Fraser ID, et al. A prospective, randomized study of the use of platelet concentrates irradiated with ultraviolet-B light in patients with hematologic malignancy. Transfusion 1996;36:296-302.
93. Snyder EL, Beardsley DS, Smith BR, et al. Storage of platelet concentrates after high-dose ultraviolet-B irradiation. Transfusion 1991;31: 491-6.
94. Bessos H, Murphy WG, Robertson A, et al. Quality of platelet concentrates irradiated with UVB light: Effect of UV dose and dose rate on glycocalcin release and correlation with other markers of the platelet storage lesions. Transfus Med 1993;3:115-21.
95. Slichter SJ, Deeg HJ, Kennedy MS. Prevention of platelet alloimmunization in dogs with systemic cyclosporin and by UV-irradiation or cyclosporin loading of donor platelets. Blood 1987;69:414-8.
96. Kao KJ. Induction of humoral immune tolerance to major histocompatibility complex antigens by transfusions of UVB-irradiated leukocytes. Blood 1996;88:4375-82.
97. Dutcher JP, Schiffer CA, Aisner J, Wiernik PH. Long-term follow-up of patients with leukemia receiving platelet transfusions: Identification of a large group of patients who do not become alloimmunized. Blood 1981;58:1007-11.
98. Holohan TV, Terasaki PI, Deisseroth AB. Suppression of transfusion-related alloimmunization in intensively treated cancer patients. Blood 1981;58:122-8.
99. Anderson CB, Sicard GA, Etheredge EE. Pretreatment of renal allograft recipients with azathioprine and donor-specific blood products. Surgery 1982;92:315-21.
100. Fujihara N, Takahashi TA, Azuma M, et al. Decreased inducible expression of CD80 and CD86 in human monocytes after ultraviolet-B: Its involvement in inactivation of alloantigenicity. Blood 1996;87:2386-93.

In: Kickler TS, and Herman JH, eds.
Current Issues in Platelet Transfusion Therapy and Platelet Alloimmunity
Bethesda, MD: AABB Press, 1999

6

Alternative Management Strategies in Alloimmunized Thrombocytopenic Patients

CLARENCE B. SARKODEE-ADOO, MD, AND
MEYER R. HEYMAN, MD

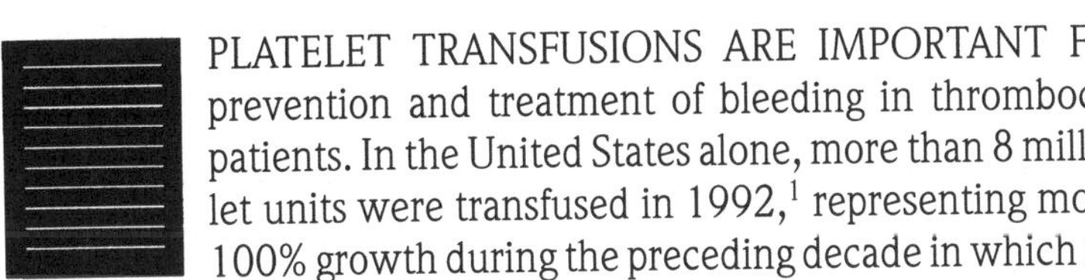

PLATELET TRANSFUSIONS ARE IMPORTANT FOR THE prevention and treatment of bleeding in thrombocytopenic patients. In the United States alone, more than 8 million platelet units were transfused in 1992,[1] representing more than a 100% growth during the preceding decade in which red blood cell transfusions increased by only 17%.[2] Tremendous improvements have been made in platelet transfusion therapy during the 3 decades that this

Clarence B. Sarkodee-Adoo, MD, Assistant Professor of Medicine, Marlene and Stewart Greenebaum Cancer Center, University of Maryland Medical System and University of Maryland School of Medicine; and Meyer R. Heyman, MD, Associate Professor of Medicine and Oncology, Marlene and Stewart Greenebaum Cancer Center, University of Maryland Medical System and University of Maryland School of Medicine, Baltimore, Maryland

modality has been available, and platelets can now be provided safely and effectively in most clinical situations where they are needed.[3,4]

However, some problems remain, one of the most serious being alloimmunization because of its association with refractoriness to platelet transfusions in patients who may be at substantial risk of severe and life-threatening bleeding from thrombocytopenia. Refractoriness to platelet transfusions is also associated with increased financial costs.[5] In a recent study in the United States,[6] average platelet transfusion costs were estimated to be $25,905 for transfusion-refractory inpatients compared with $2501 for transfusion-responsive inpatients undergoing marrow transplantation or treatment for solid tumors. In this study, the average total inpatient costs were also higher for the patients refractory to platelet transfusions ($67,128 vs $20,291).

Estimates of the incidence of alloimmunization range between 10% and 70% in different reports.[7-23] This wide variation is partly a result of the different definitions of alloimmunization and transfusion refractoriness used in these studies. It is also a result of the different proportions of individuals with previous pregnancy or blood component exposure, as well as of the distribution of underlying diseases. Alloimmunization rates may also be influenced by disparities in transfusion practice that exist among the various institutions reporting these studies, especially in terms of the use of filtration or platelets obtained by apheresis. In a recently reported, large, multi-institutional, randomized study, the incidence of alloimmune refractoriness to platelet transfusions was reduced from 13% to 3-5% by means of either leukocyte reduction or ultraviolet-B irradiation of components.[24,25] The somewhat lower incidence of alloimmune refractoriness in this study may have been related to the strict entry criteria used, with enrollment of only 603 of the 1047 patients who were screened. This study, while confirming the benefits of leukocyte reduction and ultraviolet-B irradiation, is a stark reminder that a number of individuals will develop alloimmune refractoriness despite the best preventive measures.

In addition, lymphocytotoxic antibodies, which correlate with refractoriness, are found in the sera of approximately 7-15% of patients at the time of initial presentation, before any preventive measures can be instituted.[7,9,18,23,24] Leukocyte reduction by filtration is also unsuccessful in previously sensitized individuals, and one study reports that about 45% of previously pregnant women developed lymphocytotoxic antibodies within a median of 2 weeks of the first transfusion due to an anamnestic response.[26] But although previous pregnancy and blood component exposure are the cause of prior sensitization in many patients, it is difficult to predict the development of alloimmune refractoriness in individual cases. Thus, a substantial number of thrombocytopenic patients will need measures to prevent or control bleeding complications while they are alloimmunized and refractory to platelet transfusions. This chapter focuses on alternative management strategies for the prophylaxis and treatment of bleeding in alloimmunized thrombocytopenic patients.

Selection of Donors for Alloimmunized Patients

HLA Typing and Platelet Crossmatching

In many institutions, the first step in managing the alloimmunized patient in need of platelet transfusions is the provision of single-donor platelets selected on the basis of HLA matching at the A and B loci. This requires HLA typing for a large pool of potential platelet donors as well as for all patients who might possibly develop alloimmunization. Selective mismatching, which uses known cross-compatible HLA allotypes,[27,28] extends the pool of available donors. Single HLA-antigen mismatched platelets have also been reported to provide satisfactory platelet recovery in 58-73% of alloimmunized patients.[29] In patients whose HLA type is unknown, donor units may sometimes be selected from examination of the lymphocytotoxic (LCT) antibody panel, or family members may be typed to help predict the patients' allotypes. Platelet crossmatching techniques[30-34] have also been shown to enable the selection of suitable units, some of which are poorly matched for HLA but still provide adequate increments.[35] In a study reported in 1997, 59% of refractory patients responded favorably to units selected by crossmatching even though lymphocytotoxic antibodies were not measured.[36] However, platelet crossmatching tends to be labor-intensive and does not obviate the need for a donor registry. Unfortunately, because of the widely polymorphic distribution of HLA types in the population, there are some patients for whom neither HLA typing nor crossmatching is able to identify suitable units. Furthermore, some HLA-compatible units do not provide suitable platelet recovery in alloimmunized patients, probably because these patients may be alloimmunized to platelet-specific (human platelet) antigens as well. While platelets matched for both HLA and platelet-specific antigens can be successfully used in this situation,[37] crossmatching may also be effective for the selection of units.[38,39] Matching for antigens of the blood group ABO system is also predictive of the response to transfusion in alloimmunized patients, although to a lesser degree than crossmatching and HLA matching.[40] Because single-donor apheresis platelets that are selected on the basis of HLA typing or crossmatching do not always produce an adequate posttransfusion recovery, these units may be split into two portions so that if the first portion fails to produce an adequate increment, the second can be offered to another patient.[41]

The Threshold Platelet Count for Prophylactic Transfusions

In some institutions, the prophylactic transfusion of platelets is determined by a set threshold platelet count.[1] Resetting this threshold at a lower level may extend the inventory of histocompatible units available for alloimmunized patients. Three prospective randomized studies have demonstrated that using a prophylactic platelet threshold count of 10,000/μL in selected, stable patients with acute leukemia is comparable in safety to using the value of 20,000/μL as has been done traditionally in many institutions.[42-44] Other nonrandomized studies have shown similar results using a platelet threshold of 5000/μL in patients with acute leukemia[45] and women with gynecological cancers,[46] and of 10,000/μL in patients undergoing marrow transplantation.[47] Although there is no reason to believe that the lower threshold would be less safe in alloimmunized patients, caution should be expressed in their cases because suitable platelets may not be readily available should these patients suffer hemorrhage.

Autologous Cryopreserved Platelets

Autologous platelets can be cryopreserved and will remain viable for several months or years, with posttransfusion recovery amounting to approximately one-half to two-thirds of what might be expected with fresh platelets. Because successful use of this approach requires that the period of thrombocytopenia be anticipated and finite, the approach has largely been limited to patients with acute leukemia in remission who need further myelosuppressive therapy[48,49] and to patients undergoing marrow transplantation.[50] The technique uses dimethyl sulfoxide as the cryopreservant; freezing can be accomplished in one step, simply by placing the product in the vapor phase of a liquid nitrogen freezer.[49] Washing the product prior to transfusion may not be necessary.[50] Because of concerns about tumor cell contamination, Funke et al[48] irradiated autologous units (30 Gy) before transfusion, with no apparent adverse effect on the posttransfusion platelet increment. This approach could be extended to the provision of frozen allogeneic platelets for individuals with rare HLA or platelet-specific antigen types.

Modulation of Effector Mechanisms Involved in Alloimmune Platelet Destruction

HLA Antigen Elutriation of Platelets for Transfusion

Kao reported in 1988 that HLA antigens could be stripped off platelets by means of elutriation with chloroquine diphosphate.[51] This finding sparked interest in the potential use of agents that might render platelets non-HLA antigenic in vivo. However, chloroquine treatment results in morphologic changes and loss of platelet viability and thus has not been useful in preparing components for transfusion. In contrast, acid treatment, which is also effective for the selective elutriation of HLA A and B antigens from platelets, preserves platelet viability and in-vitro function.[52] To date, however, clinical experience with acid-treated platelets is limited. Shanwell et al[53] showed that in two healthy subjects, platelet recovery was unaffected by acid treatment, and that in one patient, a crossmatch-incompatible random-donor unit was successfully transfused after acid treatment. Novotny et al[54] treated two alloimmunized patients with acid-elutriated platelets; although one patient had a severe transfusion reaction with no platelet increment, the other patient was successfully treated with repeated transfusions, which were accompanied by impressive count increments and clinical hemostasis. These initial reports are encouraging, and the technique of acid elutriation deserves further evaluation as a method for improving count recovery in alloimmunized individuals.

Reticuloendothelial Blockade: Splenectomy and Immune Globulin Infusion

It is widely held that the reticuloendothelial system is the final arbiter of platelet destruction in alloimmunized individuals. This is certainly the case in autoimmune thrombocytopenia, in which maneuvers such as splenectomy and the administration of immune globulin are effective for the treatment of immune thrombocytopenia through reticuloendothelial blockade. Splenomegaly is associated with poor responses to platelet transfusions, and splenectomized patients in general have higher count increments following platelet transfusions.[55] However, the positive influence of splenectomy on posttransfusion count recovery is not seen with the transfusion of random-donor platelets to alloimmunized patients.[56,57]

Several case reports have suggested that immune globulin infusions might be useful for the treatment of alloimmunized patients; however, larger series and one randomized study failed to show a consistent benefit.[58-62] In the first report by Zeigler et al,[58] 2-6 g/kg of immune globulin (Sandoglobulin, Sandoz Pharmaceuticals, East Hanover, NJ) was administered to 10 patients who were refractory to platelet transfusions. Six of the patients responded with improved responses to transfusion of HLA-compatible, single-donor platelets; however, random-donor platelets were still ineffective. In this study, 6 of the 10 patients had fever, and 2 had splenomegaly. In addition, all the patients had previously failed to respond to transfusions of HLA-compatible platelets. Thus, it is not clear that the cause of refractoriness in these patients was alloimmunization to HLA antigens. Zeigler et al subsequently updated their experience to a total of 19 patients, 18 of whom had fever during the time of transfusion refractoriness.[59] Interestingly, 11 of the 13 responders had less than 85% LCT reactivity, and only 2 of 8 patients with more than 85% LCT reactivity had responded favorably to immune globulin infusions. Schiffer et al reported a series of 11 patients treated with similar doses of the same immune globulin preparation.[60] In this series, all patients were refractory to random-donor platelets and responsive to HLA-matched units, and all demonstrated high titers of LCT. There were no responses in this series nor in a subsequent series of 7 similarly selected patients from the same institution who received a different preparation of immune globulin (Gammimmune, Cutter Biological, Berkeley, CA).[61] In the only randomized, placebo-controlled study of immune globulin for alloimmunized patients, Kickler et al used yet a different preparation of immune globulin (Gammagard, Baxter Healthcare, Glenside, CA), also in high doses.[62] Similar to the series reported by Schiffer et al[60] and Lee et al,[61] and in contrast to the studies by Zeigler et al,[58,59] Kickler's study enrolled patients only if they were refractory to random-donor platelets; responsive to HLA-matched platelets; reactive to LCT antibodies; and free of fever, sepsis, splenomegaly, or disseminated intravascular coagulation. In this study, although 1-hour posttransfusion corrected count increments were improved in 5 of the 7 patients who received immune globulin, this improvement was not evident 24 hours later. Thus, in the majority of patients, infusions of immune globulin appear not to be useful for the treatment of alloimmune refractoriness to platelet transfusions.

Immunosuppressive Approaches

The failure of splenectomy and immune globulin infusions to improve platelet recovery in alloimmunized patients raises important questions about the mechanism of alloimmune platelet destruction and the role of the reticuloendothelial system. Moreover, because alloimmunization is known to occur in the setting of highly myelo- and immunosuppressive therapy, it is doubtful that immunosuppressive approaches would be of major benefit in most patients. In one study,[57] high-dose therapy with prednisone failed to improve the response to random-donor platelets in alloimmunized patients, although the count recovery after transfusion of matched platelets was higher. Sporadic reports of the successful treatment of alloimmune refractoriness using such medications as vincristine[63] and cyclosporine[64,65] need to be confirmed in larger studies before these drugs can be recommended for general use.

Other investigators have attempted to interfere with the immune system by blocking the development of alloimmunization. The initiation of alloimmune response depends on the presentation of donor antigens in association with B7 costimulatory molecules, which reside on the surface of antigen-presenting cells.[66] When stimulated by donor antigens in association with B7, host T lymphocytes in turn secrete cytokines, which cause B cells to produce the antibodies that mediate alloimmunity.[67] By means of an elegant series of experiments, Ibrahim et al[68] showed that a fusion protein, CTLA4Ig, interferes with antibody formation by adhering preferentially to B7 and preventing ligation of the T-cell receptor CD28 by the antigen-presenting cell. A single dose of this protein successfully prevented IgG alloantibody response in rats when given with the first transfusion and also blunted further antibody production when given with the second transfusion. Potentially, this approach could be useful not only in preventing alloimmunization but also in abrogating the secondary, anamnestic response seen in some previously sensitized patients.

Reticuloendothelial blockade has also been studied for its potential to block the development of alloimmunization. Heddle et al[69] investigated whether treatment with anti-D might be useful in preventing at-risk patients from developing alloimmune platelet refractoriness. In this double-blind, randomized study, Rh-positive patients with acute leukemia undergoing induction therapy were allocated to weekly anti-D or placebo, initiated before their first platelet transfusion. No difference was found between the two groups in terms of refractoriness to platelet transfusions, although LCT antibodies were not evaluated in this study. This study was not designed to test whether large doses of anti-D might improve platelet recovery if administered immediately before random-donor platelets in alloimmunized Rh-positive patients. However, the lack of significant success with immune globulin infusions suggests that anti-D would not be very useful in this situation.

Plasmapheresis and the Staphylococcal Protein A Adsorption Column

Few studies have examined the role of plasma exchange in the management of alloimmune platelet transfusion refractoriness. The rationale underlying this approach is to remove the LCT antibodies that are responsible for alloimmune refractoriness. Bensinger et al applied this therapy to 18 patients and demonstrated improved posttransfusion counts in 11 of them.[70] The improvement was most prominent in those patients with LCT antibodies in whom the improved count recovery was accompanied by a decline in antibodies. In another study, improved platelet transfusion responsiveness was shown in 4 of 8 alloimmune patients whose plasma was adsorbed with a staphyloccocal protein A silica gel column and then returned to the circulation.[71] However, these studies must be interpreted with caution since LCT antibodies and refractoriness to transfusions are known to be transient in some patients.[14,23] Randomized controlled studies would be required to evaluate the role of these relatively expensive modalities in the management of the alloimmunized patient.

Marrow Stimulation by Cytokine Therapy

Several drugs have demonstrated the potential to stimulate marrow production of platelets in preclinical studies. Some of these drugs have been tested in the clinical setting of chemotherapy-induced thrombocytopenia, and one of these agents, interleukin (IL) -11, is now licensed in the United States for the prophylaxis of this disease. Phase I studies of this drug identified fatigue, arthralgia/myalgia, and hematocrit decrements as important side effects[72]; the hematocrit decrements were likely due to hemodilution secondary to fluid retention. In a randomized, placebo-controlled study of breast cancer patients receiving fairly high doses of chemotherapy, Isaacs et al found that IL-11, at a dose of 50 μg/kg given for 10-17 days after chemotherapy, resulted in only 32% of patients requiring platelet transfusions, compared with 59% of patients in the placebo group ($p=0.02$).[73] In a randomized study reported by Tepler et al,[74] patients with widely different types of cancer who had required platelet transfusions during a previous cycle of chemotherapy received placebo or IL-11 in a dose of 25 μg/kg or 50 μg/kg daily following another cycle of the same chemotherapy. A statistically significant benefit was seen only in the group treated with 50 μg/kg, in whom 70% of patients required platelet transfusions compared with 96% in the control group. In both of these studies, side effects were generally tolerable and were related in large part to fluid retention.

Other cytokines, including IL-1, IL-3, and IL-6, as well as granulocyte-macrophage colony-stimulating factor (GM-CSF) and PIXY 321, have also been evaluated in clinical trials for their effects on chemotherapy-induced thrombocytopenia. Smith et al[75] administered IL-1 alpha to patients receiving myelosuppressive doses of carboplatin and found that the mean duration of thrombocytopenia was 16 days in treated patients compared with 21 days in a (nonrandomly selected) control group. Administration of IL-1 before chemotherapy had no demonstrable effect on subsequent platelet counts. Similar findings were reported from another study, in which IL-1 administration permitted multiple cycles of carboplatin in patients with ovarian cancer.[76] In contrast, Elkordy et al[77] did not find IL-1 beta, which is active through the identical cellular receptor, to have a significantly beneficial effect on thrombocytopenia following high-dose chemotherapy and autologous marrow transplantation. In a larger study, Southwest Oncology Group investigators were also unable to find significant amelioration of chemotherapy-induced thrombocytopenia with the administration of IL-I beta.[78]

In limited studies, IL-6 administration has been reported to be associated with modest decreases in the duration of chemotherapy-induced thrombocytopenia and, perhaps, in the need for platelet transfusions.[79,80] Studies of IL-3 show similar, albeit small benefits.[81-83] Treatment with GM-CSF does not have a demonstrable benefit on chemotherapy-induced thrombocytopenia,[84] and some schedules combining GM-CSF with IL-3 may actually be detrimental.[85] PIXY 321, which is a fusion product of IL-3 and GM-CSF, was associated with some benefit when given after, but not before, chemotherapy in one study, but was found to be no better than GM-CSF alone in a larger, randomized study.[86,87] In these studies, fever, flu-like symptoms, arthralgia, and in some cases fluid retention have accompanied the administration of these cytokines, and further studies are in progress to determine the clinical usefulness of these agents relative to their toxicity. However, none of these agents is being tested on a large scale in patients with acute leukemia, who account for a significant percentage of alloimmunized thrombocytopenic patients in many institutions. In contrast, pegylated recombinant human megakaryocyte growth and development factor (PEG-rHuMGDF), which has already been shown to improve chemotherapy-related thrombocytopenia significantly in solid-tumor patients,[88,89] is being evaluated in randomized prospective trials in patients with acute myeloid leukemia. In a randomized, double-blind, placebo-controlled study of patients receiving chemotherapy for lung cancer, PEG-rHuMGDF was associated with a higher platelet count nadir as well as a faster platelet count recovery (14 days vs 21 days) than was found in the placebo-administered group.[89] Patients treated with PEG-rHuMGDF did not have an excess incidence of fever, flulike symptoms, or fluid retention, although pulmonary thromboembolism and superficial phlebitis were seen in one patient each. It is hoped that these encouraging results may eventually also be demonstrated in patients with acute leukemia without an adverse effect on the chemotherapeutic response rates.

Platelet Substitutes

The obvious problems with the procurement, storage, and side effects of platelets have led to a search for artificial or semiartificial platelet substitutes (Table 6-1). Of these agents, infusible platelet membrane (Cyplex, Cypress Bioscience Inc, San Diego, CA) is one of the best studied. The product is prepared from human platelets by means of several freeze-thaw steps followed by heat treatment and lyophilization, resulting in a virus-inactivated powder with a shelf life of at least 3 years.[90] Infusible platelet membrane appears to retain some (GPIb, IIb, IIIa) but not other (GPIa, IIa, IIIb) platelet antigenic activity, and importantly, HLA-A and -B antigens are not detectable in the product after the heating step. When reconstituted for infusion, this product is associated with significant procoagulant activity, as has been demonstrated in pilot studies by reduced bleeding time in aspirinized volunteer subjects and thrombocytopenic patients (AM Houranieh, personal communication). A Phase II study also showed reduced bleeding in 16 of 26 thrombocytopenic bleeding patients.[91] Of major interest were the responses seen in 9 of the 15 patients in this trial who had previously failed to respond to platelet transfusions. No clinically important toxic effects due to the administration of infusible platelet membrane have as yet been reported, and this product may possibly be found to be safer than platelet transfusions because it is associated with a lower incidence of infectious complications, transfusion reactions, transfusion-associated graft-vs-host disease, and alloimmunization. Studies currently under way should define the full safety profile and activity of infusible platelet membrane in thrombocytopenic patients, including those who are alloimmunized.

The process of lyophilization with the intent of extending shelf life has also been applied to whole platelets. Read et al reported extensive preclinical evaluations of such a product, showing that it possessed intact morphologic ultrastructure, antigenic profile, and the ability to participate in carotid arterial thrombus formation in normal canine subjects.[92] Lyophilized whole platelets, in contrast to infusible platelet membrane, exhibit HLA-A and -B antigens, and therefore, in order to be useful in alloimmunized recipients, they would have to be prepared from HLA-selected single donors.

Table 6-1. Platelet Substitutes in Development

Product	Potential Advantages	Potential Drawbacks
Lyophilized platelets[92]	Virus inactivated Extended shelf life Similar to natural platelets	Freezing step required Intact HLA antigens
Infusible platelet membrane[90,91]	Virus inactivated Extended shelf life May not cause alloimmunization May be useful in alloimmunized patients	Multiple daily dosing
Thromboerythrocytes[93]	Relatively simple process Autologous blood used May not cause alloimmunization May be useful in alloimmunized patients	Short shelf life Phlebotomy required
Thrombospheres[94]	Virus-free Extended shelf life May not cause alloimmunization May be useful in alloimmunized patients Extended duration of action	Studies needed to show lack of thrombogenicity

As described by Read et al, the process of preparing lyophilized platelets appears to be quite complicated and includes storage at –80 C. Thus, the logistic advantage that this product might have over frozen platelets for the treatment of alloimmunized patients is unclear. In contrast, thromboerythrocytes[93] are prepared by means of a simpler procedure using autologous red blood cells coated with a peptide that features the arginine-glycine-aspartate sequence important for interaction with platelet GPIIb/IIIa complex. In-vitro experiments have demonstrated that thromboerythrocyte binding to platelets is limited to activated platelets, suggesting that it might not be associated with spontaneous blood clotting. By binding to activated circulating and endothelium-adherent platelets, thromboerythrocytes form microaggregates that may be expected to substitute for platelets in the hemostatic process. Because of the characteristics of the thromboerythrocyte-platelet interaction, enough thromboerythrocytes could potentially be manufactured from 50 mL of autologous blood to provide the equivalent of 18 units of platelets by mass. Thus, if proved to be safe, thromboerythrocytes would be a very welcome alternative to platelet transfusions for the management of thrombocytopenic patients.

Lyophilized platelets, thromboerythrocytes, and infusible platelet membrane are all manufactured from cellular blood products. In contrast, thrombospheres, which are also being developed as a potential platelet substitute, are made from cross-linked albumin spherules coated with fibrinogen. The administration of thrombospheres to thrombocytopenic rabbits was associated with marked shortening of the bleeding time (which persisted for 72 hours) and a reduction in clinical bleeding compared with that resulting from the administration of bland albumin spherules.[94]

Thrombospheres probably exert their hemostatic activity by means of direct participation in fibrin clot formation, thus bypassing platelets as a substrate. Clinical studies are needed to define their safety and activity in thrombocytopenic patients.

Pharmacologic Agents to Reduce Bleeding Complications

Alloimmunized thrombocytopenic patients may also benefit from the judicious use of pharmacologic hemostatic agents. Tranexamic acid, epsilon aminocaproic acid (EACA), and aprotinin exert their hemostatic effects through stabilization of the fibrin clot by inhibition of fibrinolysis. Ben-Bassat et al[95] treated 54 consecutive acute myeloid leukemia patients with oral or IV tranexamic acid during the periods of thrombocytopenia that resulted from induction or consolidation therapy. In this nonrandomized study, patients were examined twice daily and transfused with platelets only if they showed signs of bleeding, irrespective of the platelet count. This approach resulted in an average of only 4.6 ± 4.1 platelet transfusions given during induction therapy and 1.7 ± 1.8 platelet transfusions given during consolidation. It is important to note that only 6 of the 78 induction courses and none of the 53 consolidation courses were complicated by major bleeding events. The investigators in this study estimated that the expected number of platelet transfusions during induction therapy was 7-12, and they therefore concluded that the administration of tranexamic acid was likely responsible for the ability to reduce safely the number of platelet transfusions given. However, because of studies that have demonstrated the safety of stringent criteria for prophylactic platelet transfusions,[42-44] it is not clear from this study that the reduced transfusion requirement was entirely attributable to the administration of tranexamic acid. This question was therefore addressed by a subsequent controlled study[96] in which these investigators showed that tranexamic acid compared with placebo reduced the need for platelet transfusions during consolidation but did not reduce the need for induction therapy in patients with acute myeloid leukemia.

The efficacy of tranexamic acid in thrombocytopenic bleeding has also been evaluated in other patient groups. Seven patients with aplastic anemia were enrolled in a prospective randomized, double-blind study using a crossover design in which each patient served as his or her own control.[97] In the 3 patients who completed the randomized portion of the study, tranexamic acid did not prevent bleeding episodes. In contrast, patients with acute promyelocytic leukemia were shown in another small, randomized study to benefit from the administration of tranexamic acid, with fewer hemorrhagic events and a decreased need for platelet transfusions.[98] In these randomized studies of tranexamic acid, as well as in the uncontrolled study, the drug appeared to be safe, with no excess thrombotic events noted; however, the safety of long-term treatment in these patient groups is not known.

Another antifibrinolytic agent, EACA, has been evaluated in uncontrolled studies in thrombocytopenic patients.[99-101] In these studies, the use of EACA resulted in a reduction in transfusion requirements in thrombocytopenic patients, and in one study, bleeding complications appeared to be reduced. In addition, Benson et al[102] reported their experience with 18 marrow transplantation patients who were treated with EACA to control severe bleeding associated with thrombocytopenia. Ten of the patients also received desmopressin. Nine of the patients in this study were alloimmunized. Bleeding ceased or decreased in 12 of the 18 patients within a median of 2 days. Roath et al[103] reported that bleeding complications were also reduced in 5 thrombocytopenic patients who were treated with aprotinin, another antifibrinolytic agent. These limited studies suggest that antifibrinolytic agents may be useful in selected thrombocytopenic patients, and they underscore the need for larger, randomized evaluations of the role of these agents in the control of thrombocytopenic bleeding.

Desmopressin administration is associated with a hemostatic effect possibly through the release of von Willebrand factor. While most useful in patients with von Willebrand disease and mild hemophilia A, this effect may also be of some benefit in thrombocytopenic patients by improving the effectiveness of the circulating platelets. Castaman et al[104] successfully controlled bleeding in all of 15 patients with thrombocytopenia who were treated with desmopressin. Among 4 of these patients whose bleeding time was also evaluated, a significant improvement was seen in 3. However, the tachyphylaxis associated with desmopressin-induced release of von Willebrand factor may limit the usefulness of this drug for the long-term control of bleeding in thrombocytopenic patients.

Other agents have been developed for their hemostatic potential when applied locally at sites of bleeding. Both EACA and tranexamic acid help to control dental bleeding when used in the form of mouthwash in patients with hemophilia or in others who are on anticoagulant therapy.[105-107] Although this has not been evaluated systematically in thrombocytopenic patients, local application of EACA is reportedly useful for the control of epistaxis due to thrombocytopenia.[108] Fibrin sealants are a heterogenous group of products developed to provide a local hemostatic or tissue adhesive effect. They generally consist of varying concentrations of fibrinogen, Factor XIII, thrombin, and sometimes antifibrinolytic agents such as tranexamic acid, EACA, or aprotinin. Many of these agents are used widely in Europe as well as in some institutions in the United States, especially in surgical practice. To date, experience with these agents in thrombocytopenia has been limited, although in one center's experience with hepatic surgery some of the patients were mildly thrombocytopenic.[109] Alloimmunized thrombocytopenic patients represent one group in which these agents might be of some potential use and in whom they could be investigated in a systematic manner. The use of bovine thrombin in many of these preparations has been found to be associated with the production of antibodies that may cross-react with human coagulation proteins, resulting in abnormal coagulation test results and potentially causing bleeding.[110-112] Anaphylactic reactions to bovine thrombin have also been reported.[113,114]

Adjunctive Measures

Several clinical factors have been shown to be associated either with an increased risk of bleeding in thrombocytopenic patients or with a decreased response to platelet transfusions in the presence or absence of alloimmunization.[55,115-119] These factors include splenomegaly, fever, sepsis, the concurrent administration of amphotericin B or certain antibiotics (ciprofloxacin and vancomycin in one study), and the use of platelets stored for a longer duration. In alloimmune patients, it is especially important to minimize the effects of factors associated with poor platelet transfusion response, thereby reducing the risk of hemorrhagic complications. Thus, fresh platelets should be used if available, and infections should be treated aggressively with the use, where possible, of antibiotics that are not associated with a deleterious effect on platelet transfusions. Fever should be controlled with antipyretic medications while aspirin and nonsteroidal anti-inflammatory drugs are avoided. Because transfusion reactions do not appear to have a significant adverse impact on platelet recovery after transfusion,[120] those transfusions that are complicated by urticarial reactions should be continued if possible. Coagulopathy, such as might be due to vitamin K deficiency or hypofibrinogenemia secondary to asparaginase, should be identified promptly and treated appropriately. A high index of suspicion should also be maintained for other causes of thrombocytopenia, such as disseminated intravascular coagulation and immune or thrombotic thrombocytopenic purpura, all of which can mimic or coexist with chemotherapy-induced or cancer- and leukemia-related thrombocytopenia.

Retinal hemorrhages are associated with severe anemia in patients with acute leukemia,[121,122] and some early evidence suggests that the correction of anemia in thrombocytopenic patients may aid the control of bleeding in general.[123-125] It must be borne in mind, however, that alloimmunization to platelets can occur through the exclusive transfusion of red blood cells,[13] and measures intended to prevent alloimmunization must also be applied to red cell transfusions.

Conclusions

Several interesting approaches are in development as alternative treatments for thrombocytopenic patients, and many of these could be adapted for alloimmunized individuals. In practice, some of these approaches might be complementary to each other, as for example in the potential use of PEG-rHuMGDF to boost platelet counts prior to collection of autologous or allogeneic platelets that could be cryopreserved and transfused later using "split apheresis" techniques. An intriguing experimental approach is the use of gene transfer techniques to insert a sequence that favorably upregulates platelet production for the prevention or treatment of thrombocytopenia. This technique has already been demonstrated in animal studies.[126] Among the most interesting advances yet to become available for general clinical use is the use of acid elutriation to render random-donor units suitable for transfusion to alloimmunized patients. Other investigators are in the process of developing platelet substitutes, and one such product, infusible platelet membrane, which is apparently free of HLA antigens, is already in clinical evaluation. These innovations are expected to translate in the near future into effective alternative management strategies for alloimmunized thrombocytopenic patients.

References

1. Wallace EL, Churchill WH, Surgenor DM, et al. Collection and transfusion of blood and blood components in the United States, 1992. Transfusion 1995;35:802-12.
2. Surgenor DM, Wallace EL, Hao SH, Chapman RH. Collection and transfusion of blood in the United States, 1982-1988. N Engl J Med 1990;322:1646-51.
3. Heyman M, Schiffer C. Platelet transfusion to patients receiving chemotherapy. In: Ross E, Simon T, Moss G, Gould S, eds. Principles of transfusion medicine. 2nd ed. Baltimore, MD: Williams and Wilkins, 1996:263-73.
4. Sarkodee-Adoo C, Schiffer CA. Platelet transfusion support for patients with cancer and hematologic malignancies. Curr Opin Hematol 1996;3:347-54.
5. Snider C, Erder H, LaBrecque J, et al. What are the true costs of platelet transfusions? A prospective time motion study of resource utilization associated with platelet transfusions at UCLA medical center (abstract). Blood 1996;88:333a.
6. Kallich J, Erder M, LaBrecque J, et al. Inpatient platelet use and costs for patients with solid tumors: A comparison between refractory and non-refractory patients. Proceedings of the American Society of Clinical Oncology 1997;16:419a.
7. Abou-Elella AA, Camarillo TA, Allen MB, et al. Low incidence of red cell and HLA antibody formation by bone marrow transplant patients. Transfusion 1995;35:931-5.
8. Legler TJ, Fischer I, Dittmann J, et al. Frequency and causes of refractoriness in multiply transfused patients. Ann Hematol 1997;74: 185-9.
9. Hogge DE, McConnell M, Jacobson C, et al. Platelet refractoriness and alloimmunization in pediatric oncology and bone marrow transplant patients. Transfusion 1995;35:645-52.

10. Williamson LM, Wimperis JZ, Williamson P, et al. Bedside filtration of blood products in the prevention of HLA alloimmunization—a prospective randomized study. Blood 1994;83:3028-35.
11. Gmur J, von Felten A, Osterwalder B, et al. Delayed alloimmunization using random single-donor platelet transfusions: A prospective study in thrombocytopenic patients with acute leukemia. Blood 1983;62:473-9.
12. Klingemann HG, Self S, Banaji M, et al. Refractoriness to random donor platelet transfusions in patients with aplastic anaemia: A multivariate analysis of data from 264 cases. Br J Haematol 1987;66:115-21.
13. Friedman DF, Lukas MB, Jawad A, et al. Alloimmunization to platelets in heavily transfused patients with sickle cell disease. Blood 1996;88:3216-22.
14. Brand A, Claas FHJ, Voogt PJ, et al. Alloimmunization after leukocyte-depleted multiple random donor platelet transfusions. Vox Sang 1988;54:160-6.
15. Godeau B, Fromont P, Seror T, et al. Platelet alloimmunization after multiple transfusions: A prospective study of 50 patients. Br J Haematol 1992;81:395-400.
16. Holohan TV, Terasaki PI, Deisseroth AB. Suppression of transfusion-related alloimmunization in intensively treated cancer patients. Blood 1981;58:122-8.
17. Howard JE, Perkins HA. The natural history of alloimmunization to platelets. Transfusion 1978;18:496-503.
18. Novotny V, van Doorn R, Witvliet M, et al. Occurrence of allogeneic HLA and non-HLA antibodies after transfusion of prestorage filtered platelets and red blood cells: A prospective study. Blood 1995;85:1736-41.
19. Murphy MF, Metcalfe P, Thomas H, et al. Use of leucocyte-poor blood components and HLA-matched-platelet donors to prevent HLA alloimmunization. Br J Haematol 1986;62:529-34.
20. Murphy MF, Metcalfe P, Ord J, et al. Disappearance of HLA and platelet-specific antibodies in acute leukaemia patients alloimmunized by multiple transfusions. Br J Haematol 1987;67:255-60.
21. Schiffer CA, Dutcher JP, Aisner J, et al. A randomized trial of leukocyte-depleted platelet transfusion to modify alloimmunization in patients with leukemia. Blood 1983;62:815-20.

22. van Marwijk Kooij M, van Prooijen HC, Moes M, et al. Use of leukocyte-depleted platelet concentrates for the prevention of refractoriness and primary HLA alloimmunization: A prospective, randomized trial. Blood 1991;77:201-5.
23. Dutcher JP, Schiffer CA, Aisner J, Wiernik P. Long-term follow-up of patients with leukemia receiving platelet transfusions: Identification of a large group of patients who do not become alloimmunized. Blood 1981;58:1007-11.
24. Trial to Reduce Alloimmunization to Platelets (TRAP) Study Group. Leukocyte reduction and ultraviolet B irradiation of platelets to prevent alloimmunization and refractoriness to platelet transfusions. N Engl J Med 1997;337:1861-9.
25. Kao KJ, Mickel M, Braine HG, et al. White cell reduction in platelet concentrates and packed red cells by filtration: A multicenter clinical trial. Transfusion 1995;35:13-9.
26. Sintnicolaas K, van Marwijk Kooij M, van Prooijen HC, et al. Leukocyte depletion of random single-donor platelet transfusion does not prevent secondary human leukocyte antigen-alloimmunization and refractoriness: A randomized prospective study. Blood 1995;85: 824-8.
27. Dahlke MB, Weiss KL. Platelet transfusion from donors mismatched for crossreactive HLA antigens. Transfusion 1984;24:299-302.
28. Dusquenoy R, Filip D, Rodey G. Successful transfusion of platelets "mismatched" for HLA antigens to alloimmunized thrombocytopenic patients. Am J Hematol 1977;2:219-26.
29. Hussein M, Lee E, Fletcher R, Schiffer C. The effect of lymphocytotoxic antibody reactivity on the results of single antigen mismatched platelet transfusions to alloimmunized patients. Blood 1996;87: 3959-62.
30. Sintnicolaas K, Lowenberg B. A flow cytometric platelet immunofluorescence crossmatch for predicting successful HLA matched platelet transfusions. Br J Haematol 1996;92:1005-10.
31. Brubaker DB, Duke JC, Romine M. Predictive value of enzyme-linked immunoassay platelet crossmatching for transfusion of platelet concentrates to alloimmunized recipients. Am J Hematol 1987; 24:375-87.
32. O'Connell BA, Schiffer CA. Donor selection for alloimmunized patients by platelet crossmatching of random-donor platelet concentrates. Transfusion 1990;30:314-7.

33. Kickler TS, Braine HG, Ness PM, et al. A radiolabeled antiglobulin test for crossmatching platelet transfusions. Blood 1983;61:238-42.
34. Ogden DM, Asfour A, Koller C, Lichtiger B. Platelet crossmatches of single-donor platelet concentrates using a latex agglutination assay. Transfusion 1993;33:644-50.
35. Friedberg RC, Donnelly SF, Mintz PD. Independent roles for platelet crossmatching and HLA in the selection of platelets for alloimmunized patients. Transfusion 1994;34:215-20.
36. Gelb AB, Leavitt AD. Crossmatch-compatible platelets improve corrected count increments in patients who are refractory to randomly selected platelets. Transfusion 1997;37:624-30.
37. Kekomaki S, Volin L, Koistinen P, et al. Successful treatment of platelet transfusion refractoriness: The use of platelet transfusions matched for both human leucocyte antigens (HLA) and human platelet alloantigens (HPA) in alloimmunized patients with leukaemia. Eur J Haematol 1998;60:112-8.
38. Brand A, van Leeuwen A, Eernisse JG, van Rood JJ. Platelet transfusion therapy. Optimal donor selection with a combination of lymphocytotoxicity and platelet fluorescence tests. Blood 1978;51: 781-8.
39. Kohler M, Dittmann J, Legler TJ, et al. Flow cytometric detection of platelet-reactive antibodies and application in platelet crossmatching. Transfusion 1996;36:250-5.
40. Heal JM, Blumberg N, Masel D. An evaluation of crossmatching, HLA, and ABO matching for platelet transfusions to refractory patients. Blood 1987;70:23-30.
41. Gharpure V, Norris D, Lee E, Schiffer C. Use of "split" plateletpheresis products for alloimmunized patients. Vox Sang 1994;67:272-4.
42. Wandt H, Frank M, Ehninger G, et al. Safety and cost effectiveness of a 10×10^9/L trigger for prophylactic platelet transfusions compared with the traditional 20×10^9/L trigger: A prospective comparative trial in 105 patients with acute myeloid leukemia. Blood 1998;91: 3601-6.
43. Rebulla P, Finazzi G, Marangoni F, et al. A multicenter randomized study of the threshold for prophylactic platelet transfusions in adults with acute myeloid leukemia. Gruppo Italiano Malattie Ematologiche Maligne dell'Adulto. N Engl J Med 1997;337:1870-5.
44. Heckman KD, Weiner GJ, Davis CS, et al. Randomized study of prophylactic platelet transfusion threshold during induction therapy for

adult acute leukemia: 10,000/microL versus 20,000/microL. J Clin Oncol 1997;15:1143-9.

45. Gmur J, Burger J, Schanz U, et al. Safety of stringent prophylactic platelet transfusion policy for patients with acute leukaemia. Lancet 1991;338:1223-6.
46. Fanning J, Hilgers RD, Murray KP, et al. Conservative management of chemotherapeutic-induced thrombocytopenia in women with gynecologic cancers. Gynecol Oncol 1995;59:191-3.
47. Gil-Fernandez JJ, Alegre A, Fernandez-Villalta MJ, et al. Clinical results of a stringent policy on prophylactic platelet transfusion: Non-randomized comparative analysis in 190 bone marrow transplant patients from a single institution. Bone Marrow Transplant 1996;18:931-5.
48. Funke I, Wiesneth M, Koerner K, et al. Autologous platelet transfusion in alloimmunized patients with acute leukemia. Ann Hematol 1995;71:169-73.
49. Schiffer CA, Aisner J, Wiernik PH. Frozen autologous platelet transfusion for patients with leukemia. N Engl J Med 1978;299:7-12.
50. Mulder PO, Maas A, de Vries EG, et al. Bleeding prophylaxis in autologous bone marrow transplantation for solid tumors. Comparison of cryopreserved autologous and fresh allogeneic single-donor platelets. Haemostasis 1989;19:120-4.
51. Kao KJ. Selective elution of HLA antigens and beta 2-microglobulin from human platelets by chloroquine diphosphate. Transfusion 1988;28:14-7.
52. Sugawara S, Abo T, Kumagai K. A simple method to eliminate the antigenicity of surface Class I MHC molecules from the membrane of viable cells by acid treatment at pH 3. J Immunol Methods 1987; 100:83-90.
53. Shanwell A, Sallander S, Olsson I, et al. An alloimmunized, thrombocytopenic patient successfully transfused with acid-treated, random-donor platelets. Br J Haematol 1991;79:462-5.
54. Novotny VM, Huizinga TW, van Doorn R, et al. HLA Class I-eluted platelets as an alternative to HLA-matched platelets. Transfusion 1996;36:438-44.
55. Bishop JF, McGrath K, Wolf MM, et al. Clinical factors influencing the efficacy of pooled platelet transfusions. Blood 1988;71:383-7.
56. Hogge DE, Dutcher JP, Aisner J, Schiffer CA. The ineffectiveness of random donor platelet transfusion in splenectomized, alloimmunized recipients. Blood 1984;64:253-6.

57. Grumet FC, Yankee RA. Long-term platelet support of patients with aplastic anemia. Effect of splenectomy and steroid therapy. Ann Intern Med 1970;73:1-7.
58. Zeigler ZR, Shadduck RK, Rosenfeld CS, et al. High-dose intravenous gamma globulin improves responses to single-donor platelets in patients refractory to platelet transfusion. Blood 1987;70:1433-6.
59. Zeigler ZR, Shadduck RK, Rosenfeld CS, et al. Intravenous gamma globulin decreases platelet-associated IgG and improves transfusion responses in platelet refractory states. Am J Hematol 1991;38:15-23.
60. Schiffer CA, Hogge DE, Aisner J, et al. High-dose intravenous gammaglobulin in alloimmunized platelet transfusion recipients. Blood 1984;64:937-40.
61. Lee EJ, Norris D, Schiffer CA. Intravenous immune globulin for patients alloimmunized to random donor platelet transfusion. Transfusion 1987;27:245-7.
62. Kickler T, Braine HG, Piantadosi S, et al. A randomized, placebo-controlled trial of intravenous gammaglobulin in alloimmunized thrombocytopenic patients. Blood 1990;75:313-6.
63. Bruggers CS, Kurtzberg J, Friedman HS. Vincristine therapy for severe platelet alloimmunization. Am J Pediatr Hematol Oncol 1991; 13:300-4.
64. Tilly H, Azagury M, Bastit D, et al. Cyclosporin for treatment of life-threatening alloimmunization. Am J Hematol 1990;34:75-6.
65. Yamamoto M, Ideguchi H, Nishimura J, et al. Treatment of platelet-alloimmunization with cyclosporin A in a patient with aplastic anemia. Am J Hematol 1990;33:220-1.
66. Guinan EC, Gribben JG, Boussiotis VA, et al. Pivotal role of the B7:CD28 pathway in transplantation tolerance and tumor immunity. Blood 1994;84:3261-82.
67. Schwartz RH. Costimulation of T lymphocytes: The role of CD28, CTLA-4, and B7/BB1 in interleukin-2 production and immunotherapy. Cell 1992;71:1065-8.
68. Ibrahim S, Jakobs F, Kittur D, et al. CTLA4Ig inhibits alloantibody responses to repeated blood transfusions. Blood 1996;88:4594-600.
69. Heddle NM, Klama L, Kelton JG, et al. The use of anti-D to improve post-transfusion platelet response: A randomized trial. Br J Haematol 1995;89:163-8.

70. Bensinger WI, Buckner CD, Clift RA, et al. Plasma exchange for platelet alloimmunization. Transplantation 1986;41:602-5.
71. Christie DJ, Howe RB, Lennon SS, Sauro SC. Treatment of refractoriness to platelet transfusion by protein A column therapy. Transfusion 1993;33:234-42.
72. Gordon MS, McCaskill-Stevens WJ, Battiato LA, et al. A Phase I trial of recombinant human interleukin-11 (Neumega rhIL-11 growth factor) in women with breast cancer receiving chemotherapy. Blood 1996;87:3615-24.
73. Isaacs C, Robert NJ, Bailey FA, et al. Randomized placebo-controlled study of recombinant human interleukin-11 to prevent chemotherapy-induced thrombocytopenia in patients with breast cancer receiving dose-intensive cyclophosphamide and doxorubicin. J Clin Oncol 1997;15:3368-77.
74. Tepler I, Elias L, Smith JW 2d, et al. A randomized placebo-controlled trial of recombinant human interleukin-11 in cancer patients with severe thrombocytopenia due to chemotherapy. Blood 1996;87:3607-14.
75. Smith JW 2d, Longo DL, Alvord WG, et al. The effects of treatment with interleukin-1 alpha on platelet recovery after high-dose carboplatin. N Engl J Med 1993;328:756-61.
76. Vadhan-Raj S, Kudelka AP, Garrison L, et al. Effects of interleukin-1 alpha on carboplatin-induced thrombocytopenia in patients with recurrent ovarian cancer. J Clin Oncol 1994;12:707-14.
77. Elkordy M, Crump M, Vredenburgh J, et al. A phase I trial of recombinant human interleukin-1 beta (OCT-43) following high-dose chemotherapy and autologous bone marrow transplantation. Bone Marrow Transplant 1997;19:315-22.
78. Rinehart J, Hersh E, Issell B, et al. Phase I trial of recombinant human interleukin-1 beta (rhIL-1 beta), carboplatin, and etoposide in patients with solid cancers: Southwest Oncology Group Study 8940. Cancer Invest 1997;15:403-10.
79. Gordon MS, Nemunaitis J, Hoffman R, et al. A phase I trial of recombinant human interleukin-6 in patients with myelodysplastic syndromes and thrombocytopenia. Blood 1995;85:3066-76.
80. D'Hondt V, Humblet Y, Guillaume T, et al. Thrombopoietic effects and toxicity of interleukin-6 in patients with ovarian cancer before and after chemotherapy: A multicentric placebo-controlled, randomized phase Ib study. Blood 1995;85:2347-53.

81. D'Hondt V, Weynants P, Humblet Y, et al. Dose-dependent interleukin-3 stimulation of thrombopoiesis and neutropoiesis in patients with small-cell lung carcinoma before and following chemotherapy: A placebo-controlled randomized phase Ib study. J Clin Oncol 1993;11:2063-71.
82. Ganser A, Seipelt G, Lindemann A, et al. Effects of recombinant human interleukin-3 in patients with myelodysplastic syndromes. Blood 1990;76:455-62.
83. Tepler I, Elias A, Kalish L, et al. Effect of recombinant human interleukin-3 on haematological recovery from chemotherapy-induced myelosuppression. Br J Haematol 1994;87:678-86.
84. Chambers L, Garcia L. Lack of effect on platelet increments of granulocyte-macrophage-colony-stimulating factor following autologous bone marow transplantation for malignant lymphoma. Transfusion 1994;34:221-5.
85. O'Shaughnessy JA, Venzon DJ, Gossard M, et al. A phase I study of sequential versus concurrent interleukin-3 and granulocyte-macrophage colony-stimulating factor in advanced breast cancer patients treated with FLAC (5-fluorouracil, leucovorin, doxorubicin, cyclophosphamide) chemotherapy. Blood 1995;86:2913-21.
86. Runowicz CD, Mandeli J, Speyer JL, et al. Phase I/II study of PIXY 321 in combination with cyclophosphamide and carboplatin in the treatment of ovarian cancer. Am J Obstet Gynecol 1996;174:1151-60.
87. O'Shaughnessy JA, Tolcher A, Riseberg D, et al. Prospective, randomized trial of 5-fluorouracil, leucovorin, doxorubicin, and cyclophosphamide chemotherapy in combination with the interleukin-3/granulocyte-macrophage colony-stimulating factor (GM-CSF) fusion protein (PIXY 321) versus GM-CSF in patients with advanced breast cancer. Blood 1996;87:2205-11.
88. Basser RL, Rasko JE, Clarke K, et al. Randomized, blinded, placebo-controlled phase I trial of pegylated recombinant human megakaryocyte growth and development factor with filgrastim after dose-intensive chemotherapy in patients with advanced cancer. Blood 1997;89:3118-28. [Published erratum appears in Blood 1997;90: 2513.]
89. Fanucchi M, Glaspy J, Crawford J, et al. Effects of polyethylene glycol-conjugated recombinant human megakaryocyte growth and development factor on platelet counts after chemotherapy for lung cancer. N Engl J Med 1997;336:404-9.

90. Chao FC, Kim BK, Houranieh AM, et al. Infusible platelet membrane microvesicles: A potential transfusion substitute for platelets. Transfusion 1996;36:536-42.
91. Scigliano, Enright H, Telen M, et al. Infusible platelet membrane for control of bleeding in thrombocytopenic patients (abstract). Blood 1997;10:267.
92. Read MS, Reddick RL, Bode AP, et al. Preservation of hemostatic and structural properties of rehydrated lyophilized platelets: Potential for long-term storage of dried platelets for transfusion. Proc Natl Acad Sci U S A 1995;92:397-401.
93. Coller BS, Springer KT, Beer JH, et al. Thromboerythrocytes. In vitro studies of a potential autologous, semi-artificial alternative to platelet transfusions. J Clin Invest 1992;89:546-55.
94. Yen R, Ho T, Blajchman M. A novel approach to correcting the bleeding associated with thrombocytopenia (abstract). Transfusion 1996; 35(suppl):41S.
95. Ben-Bassat I, Douer D, Ramot B. Tranexamic acid therapy in acute myeloid leukemia: Possible reduction of platelet transfusions. Eur J Haematol 1990;45:86-9.
96. Shpilberg O, Blumenthal R, Sopher O, et al. A controlled trial of tranexamic acid therapy for the reduction of bleeding during treatment of acute myeloid leukemia. Leuk Lymphoma 1995;19:141-4.
97. Fricke W, Alling D, Kimball J, et al. Lack of efficacy of tranexamic acid in thrombocytopenic bleeding. Transfusion 1991;31:345-8.
98. Avvisati G, ten Cate JW, Buller HR, Mandelli F. Tranexamic acid for control of haemorrhage in acute promyelocytic leukaemia. Lancet 1989;2:122-4.
99. Garewal HS, Durie BG. Anti-fibrinolytic therapy with aminocaproic acid for the control of bleeding in thrombocytopenic patients. Scand J Haematol 1985;35:497-500.
100. Bartholomew JR, Salgia R, Bell WR. Control of bleeding in patients with immune and nonimmune thrombocytopenia with aminocaproic acid. Arch Intern Med 1989;149:1959-61.
101. Gardner FH, Helmer RE 3d. Aminocaproic acid. Use in control of hemorrhage in patients with amegakaryocytic thrombocytopenia. JAMA 1980;243:35-7.
102. Benson K, Fields K, Hiemenz J, et al. The platelet-refractory bone marrow transplant patient: Prophylaxis and treatment of bleeding. Semin Oncol 1993;20:102-9.

103. Roath OS, Majer RV, Smith AG. The use of aprotinin in thrombocytopenic patients: A preliminary evaluation. Blood Coagul Fibrinolysis 1990;1:235-7.
104. Castaman G, Bona ED, Schiavotto C, et al. Pilot study on the safety and efficacy of desmopressin for the treatment or prevention of bleeding in patients with hematologic malignancies. Haematologica 1997;82:584-7.
105. Borea G, Montebugnoli L, Capuzzi P, Magelli C. Tranexamic acid as a mouthwash in anticoagulant-treated patients undergoing oral surgery. An alternative method to discontinuing anticoagulant therapy. Oral Surg Oral Med Oral Pathol 1993;75:29-31.
106. Forbes CD, Barr RD, Reid G, et al. Tranexamic acid in control of haemorrhage after dental extraction in haemophilia and Christmas disease. Br Med J 1972;2:311-3.
107. Sindet-Pedersen S, Stenbjerg S. Effect of local antifibrinolytic treatment with tranexamic acid in hemophiliacs undergoing oral surgery. J Oral Maxillofac Surg 1986;44:703-7.
108. Berkstein A. Aminocaproic acid as a local hemostatic agent in epistaxis. Arch Otolaryngol 1971;93:456-7.
109. Ochsner MG, Maniscalco-Theberge ME, Champion HR. Fibrin glue as a hemostatic agent in hepatic and splenic trauma. J Trauma 1990;30:884-7.
110. Israels SJ, Israels ED. Development of antibodies to bovine and human factor V in two children after exposure to topical bovine thrombin. Am J Pediatr Hematol Oncol 1994;16:249-54.
111. Banninger H, Hardegger T, Tobler A, et al. Fibrin glue in surgery: Frequent development of inhibitors of bovine thrombin and human factor V. Br J Haematol 1993;85:528-32.
112. Muntean W, Zenz W, Edlinger G, Beitzke A. Severe bleeding due to factor V inhibitor after repeated operations using fibrin sealant containing bovine thrombin (letter; comment). Thromb Haemost 1997;77:1223.
113. Mitsuhata H, Horiguchi Y, Saitoh J, et al. An anaphylactic reaction to topical fibrin glue. Anesthesiology 1994;81:1074-7.
114. Milde LN. An anaphylactic reaction to fibrin glue. Anesth Analg 1989;69:684-6.
115. Bock M, Muggenthaler KH, Schmidt U, Heim MU. Influence of antibiotics on posttransfusion platelet increment. Transfusion 1996;36:952-4.

116. Doughty HA, Murphy MF, Metcalfe P, et al. Relative importance of immune and non-immune causes of platelet refractoriness. Vox Sang 1994;66:200-5.
117. McFarland JG, Anderson AJ, Slichter SJ. Factors influencing the transfusion response to HLA-selected apheresis donor platelets in patients refractory to random platelet concentrates. Br J Haematol 1989;73:380-6.
118. Alcorta I, Pereira A, Ordinas A. Clinical and laboratory factors associated with platelet transfusion refractoriness: A case-control study. Br J Haematol 1996;93:220-4.
119. Schiffer CA, Lee EJ, Ness PM, Reilly J. Clinical evaluation of platelet concentrates stored for one to five days. Blood 1986;67:1591-4.
120. Sarkodee-Adoo CB, Kendall JM, Sridhara R, et al. The relationship between the duration of platelet storage and the development of transfusion reactions. Transfusion 1998;38:229-35.
121. Guyer DR, Schachat AP, Vitale S, et al. Leukemic retinopathy. Relationship between fundus lesions and hematologic parameters at diagnosis. Ophthalmology 1989;96:860-4.
122. abu el-Asrar AM, al-Momen AK, Kangave D, et al. Correlation of fundus lesions and hematologic findings in leukemic retinopathy. Eur J Ophthalmol 1996;6:167-72.
123. Ho CH. The hemostatic effect of adequate red cell transfusion in patients with anemia and thrombocytopenia (letter). Transfusion 1996;36:290.
124. Escolar G, Garrido M, Mazzara R, et al. Experimental basis for the use of red cell transfusion in the management of anemic-thrombocytopenic patients. Transfusion 1988;28:406-11.
125. Blajchman MA, Bordin JO, Bardossy L, Heddle NM. The contribution of the haematocrit to thrombocytopenic bleeding in experimental animals. Br J Haematol 1994;86:347-50.
126. Konishi H, Ochiya T, Sakamoto H, et al. Effective prevention of thrombocytopenia using adenovirus-mediated transfer of HST-11FGF-4 gene: In vivo and in vitro studies. Leukemia 1997;11 (suppl)3:530-2.

In: Kickler TS, and Herman JH, eds.
Current Issues in Platelet Transfusion Therapy and Platelet Alloimmunity
Bethesda, MD: AABB Press, 1999

7

Antenatal Immune Thrombocytopenia: A Case Study Approach to Current Issues

JAMES B. BUSSEL, MD

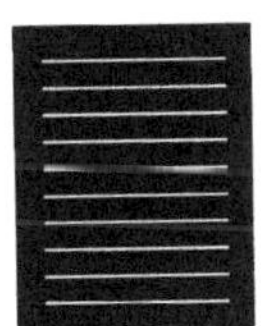

ANTENATAL IMMUNE THROMBOCYTOPENIA (AIT) IS A major cause of morbidity and mortality in the thrombocytopenic fetus and neonate. The basic pathophysiology of AIT has been well understood for more than 30 years, since the seminal work of von Loghem et al[1] and Pearson et al,[2] and there has been considerable recent evolution in the approach to this disease.[3,4] This review briefly summarizes the state of knowledge in AIT and

James B. Bussel, MD, Associate Professor of Pediatrics, Weill Medical College of Cornell University, Department of Pediatrics, Division of Pediatric Hematology/Oncology, New York, New York

(This chapter was partially supported by the ITP Society of the Children's Blood Foundation and by Alpha Therapeutics Inc.)

then uses two cases to highlight current approaches and point out areas in which our understanding is still incomplete.

Overview

AIT results from parental platelet antigen incompatibility and may occur in approximately 1 in 1000 deliveries among Caucasians.[5] The mother lacks a "platelet-specific" antigen that is expressed on paternal platelets. She becomes sensitized to this antigen and develops antibody, which crosses the placenta and mediates the destruction of fetal platelets that express the antigen in question via inheritance from the father. Although the most common antigen causing severe disease is P^{A1} (HPA-1a), up to 14 platelet-specific antigens have been reported to cause AIT (Table 7-1). Some are restricted to certain ethnic groups and others are generally known to result in milder thrombocytopenia than is seen with P^{A1} incompatibility; the last nine antigens in Table 1 are not yet well characterized as to how often they are the cause of AIT. Given such variability, laboratory testing for AIT may be quite complicated.

Fetal thrombocytopenia as a result of P^{A1} incompatibility often occurs early in gestation and often is severe; in 50% of cases, the initial fetal blood sampling (FBS) reveals a platelet count of no more than 20,000/μL.[3] The primary identifier of AIT in a thrombocytopenic newborn is a platelet count of below 30,000-50,000/μL within 24 hours of birth (unpublished observation); other factors include a term infant with unexplained thrombocytopenia, a family history of transient neonatal thrombocytopenia, and an intraparenchymal (instead of intraventricular) intracranial hemorrhage (ICH) in the setting of thrombocytopenia.

Fetal and neonatal thrombocytopenia may result in hemorrhage, including spontaneous ICH in utero as well as in the perinatal period.[3,6] The thrombocytopenia spontaneously resolves in the newborn, usually within 2 weeks, but in rare circumstances, may last as long as 2-3 months. Several treatments are available for the newborn, especially antigen-negative, usually maternal, platelets[7] and/or intravenous immunoglobulin (IVIG).[8] Random-platelet transfusion, exchange transfusion, and steroids can all be used as adjunctive treatments. Exchange transfusion followed by platelet transfusion is a highly effective treatment, but it is relatively difficult to deliver and is therefore not widely used.

Antenatal management of subsequent pregnancies or, at the very least, a careful assessment of the situation, may be required in a woman who has had a previous infant affected by AIT. The subsequent affected sibling is typically more severely affected than the previous affected sibling. Pro-

Table 7-1. Platelet-Specific Antigens

Antigen	Synonym	Glyco-protein Location	Nucleo-tide Substitu-tion	Amino-Acid Substitu-tion	Refer-ence
HPA-1a	Zw^{3}, Pl^{A1}	GPIIIa	T_{196}	Leu_{33}	9
HPA-1b	Zw^{b}, Pl^{A2}		C_{196}	Pro_{33}	
HPA-2a	Ko^{b}	GPIbα	C_{524}	Thr_{145}	10
HPA-2b	Ko^{a}, Sib^{a}		T_{524}	Met_{145}	
HPA-3a	Bak^{a}, Lek^{a}	GPIIb	T_{2622}	Ile_{843}	11
HPA-3b	Bak^{b}		C_{2622}	Ser_{843}	
HPA-4a	Yuk^{b}, Pen^{a}	GPIIIa	G_{526}	Arg_{143}	12
HPA-4b	Yuk^{a}, Pen^{b}		A_{526}	Gln_{143}	
HPA-5a	Br^{b}, Zav^{b}	GPIa	G_{1648}	Glu_{505}	13
HPA-5b	Br^{a}, Zav^{a}, Hc^{a}		A_{1648}	Lys_{505}	
HPA-6bW	Ca^{a}, Tu^{a}	GPIIIa	A_{1564}	Gln_{489}	14
			G_{1564}	Arg_{489}	
HPA-7bW	Mo^{a}	GPIIIa	G_{1317}	Ala_{407}	15
			C_{1317}	Pro_{407}	
HPA-8bW	Sr^{a}	GPIIIa	T_{2004}	Cys_{636}	16
			C_{2004}	Arg_{636}	
HPA-9bW	Max^{a}	GPIIb	A_{2603}	Met_{837}	17
			G_{2603}	Val_{837}	
HPA-10bW	La^{a}	GPIIIa	A_{281}	Gln_{62}	18
			G_{281}	Arg_{62}	
HPA-11bW	Gro^{a}	GPIIIa	A_{1996}	His_{633}	19
			G_{1996}	Arg_{633}	
HPA-12bW	Iy^{a}	$GPIb_{b}$	A_{141}	Glu_{15}	20
			G_{141}	Gly_{15}	
HPA-13bW	Sit^{a}	GPIa	T_{2531}	Met_{799}	21
			C_{2531}	Thr_{799}	

Source: S. Santoso, Giessen, Germany

grams have therefore been instituted to provide treatment to increase the fetal platelet count and avoid fetal and neonatal ICH.[3,9]

How can this and other information be integrated into the management of a typical patient?

Case Study #1

Initial Presentation

Mrs. Smith was a healthy 27-year-old G1P0 woman who had an uneventful pregnancy. At term she went into spontaneous labor and delivered an apparently well 3700-g boy with Apgar scores of 8 and 9. At 4 hours of age, the infant revealed diffuse petechiae and a platelet count of 7000/μL. On physical examination the infant was otherwise normal and in no distress. However, his anterior fontanel was flat and soft, and ultrasound of the head revealed a 1-cm by 1-cm left parietal hemorrhage. Random-donor platelets were infused; the platelet count increased to 38,000/μL but then decreased to 12,000/μL several hours later. IVIG was begun, and arrangements were made to have Mrs. Smith donate platelets. The platelets were spun down once after collection, reconstituted in plasma, and infused. The infant's platelet count increased to 186,000/μL and remained above 80,000/μL. It then became normal 2 weeks after birth and remained so.

This case has many features typical of neonatal AIT, including the following:

1. An otherwise completely well child
2. Severe thrombocytopenia close to the time of birth
3. A normal physical examination other than signs of hemorrhage
4. No obvious explanation for the thrombocytopenia
5. Occurrence in the first child
6. The presence of an intraparenchymal ICH
7. Failure to respond well to random-donor platelets

These points are discussed in full below.

First, there are many causes of neonatal thrombocytopenia. Almost anything that makes a neonate sick can make the infant thrombocytopenic.[6,10] In a child without other medical problems who has a totally unexplained thrombocytopenia, it is appropriate to think of AIT.

Second, studies have shown that AIT is a cause of disproportionately severe thrombocytopenia, which is especially evident close to (ie, within hours of) birth. The single most diagnostic feature of AIT is a platelet count of less than 20,000/μL within hours of birth (unpublished observation).

Testing for AIT has been recommended for all cases of neonatal thrombocytopenia in which the platelet count within 24 hours of birth is below 50,000/μL (unpublished observation).

Third, physical examination for thrombocytopenia could reveal hepatosplenomegaly and/or adenopathy, which might suggest TORCH syndrome or other infection. In addition, congenital hereditary thrombocytopenias, which may also be associated with severe neonatal thrombocytopenia, typically have abnormalities of the radial ray (thrombocytopenia-absent radius); other anomalies are seen with trisomies 13 and 18. Wiskott-Aldrich syndrome would primarily be detected by a review of the blood smear that revealed very small platelets.[11]

Fourth, the normal labor and delivery without fetal or neonatal distress and with good Apgar scores in the absence of any signs of distress in the nursery are very consistent with AIT.

Fifth, unlike hemolytic disease of the newborn, in which the first child is virtually never affected,[12] AIT is identified in the first child of a family in approximately 40-50% of cases.[13]

Sixth, ICH occurs in approximately 10-20% of cases of AIT that have been diagnosed because of signs and symptoms of neonatal thrombocytopenia (unpublished observation). Because an infant's behavior and a soft fontanel are not adequate to exclude ICH, it was very appropriate in the case cited to perform an urgent head sonogram to include or exclude ICH. Management needs to be more aggressive if an ICH is present.

Seventh, because of the platelet antibodies present in the neonate, random-donor platelets are generally unlikely to be effective.[3] While there may be an immediate postinfusion peak in the platelet count,[6] the effects are typically short-lived, as seen in this case, and other therapy (ie, matched platelets or IVIG) is almost always required in addition. Nonetheless, in a case such as this, in which there is an ICH, it is very appropriate to attempt to curtail the hemorrhage by infusing matched, usually maternal platelets while administering IVIG, which has a 24- to 72-hour onset of effect. The random-platelet transfusion has also been thought to confirm the diagnosis of AIT, but a study reported in 1997 has called this into question.[4]

A critical unanswered question is the appropriate way to prepare maternal platelets. The objective is to "concentrate" the platelets as much as possible to minimize the transfusion of maternal P^{A1} antibody with the platelets. The downside to doing this is that extra handling of maternal platelets runs the risk of damaging them. Also, if the platelets are to be concentrated, it is unclear what they should be reconstituted in: plasma, albumin, buffer, saline, or something else. Centers that have been able to collect concentrated platelets have used them without further handling.

While the neonatal thrombocytopenia is being managed, testing for AIT should be performed on the mother and the father but not usually on the neonate.[14] This presumes that the mother has no history of idiopathic thrombocytopenic purpura (ITP) or of unexpected severe thrombocytopenia compatible with ITP. Gestational thrombocytopenia can occur in up to 5% of otherwise normal deliveries, so it should not be assumed that neonatal thrombocytopenia in the infant of a woman with a platelet count of 100,000/μL at delivery is caused by ITP.

Laboratory Testing

Testing revealed that Mrs. Smith was Pl^{A1-} (Pl^{A2}/Pl^{A2}) with strong Pl^{A1} antibodies and that her husband was Pl^{A1+}.

This is a classic test result, confirming the diagnosis of AIT. It is not surprising that the father was Pl^{A1+} since Pl^{A1} is expressed by 97-98% of the population. However, crucial to the laboratory evaluation are the methods. Antibody must be demonstrated to have specificity to Pl^{A1} and not just reactivity to paternal but not maternal platelets. Ideally, this involves the use not only of typed controls but also of antigen capture assays to determine that binding is to platelet glycoprotein IIIa.

Consultations

Mr. and Mrs. Smith were referred to an obstetrician who specialized in high-risk fetomaternal medicine. They wanted to know whether their next child would be affected and, if so, whether there would be another ICH.

The first issue was to determine the father's zygosity. Approximately one in four Pl^{A1+} fathers are heterozygotes. If the father was Pl^{A1}/Pl^{A1} (homozygous), the next infant would always be at least as affected as the previous one.

There were insufficient data to know the recurrence rate of ICH per se. If the ICH was antenatal, the presumed recurrence rate would be very high (100% without as much as intervention); if it was not antenatal, the rate of recurrence would be lower but probably still high. A key step, then, would involve careful review of the cranial ultrasound to ensure that there were no signs of an antenatal ICH.

Testing revealed that the father was heterozygote $P1^{A1/A2}$. This meant that there would be a 50:50 chance that the next infant would be affected. To avoid an FBS, the fetal platelet type can be determined by DNA-based platelet typing on cells obtained by amniocentesis.[15]

Mrs. Smith returned to the fetomaternal medicine specialist for amniocentesis when she was 14 weeks pregnant. The amniocentesis showed that the fetus was Pl^{A1+}*. The ultrasound of the previous sibling was discussed, and Mrs. Smith was assured that there was no reason to suspect that the previous ICH had occurred antenatally.*

Mrs. Smith returned again to ask whether there could have been an error in the typing and, if the typing was correct and the fetus was affected, how affected the fetus would be and what, if anything, could be done.

When performed by an experienced laboratory with the appropriate controls, the typing should not have resulted in any errors. The blood center reported on its first series of testings of more than 200 patients and found perfect concordance between DNA-based typing and serologic typing of both neonatal and fetal platelets. To avoid falsely identifying the fetal platelets as Pl^{A1-} negative by accidentally studying maternal DNA instead of fetal DNA, variable number tandem repeat (VNTR) analysis is used to confirm the source of the specimen studied.[16] The results allowed the fetomaternal specialist to assure Mrs. Smith that her fetus was very likely to be Pl^{A1+} and therefore affected.

The next issue was the extent to which the fetus would be affected. This was difficult to determine with certainty because past records had relatively few families in which two successive infants could be compared as to their relative severity of disease, especially in regard to ICH. In any event, such infants could only have been compared as neonates, since FBS was rarely performed until relatively recently and, when performed, was typically accompanied by intervention. Radiologic evaluation of the neonatal head was not routine either, so the presence or absence of ICH was often uncertain. The only large-scale set of data compared the initial fetal platelet counts of 98 fetuses prior to treatment with the counts recorded in the birth history of the previous siblings.[3] Surprisingly, these data showed no relationship between the initial fetal platelet counts and either the previous siblings' birth platelet counts or the presence or absence of sibling ICH. The only predictor of a lower initial fetal platelet count was an *antenatal* ICH in the previous sibling. On the basis of a comparison of the birth platelet count with the initial fetal platelet count, however, it appeared that the subsequent affected sibling (fetus) would be at least as affected as the previous affected sibling. Also, there is a clear tendency of the fetal platelet count to decrease or remain very low as gestation progresses. Institution of treatment after the initial FBS has prevented further observation of the natural history of the second affected fetus as compared with that of the first.

While reports of antenatal ICH have often involved two siblings in a family (reviewed by Herman et al[6]), it is unclear whether the same is true of

ICH that is not antenatal. Therefore, according to our current stratification, if the ICH that occurred in the previous sibling was not at least suggestive of having occurred prior to birth, this fetus would be stratified as high risk but not very high risk.

Treatment Options

What treatment could be offered?

The initial treatment of fetal AIT was reported by Daffos, Forestier, and Muller in 1984 as a fetal platelet transfusion prior to delivery to allow a vaginal birth.[16] Since then, two primary lines of investigation have been pursued. European work has been more divergent than work in the United States since it has emanated from several centers. In England, IVIG was found to be insufficiently effective in a very high risk group of patients, so the focus became the use of weekly fetal platelet transfusions.[17] In France, initial studies focused on low-dose prednisone (10-20 mg/day)[18] as had been modeled for ITP in pregnancy[19]; efficacy was demonstrated but only in a limited number of cases, and therefore this treatment was largely abandoned as the sole modality. In Germany, a series was performed first with IVIG administered to the mother and then with IVIG administered in utero; both treatments, especially the latter, were relatively ineffective, and one fetus whose mother received IVIG suffered an in-utero ICH.[20]

In the United States, there has primarily been one coordinating center for multicenter protocols; as of April 1998, the third study is ongoing and has 53 patients enrolled. All protocols have used the model of an FBS performed prior to treatment and then repeated 4-6 weeks later to determine the effect of treatment; in addition, all protocols have used the IVIG dose of 1 g/kg per week administered to the mother.

In brief, the first protocol enrolled 18 mother-infant pairs in a pilot study of IVIG treatment administered to the mother at a dose of 1 g/kg per week.[9,21] The initial five patients also received 5 mg and then 3 mg daily of dexamethasone, which was not used further because oligohydramnios developed in 4 of the 5 patients. Subsequent treatment with IVIG alone appeared to be less effective when 5 patients treated with "high-dose" dexamethasone (3-5 mg/day) were compared with 6 patients treated with IVIG alone. Therefore, after piloting 2 patients with 1.5 mg per day of "low-dose" dexamethasone, researchers instituted a second study.

The second study compared IVIG alone (1 g/kg/week) against IVIG at the same dose plus 1.5 mg per day of dexamethasone in a randomized fashion to see if there would be an additive effect of the two treatments.[22] Furthermore, it had a "salvage" arm of IVIG plus 60 mg per day of prednisone at the time of the second FBS for nonresponders who could not be delivered. Criteria for response were twofold because patients with an initial fetal platelet count below 100,000/μL would be treated. Response was defined as either 1) a fetal platelet count of at least 25,000/μL *and* an increase in the fetal platelet count, **or** 2) a fetal platelet count of at least 40,000/μL *and* a decrease in the fetal platelet count of not more than 10,000/μL. The conclusions of this 55-patient second study were as follows:

First, low-dose dexamethasone, at 1.5 mg per day, added nothing to the effect of IVIG alone.

Second, the mean increase of the birth platelet count of the treated siblings compared with either the initial fetal platelet count prior to treatment or to the birth platelet count of the previous sibling was more than 60,000/μL. Individual response, which was assessed by six different criteria, revealed a range of response from 59% to 85%, depending on both the criterion and the timing of the assessment (at the second FBS or at birth).

Third, the salvage arm demonstrated response to the addition of 60 mg of prednisone per day to the IVIG in 5 of 10 cases without the development of oligohydramnios. In 4 of the other 5 cases, there were possible reasons for failure of the salvage arm to be more effective: underdosage of prednisone in 2 cases and weekly fetal sampling in 2 cases may have caused increased sensitization.

Fourth, of special note, none of the 73 fetuses or neonates in the first two studies had an ICH even though more than 16 of their siblings did have an ICH, including a number with definite antenatal ICH.

Fifth, as was reported in 1995, there were increased problems with bleeding at the time of FBS in the setting of severe thrombocytopenia. When this was recognized during the study, it was rectified by transfusion of maternal platelets during sampling.[23]

Overall, these results were very encouraging, and the following ongoing study was developed. The standard risk arm in this study is for families in which the previous sibling did not have an ICH and in which the initial fetal platelet count is above 20,000/μL. This risk arm compares the maximum "tolerable" daily dose of prednisone (0.5 mg/kg) with IVIG to see if prednisone will be sufficiently effective and allow the avoidance of an expensive blood product in the least severely affected cases. Since Mrs. Smith's previous fetus had an ICH, she would not qualify for this arm.

It was further recognized that families in whom the previous affected sibling had had an antenatal ICH were at the highest risk of having another child with hemorrhage and that the infant might respond least well to IVIG alone. Moreover, these families were the group in whom the initial fetal platelet count was known to be very low. Therefore, they were assigned to the very high risk group. They were the only patients in whom IVIG was started at 12-14 weeks prior to initial FBS, which occurred at approximately 20-22 weeks of gestation. Subsequent treatment was adjusted as needed and included the addition of 1 mg/kg of prednisone and, as a second salvage arm, the dose of IVIG doubled to 2 g/kg per week. Mrs. Smith's infant would not be in this arm because, as best as it could be determined from the neonatal ultrasound, the ICH in the previous sibling was not antenatal.

The high-risk arm is for fetuses with a sibling who had an ICH not suspected to be antenatal or whose initial fetal platelet count is not more than 20,000/μL. The treatment randomization compares IVIG alone with IVIG plus 1 mg/kg per day of prednisone. From the salvage arm, the combination of prednisone and IVIG appears to be superior to IVIG alone, but it will be more toxic for the mother. The questions being asked are, how much more effective and how much more toxic?

Followup and Evaluation

Initial fetal sampling of Mrs. Smith's fetus revealed a platelet count of 18,000/μL at 22 weeks' gestation. The family was randomly assigned to IVIG alone and begun on 1 g/kg IVIG infusion once per week, 2 infusions in the first week. At 27 weeks' gestation, the repeat FBS revealed a fetal platelet count of 16,000/μL, and prednisone 65 mg per day (1 mg/kg) was begun. At 32 weeks' gestation, the repeat fetal platelet count was 48,000/μL. Prednisone was tapered down slowly by 10 mg per day each week. At 37 weeks, an elective cesarean section was performed. A 3100-g female infant was delivered with Apgar scores of 8 and 9. The neonatal platelet count was 42,000/μL and no further treatment was required. Cranial ultrasound was normal.

This case illustrates several features of treatment. First, it is impossible to predict exactly what the fetal platelet count will be in a specific fetus. Sampling of 107 cases has revealed that fully 50% of the time the initial fetal platelet count will be less than 20,000/μL, but the level of the fetal platelet count is not correlated with the level of the sibling birth platelet count.[3] Second, before treatment and then again after treatment, FBS is required to monitor treatment. Response to any treatment is not universal, so intensification of treatment as appropriate, depending on the fetal platelet count, is critical to the successful avoidance of ICH. Third, it appears that weekly fetal platelet transfusion as an alternative to medical therapy administered to the mother has a very high risk of fetal mortality over time and should be reserved for cases that are unresponsive to medical treatment.

Discussion

What if the case is not as clear as the one described?

Clinical ambiguity for the initial testing can be created by *alternative neonatal causes of thrombocytopenia*, such as asphyxia, hepatosplenomegaly, and infection. In bona fide cases of AIT, these other entities can make it less clear that the neonatal thrombocytopenia is caused by AIT. Again, severe neonatal thrombocytopenia or ICH should suggest this diagnosis. If it is ever uncertain whether the patient has AIT, testing should be performed because of the important implications of diagnosing AIT for future pregnancies and for female relatives of the mother.

Another ambiguity occurs when the *thrombocytopenia is milder*—that is, the birth platelet count is 70,000/μL. If there is a "reasonable explanation" for the thrombocytopenia, the need to test is less clear. Mild but unexplained thrombocytopenia could be AIT secondary to Pl^{A1} incompatibility. This is important because the "mildness" of the first sibling's AIT does not predict a high fetal platelet count in the subsequent fetus; that count could be 10,000/μL at 20 weeks' gestation.

What if testing in a case of (mild) neonatal thrombocytopenia reveals Br^a (HPA-5b) incompatibility? On the one hand, the only large study of more than 30 patients with Br^a incompatibility demonstrated that, on average, cases of this incompatibility appear to be substantially milder than cases of Pl^{A1} incompatibility.[24] On the other hand, there were two cases of ICH, of which at least one occurred antenatally. Cases reported more recently seem without exception to be mild. Therefore, the optimal approach to making a diagnosis of Br^a incompatibility and then providing treatment remains very unclear.

A third form of ambiguity involves the serologic testing itself. The assumption thus far has been that if the testing was performed, it would confirm or reject the diagnosis of AIT. In fact, the most common ambiguity is not clinical but rather occurs when the testing itself provides ambiguous results. Usually this takes the form of the identification of a platelet antigen incompatibility without any platelet antibody, but may also be the converse: platelet antibody identified without any antigen incompatibility. In the former case, uncertainty may exist as to whether there is antibody because it is undetectable. In the latter case, the antibody can be studied to determine its specificity, which may clarify the diagnosis. However, with the now overwhelming number of platelet antigens that have been identified, this may be quite confusing as well.

Case Study #2

Initial Presentation

A 36-week-old infant that is small for its gestational age is born following maternal fever of 101 C 5 hours prior to delivery, for which the mother received antibiotics. As part of a sepsis workup, the complete blood count revealed a platelet count of 43,000/µL. The thrombocytopenia resolved, and the workup revealed that the mother is Bak^{a-} (Bak$^{b/b}$) and the father is Bak^{a+} although no antibody is seen.

Discussion

Approximately 9% of all pregnancies involve Bak^{a} incompatibility. Therefore, it is not infrequent that a workup will reveal this incompatibility; without identification of Bak^{a} antibody, this is *not* AIT. The judgment should be clinical at this point. If more severe thrombocytopenia is revealed closer to birth, the suspicion of AIT becomes higher. In such a case, additional studies could be pursued, including workup for other antigen incompatibilities, and antibody studies could be repeated 2-4 weeks and/or early in the next pregnancy.

This situation assumes clinical importance in the decision of whether to perform FBS with the next fetus. Cases need to be handled on an individual basis, but a case like the one present here probably does not warrant FBS for the next pregnancy if there is persistently negative antibody included in that pregnancy. For the time being, it appears appropriate in these cases to test for antibody frequently (perhaps monthly) in the next pregnancy to be sure that it does not develop later in the pregnancy,[25] allowing clarification of the diagnosis.

If an antibody is identified without an antigen incompatibility, the same logic applies. The first task is to identify the specificity of the antibody. This often may not be possible, but it includes testing for HLA specificity. Identification does not mean that the antibody is an anti-HLA antibody responsible for the neonatal thrombocytopenia; at least 14 platelet-specific antigen incompatibilities have been reported to cause AIT (Table 7-1). If the clinical suspicion is high, workup of these incompatibilities has to be pursued as much as possible.

A crucial feature is to have the testing performed in the most experienced, competent laboratory possible. As little as possible of the "confusion" in the case should come from uncertainties about the testing.

Summary

In summary, AIT is complicated by a number of issues that make it far less straightforward than Rh disease. All of the following are currently lacking in regard to AIT: 1) routine screening, 2) the ability to prevent the disease if it were identified by administration of a Pl^{A1} antibody, 3) an easy and reliable antibody test available in any blood bank, and 4) well-defined antigen systems that can be easily tested if required. These are all items that contribute to the disease being more of a black box and harder to manage. Clearly, identification of the newborn is feasible, as is maternally administered antenatal treatment to prevent ICH. With new developments in diagnosis and treatment, maternal screening for Pl^{A1} should be able to further reduce morbidity and mortality of the newborn. Simultaneously, better education of clinicians is required so that appropriate patients, both neonates and pregnant women, can be referred for serologic testing.

References

1. Von Loghem JJ, Dormeijer H, van der Hart M, et al. Serological and genetical studies on a platelet antigen (Zw). Vox Sang 1959;4:161-9.
2. Pearson HA, Shulman NR, Marder VJ, Cone TE Jr. Isoimmune neonatal thrombocytopenic purpura: Clinical and therapeutic considerations. Blood 1964;23:154-77.
3. Bussel JB, Zabusky MR, Berkowitz RL, McFarland JG: Fetal alloimmune thrombocytopenia. N Engl J Med 1997;337:22-6.
4. Bussel JB. Immune thrombocytopenia pregnancy: Autoimmune and alloimmune. J Reprod Immunol 1997;37:35-61.
5. Williamson LM, Hackett G, Rennie J, et al. The natural history of fetomaternal alloimmunization to the platelet-specific antigen HPA-1a ($Pl^{A1}Zw^{a}$) as determined by antenatal screening. Blood 1998;92: 2280-7.
6. Herman JH, Jumbelic MI, Ancona RJ, Kickler TS. In utero cerebral hemorrhage in alloimmune thrombocytopenia. Am J Pediatr Hematol Oncol 1986;8:312-17.
7. McIntosh S, O'Brien RT, Schwartz AD, Pearson HA. Neonatal isoimmune purpura: Response to platelet infusions. J Pediatr 1973; 82:1020-7.
8. Mueller-Eckhardt C, Kiefel V, Grubert A, et al. 348 cases of suspected neonatal alloimmune thrombocytopenia. Lancet 1989;1:363-6.

9. Bussel JB, Berkowitz RL, McFarland JG, et al. Antenatal treatment of neonatal alloimmune thrombocytopenia. N Engl J Med 1988;319: 1374-8.
10. Hohlfeld P, Forestier F, Kaplan C, et al. Fetal thrombocytopenia: A retrospective survey of 5,194 fetal blood samplings. Blood 1994;84: 1851-6.
11. Greinacher A, Mueller-Eckhardt C. Hereditary types of thrombocytopenia, an important differential diagnosis of chronic thrombocytopenia. Semin Thromb Hemost 1995;3:191-8.
12. Skupski D, Wolf C, Bussel JB. Fetal and perinatal transfusion therapy. In: Petz LD, Swisher SN, Kleinman S, et al, eds. Clinical practice of transfusion medicine. 3rd ed. New York: Churchill Livingstone, 1995:607-31.
13. Shulman NR, Jordan JV Jr. Platelet immunology. In: Colman RW, Hirsh I, Marder VI, Saltzman FW, eds. Hemostasis and thrombosis: Basic principles and clinical practice. 2nd ed. Philadelphia: J.B. Lippincott, 1987:452-529.
14. Bussel JB, Kaplan C, McFarland JG. The Working Party on Neonatal Immune Thrombocytopenia of the Neonatal Hemostasis Subcommittee of the Scientific and Standardization Committee of the ISTH. Recommendations for the evaluation and treatment of neonatal autoimmune and alloimmune thrombocytopenia. Thromb Hemost 1991;65:631-4.
15. McFarland JG, Aster RH, Bussel JB, et al. Prenatal diagnosis of neonatal alloimmune thrombocytopenia using allele-specific oligonucleotide probes. Blood 1991;78:2276-82.
16. Daffos F, Forestier F, Muller JY, et al. Prenatal treatment of alloimmune-thrombocytopenia (letter). Lancet 1984;2:632.
17. Murphy MF, Waters AH, Doughty HA, et al. Antenatal management of fetomaternal alloimmune thrombocytopenia—report of 15 affected pregnancies. Transfus Med 1994;4:281-92.
18. Daffos F, Forestier F, Kaplan C. Prenatal treatment of fetal alloimmune thrombocytopenia. Lancet 1988;2:910.
19. Karpatkin M, Porges RF, Karpatkin S. Platelet counts in infants of women with autoimmune thrombocytopenia. N Engl J Med 1981; 305:936-9.
20. Kroll H, Kiefel V, Giers G, et al. Maternal intravenous immunoglobulin treatment does not prevent intracranial haemorrhage in fetal alloimmune thrombocytopenia. Transfus Med 1994;4:293-6.
21. Lynch L, Bussel JB, McFarland JG, et al. Antenatal treatment of alloimmune thrombocytopenia. Obstet Gynecol 1992;80:67-71.

22. Bussel JB, Berkowitz RL, Lynch L, et al. Antenatal management of alloimmune thrombocytopenia with intravenous gamma-globulin: A randomized trial of the addition of low-dose steroid to intravenous gammaglobulin. Am J Obstet Gynecol 1996;174:1414-23.
23. Paidas MJ, Berkowitz RL, Lynch L, et al. Alloimmune thrombocytopenia: Fetal and neonatal losses related to cordocentesis. Am J Obstet Gynecol 1995;78:425-9.
24. Kaplan C, Morel-Kopp MC, Kroll H, et al. HPA-5b (Br^a) neonatal alloimmune thrombocytopenia: Clinical and immunological analysis of 39 cases. Br J Haematol 1991;78:425-9.
25. McFarland JG, Frenzke M, Aster RH. Prenatal testing of maternal sera in pregnancies at risk for neonatal alloimmune thrombocytopenia. Transfusion 1989;29:128-33.

In: Kickler TS, and Herman JH, eds.
Current Issues in Platelet Transfusion Therapy and Platelet Alloimmunity
Bethesda, MD: AABB Press, 1999

8

Platelet Transfusion Therapy in Infants and Children

VICTOR S. BLANCHETTE, FRCP; MARGARET L. RAND, PhD; MANUEL D. CARCAO, MD, FRCP(C); AND HEATHER HUME, MD, FRCP(C)

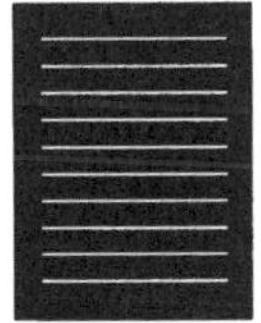

GUIDELINES FOR PLATELET TRANSFUSION THERAPY have been proposed by various groups.[1-3] Although there is adequate evidence for some elements of these proposed guidelines, recommendations for children are often based on expert opinion without the support of adequate laboratory studies or well-designed clinical trials conducted in an appropriate pediatric population.

Victor S. Blanchette, FRCP, Chief, Division of Haematology/Oncology; Margaret L. Rand, PhD, Division of Haematology/Oncology; Manuel D. Carcao, MD, FRCP(C), Division of Haematology/Oncology, The Hospital for Sick Children, Toronto, Ontario, Canada; and Heather Hume, MD, FRCP(C), Service d'Hematologie-Oncologie, Hôpital Sainte-Justine, Montreal, Quebec, Canada

This chapter focuses on platelet transfusion therapy in neonates (infants up to 4 months of age) and older children up to 18 years of age; emphasis is given to areas where pediatric and adult practices differ. The review is divided into 3 parts: guidelines for platelet transfusion therapy in neonates; guidelines for platelet transfusion therapy in older children; and product-related issues, including a review of volume-reduced platelet concentrates and of selected adverse reactions following platelet transfusion.

Guidelines for Platelet Transfusion Therapy in Neonates

The decision to transfuse platelets to a newborn infant should be made only after careful consideration of the risks and benefits of transfusion as well as of the alternatives, if any. Except in life-threatening emergency situations, these considerations should be discussed with the parents or guardians of the infant before the transfusion is given.

Guidelines for platelet transfusion of neonates, such as those guidelines used in the neonatal intensive care unit at the Hospital for Sick Children in Toronto, Canada (Table 8-1), are based on limited data in neonates and are largely extrapolated from experiences in older children and adults. These guidelines are consistent with neonatal transfusion practices in the United States, at least as reported in a survey conducted by the American Association of Blood Banks (AABB) Pediatric Hemotherapy Committee in 1989-1990.[4] In this survey, 71% of neonatal units indicated that it was their policy to transfuse platelets prophylactically to stable, nonbleeding neonates when the platelet counts fell below 20,000/µL, and only rarely (in less than 1% of cases) when counts exceeded 50,000/µL. Faced with a bleeding neonate, 78% of neonatal units would transfuse platelets if the infant's platelet count was less than 50,000/µL, whereas only 0.9% of units would transfuse such infants if the circulating count was greater than 100,000/µL.

Decisions about platelet transfusion therapy in neonates should take into consideration both the etiology and the natural history of thrombocytopenia in this age group. Causes may be congenital or acquired, and thrombocytopenia may reflect decreased platelet production, increased platelet destruction, or a combination of both mechanisms (Table 8-2). The role of platelet transfusion therapy in this diverse group of disorders varies from significant and almost always indicated (eg, in neonatal alloimmune thrombocytopenia) to insignificant and almost never indicated (eg, in neonatal autoimmune thrombocytopenia). The discussion begins with a con-

Table 8-1. Guidelines for Platelet Transfusion Support of Neonates

Platelet Transfusion Thresholds for Bleeding Prophylaxis

- Stable premature neonates with platelet counts < 30,000/mL
- Stable term neonates with platelet counts < 20,000/mL
- Sick premature neonates* with platelet counts < 50,000/mL
- Sick term neonates with platelet counts < 30,000/mL
- Preparation for an invasive procedure (eg, lumbar puncture) or minor surgery in neonates with platelet counts < 50,000/mL, and for major surgery in neonates with platelet counts < 100,000/mL

Platelet Transfusion Threshold in Neonates with Clinically Significant Bleeding

- Neonates with platelet counts < 50,000/mL
- Neonates with conditions that enhance the risk of bleeding (eg, disseminated intravascular coagulation or other significant coagulopathy) and platelet counts < 100,000/mL
- Neonates with documented significant platelet functional disorders (eg, Glanzmann's thrombasthenia) irrespective of the circulating platelet count

*The term *sick premature neonates* includes those infants with a history of perinatal asphyxia, extremely low birthweight (< 1000 g), and the need for ventilatory assistance with an inspired oxygen control greater than 40%; those who are clinically unstable or who show signs of sepsis; and those who require numerous invasive interventions (eg, placement of indwelling catheters).

sideration of the role of prophylactic platelet transfusions in infants, given that this is the most controversial of all the management issues.

Prophylactic Platelet Transfusions in Neonates

Thrombocytopenia is common in low-birthweight infants (ie, infants weighing less than 1500 g at birth), and the issue of prophylactic platelet transfusion arises most often in this subgroup of neonates. In the prospective study reported by Castle et al,[5] 22% of 807 consecutive admissions to a regional neonatal intensive care unit manifested platelet counts of less than

Table 8-2. Causes of Neonatal Thrombocytopenia

Decreased Platelet Production
- Amegakaryocytic thrombocytopenia
  - Thrombocytopenia-absent radius syndrome
  - Amegakaryocytic thrombocytopenia without limb abnormalities
- Wiskott-Aldrich syndrome
- Marrow infiltrative disorders (eg, congenital leukemia, neuroblastoma)
- Osteopetrosis

Increased Platelet Destruction
- Immune-mediated
  - Neonatal alloimmune thrombocytopenia
  - Neonatal autoimmune thrombocytopenia
- Intravascular platelet consumption
  - Disseminated intravascular coagulation
  - Giant hemangioma (Kasabach-Merritt syndrome)
  - Maternal eclampsia/HELLP syndrome
  - Necrotizing enterocolitis

Mixed Origin
- Infection
  - Congenital (eg, TORCH syndrome)
  - Acquired (eg, bacterial sepsis)
  - Erythroblastosis fetalis

Miscellaneous
- Exchange transfusion
- Extracorporeal membrane oxygenation (ECMO)
- Polycythemia
- Chromosome abnormalities (eg, Down syndrome)

150,000/µL during the first week of life. Thrombocytopenia was principally caused by increased platelet destruction, was associated with birth asphyxia and disseminated intravascular coagulation (DIC), and resolved by day 10 of life in 80% of cases. The investigators subsequently reported that the subgroup of infants with platelet counts of less than 100,000/µL were significantly more likely to experience an intraventricular hemorrhage (IVH) than were control infants without thrombocytopenia (78% versus 50%).[6] Of infants with thrombocytopenia, 44% had the most severe forms of hemorrhage (Grade III or IV) as compared with 16% of the control nonthrombocytopenic infants, and there was a higher incidence of serious long-term neurologic sequelae in infants with thrombocytopenia (41% versus 7%). The impact of thrombocytopenia was enhanced by the presence of DIC.

Prompted by these observations, Andrew et al[7] conducted a randomized controlled study of prophylactic platelet transfusions in low-birthweight premature infants. Inclusion criteria for the randomized trial included a birthweight of 500-1500 g, a gestational age of less than 33 weeks, and a platelet count of at least 50,000/µL but not more than 150,000/µL during the first 72 hours of life. Infants randomly assigned to the prophylactic platelet transfusion treatment arm of the study received blood-group-matched platelet concentrates (10 mL/kg) in an attempt to maintain the circulating platelet count at 150,000/µL or above. Infants in the control group did not receive platelet transfusions unless their platelet counts fell below 50,000/µL or they had clinical bleeding. Prophylactic platelet transfusions did not influence the frequency or severity of IVH; however, infants in the control group with platelet counts below 60,000/µL received significantly more Red Blood Cells (RBCs) and Fresh Frozen Plasma than did infants who received prophylactic platelet transfusion support. The investigators concluded that premature infants who have platelet counts above 60,000/µL and who are stable and not bleeding do not require prophylactic platelet transfusions.

Lupton et al[8] reported similar conclusions on the basis of a prospective but nonrandomized study of 302 consecutive premature infants (below 1500 g birthweight) admitted to a regional neonatal intensive care unit. Platelet counts below 100,000/µL were found in 9% of infants, and IVH was documented by ultrasound scanning in 29.8% of infants; in 16.6% of all infants, the severity of IVH was Grade III or IV. There was no statistically significant association between IVH and the presence of thrombocytopenia, and the severity of IVH did not correlate with the severity of thrombocytopenia. The investigators concluded that "treatment of moderate thrombocytopenia (platelet count >50,000/µL) is unlikely to decrease the incidence of IVH in infants of very low birthweight."[8(p1224)]

It is important to emphasize that data for the group of infants at highest risk for IVH—namely, very low birthweight infants with platelet counts of less than 50,000/µL—do not exist. The study by Lupton et al[8] contained too small a number of such infants to establish whether very low platelet counts are causally related to IVH, and premature infants with platelet counts below 50,000/µL were excluded from the randomized trial conducted by Andrew et al.[7]

Accordingly, evidence-based guidelines for platelet transfusion therapy of neonates cannot be provided because adequate data are lacking. Until such data are available, it seems reasonable to recommend that sick, low-birthweight infants receive prophylactic platelet transfusions to maintain a circulating platelet count above 50,000/µL, particularly during the first 72 hours of life when they are at highest risk for IVH. For stable premature and term infants, a platelet threshold of 20-30,000/µL is appropriate. This threshold should be adjusted upwards in the presence of conditions likely to increase the risk of hemorrhage—for example, DIC, necrotizing enterocolitis, and administration of drugs or anticoagulants (eg, heparin) that would tend to increase the risk of bleeding. An adjusted platelet threshold should also be considered for those infants with thrombocytopenia who must undergo an invasive procedure, such as a lumbar puncture, the placement of a central venous line, or surgery. For such infants, a threshold of 50,000/µL is probably reasonable. For major surgical procedures, the circulating platelet count should be maintained near to or above 100,000/µL.

Platelet Transfusion Support for Selected Neonatal Disorders

Sepsis

Thrombocytopenia is common in neonates with systemic infections that may be congenital or acquired and may be caused by bacteria, viruses, or other organisms. In a study of 49 premature infants, Zipursky et al[9] reported thrombocytopenia in seven of 15 infants with proven sepsis, compared with two of 34 infants in whom sepsis was either suspected but not proven or unlikely. All neonates with thrombocytopenia in the sepsis-proven group had platelet counts below 70,000/µL; in 5 of these infants, the platelet counts were below 30,000/µL. The average duration of thrombocytopenia was 6.6 days (range = 3-17 days). Although abnormalities in the coagulation system—in particular, a reduction in the level of Factor XII—are common in neonates with proven sepsis, laboratory evidence of DIC is uncommon. Despite the presence of severe thrombocytopenia in many septic neonates, clinically significant hemorrhage is uncommon. This may reflect the presence of hemostatically active young platelets, a response to the increased platelet destruction that is characteristic of this clinical entity. Platelet transfusion therapy should be reserved for those infants with severe thrombocytopenia or clinically significant bleeding. A shortened survival of infused donor platelets should be anticipated.[10]

Disseminated Intravascular Coagulation

The most frequent cause of severe DIC in newborns is an episode of cardiovascular collapse in the form of either cardiac arrest or profound shock.[10] Affected infants often manifest a hemorrhagic diathesis with a high mortality rate. Laboratory features of the disorder include prolongation of the thrombin time, profound hypofibrinogenemia, and mild or moderate thrombocytopenia. The hemorrhagic diathesis can be corrected with exchange transfusion, and it seldom recurs.

Localized Intravascular Coagulation

Necrotizing enterocolitis. Thrombocytopenia is common in neonates with necrotizing enterocolitis. In a study of 40 ill neonates, Hutter et al[11] reported platelet counts of less than 150,000/µL in 35 infants. Twelve infants had platelet counts of less than 50,000/µL, and in 4 infants, thrombocytopenia-related bleeding was of sufficient severity to have contributed to death. The cause of necrotizing enterocolitis is likely multifactorial and remains incompletely understood. Survival of infused platelets is often short. It is possible that localized intravascular coagulation plays a significant part in the development of thrombocytopenia. In the study reported by Hutter et al,[11] the median time to recovery of a normal platelet count was 7 days (range = 1-31 days). During the period of clinically significant thrombocytopenia, platelet transfusion therapy may be indicated; it should be anticipated, however, that the survival of infused platelets will be short in patients with severe necrotizing enterocolitis.

Kasabach-Merritt syndrome. The association of capillary hemangiomas with a consumptive coagulopathy defines a syndrome first described by Kasabach and Merritt in 1940.[12] In some infants, a microangiopathic hemolytic anemia also occurs. Thrombocytopenia results from platelets being trapped within the hemangioma; the survival of infused platelets is often short. Nonetheless, transfusions are indicated in those neonates with severe thrombocytopenia (platelet counts less than 10,000/µL) and/or clinically significant bleeding while awaiting the spontaneous resolution of the lesion or a response to various therapeutic interventions, including corticosteroids, alpha interferon, antiplatelet drugs, antifibrinolytic agents, or embolization.[13]

Pre-eclampsia and the HELLP syndrome. Infants of mothers with either pre-eclampsia or the HELLP syndrome (hemolysis, elevated liver enzymes, and low platelet count) may develop thrombocytopenia, although the incidence of this complication appears to be substantially lower among these infants than it is among infants of mothers with immune thrombocytopenic purpura (ITP).[14] Little information about the pathogenesis of thrombocytopenia in infants of mothers with pre-eclampsia is available, although platelet activation and increased clearance are thought to play a role.

Immune Thrombocytopenia

Neonatal autoimmune thrombocytopenia. Approximately 40% of infants of mothers with ITP will manifest transient thrombocytopenia secondary to transplacental passage of IgG platelet autoantibodies from mother to fetus. In approximately one-half of thrombocytopenic infants, platelet counts are less than 50,000/μL.[15-18] Because the platelet count in neonates with passively acquired ITP may be normal at birth but may fall in the first few days after delivery,[19] serial platelet counts should be obtained from affected or at-risk infants for a few days after delivery.

The incidence of major hemorrhage—particularly of intracranial hemorrhage—in neonates with passively acquired ITP is low and less than that in infants with alloimmune thrombocytopenia. The incidence is likely similar to that observed in older children with ITP, in whom intracranial hemorrhage occurs in 1% or less of cases and appears to be confined to those with platelet counts of less than 20,000/μL.[20,21] The recovery and survival of random-donor platelets in infants with neonatal ITP is poor, reflecting the broad reactivity of platelet autoantibodies for target platelet antigens. As a result, platelet transfusions should be reserved for affected neonates with extreme thrombocytopenia and overt life-threatening hemorrhage. Therapy for neonates with ITP and clinically significant thrombocytopenia (platelet counts less than 50,000/μL) should initially involve intravenous infusion of high doses of IgG, corticosteroids, or a combination of both therapies. If intravenous IgG (IVIgG) is the treatment selected, administration of 1 g/kg of body weight intravenously for 2 consecutive days is recommended. A successful response, defined as an increase in the circulating platelet count to above 50,000/μL and at least twice the pretreatment value, can be anticipated in at least 75% of neonates.[22] Careful follow-up is recommended since some neonates will experience a recurrence of thrombocytopenia and require retreatment.[23]

An alternative to IVIgG is corticosteroid therapy. If corticosteroids are selected for use, a starting dose of 3-4 mg/kg per day of prednisone (or its equivalent) is recommended, tapering the dose once a platelet response is observed. This higher-than-usual dose of prednisone has proven to be very effective in young children with acute ITP and marked thrombocytopenia.[24-26] Corticosteroids should also be considered for infants who fail to respond to high-dose IVIgG; the combination of high-dose IVIgG and corticosteroids should be reserved for those neonates with severe thrombocytopenia (platelet counts <10,000/µL) and/or clinically significant bleeding. For these infants, a trial of random-donor platelets should also be considered, as improved survival of donor platelets may occur in association with high-dose IVIgG therapy.[27]

Additional therapies include splenectomy and exchange transfusion. Splenectomy is rarely, if ever, indicated in neonates with ITP. Exchange transfusion will remove pathologic platelet autoantibodies, but it is an invasive procedure that is not technically easy in infants with thrombocytopenia unless an umbilical catheter is in place or can easily be put in place.

Neonatal alloimmune thrombocytopenia. Neonatal alloimmune thrombocytopenia is caused by the transplacental passage of maternal IgG platelet alloantibodies into the fetal circulation with subsequent accelerated destruction of fetal platelets. Alloantibodies develop following maternal sensitization to paternally derived antigens present on fetal cells but absent on maternal cells. Immunization generally occurs as a result of the exposure of an antigen-negative mother to antigen-positive fetal platelets during pregnancy or at the time of delivery. In a minority of cases, the trigger for maternal sensitization is an incompatible blood transfusion.

The incidence of neonatal alloimmune thrombocytopenia is approximately 1 per 3000-5000 live births.[28,29] In a Caucasian-based population, more than 80% of serologically confirmed cases reflect fetomaternal incompatibility for the platelet-specific antigen HPA-1a (Pl^{A1}). In a series of 348 infants with suspected neonatal alloimmune thrombocytopenia, Mueller-Eckhardt et al[30] reported the following antibody specificities: anti-Pl^{A1} (94 cases), anti-Pl^{A2} (1 case), anti-Br^{a} (6 cases), anti-HLA (10 cases), anti-A (1 case), anti-B (1 case), and mixed alloantibodies (17 cases). No alloantibodies were found in the remaining 218 infants. The severity of thrombocytopenia was most marked in those infants with neonatal alloimmune thrombocytopenia caused by HPA-1a alloantibodies; 14% of such infants were reported to have had intracranial hemorrhages. ABO and HLA alloantibodies are an infrequent cause of neonatal alloimmune thrombocytopenia.[31]

Laboratory evaluation of infants with suspected neonatal alloimmune thrombocytopenia should include platelet-antigen phenotyping of both biologic parents and the screening of a maternal serum sample for evidence of platelet-specific HLA and ABO alloantibodies. These tests may be available only in reference laboratories and may take some time to complete. It is important to emphasize, however, that a complete serologic evaluation is not essential for immediate management of affected infants. Because fetomaternal incompatibility for the platelet-specific antigen HPA-1a is the most frequent cause of neonatal alloimmune thrombocytopenia, it is useful to arrange for urgent HPA-1a phenotyping of the mother and screening of a maternal serum sample for evidence of HPA-1a alloantibodies. Blood banks or blood centers that service large neonatal units should provide such testing as a routine service, since the test results are clinically useful and may serve as an important guide to platelet support of affected infants.

Postnatal management. Infants with neonatal alloimmune thrombocytopenia are at significant risk for life-threatening—particularly intracranial—hemorrhage. The incidence of this complication has been estimated to be as high as 12%[28]; there is, therefore, an urgency about diagnosis and initiation of appropriate management of this neonatal disorder.[32] The key aspect of management is the provision of compatible antigen-negative platelets, a useful source of which is the mother because she will always be negative for the involved antigen. Maternal platelets can be prepared from a whole blood donation or by apheresis. If a whole blood donation is obtained, it is important that the mother get back her unused RBCs. The advantage of a plateletpheresis concentrate is that this product, which can be stored for up to 5 days, can provide more than one platelet transfusion for an affected infant. Plasma should be removed from maternal platelets by washing or centrifugation to eliminate pathologic platelet alloantibodies before transfusion.[33,34] Failure of a compatible platelet transfusion is extremely rare; however, the presence of hidden maternal autoantibodies may result in the poor survival of apparently compatible donor platelets in an occasional infant.[35]

Before transfusion, maternal platelets must be irradiated (at ≥ 2500 cGy) to prevent graft-vs-host disease (GVHD). An alternative to maternal platelets is a compatible antigen-negative platelet product harvested from a blood donor known to be negative for the pathologic platelet antigen. Because of the high incidence of HPA-1a incompatibility as the cause of neonatal alloimmune thrombocytopenia, blood banks that service large neonatal intensive care units should maintain a registry of HPA-1a-negative donors who are available on short notice to donate platelets for affected infants. An alternate source of compatible donors is an antigen-negative family member. For infants in whom neonatal alloimmune thrombocytopenia can be anticipated because of the history of a previously affected sibling or the finding of platelet-specific alloantibodies in a maternal serum sample before delivery, compatible antigen-negative platelets should be available at the time of delivery. In rare situations in which the mother cannot act as a platelet donor for her infant (eg, when the mother is a chronic carrier for the hepatitis B virus) and where rapid access to an antigen-negative donor is problematic, the collection of compatible antigen-negative platelets that are stored frozen before delivery should be considered.[36]

In approximately 50% of cases of neonatal thrombocytopenia, the condition occurs unexpectedly. In neonates with suspected alloimmune thrombocytopenia and platelet counts of less than 30,000/μL or clinical bleeding, and during the period when serologic tests are being performed and when antigen-negative platelets are being prepared and tested for viral markers such as human immunodeficiency virus and hepatitis B and C, a trial of random-donor platelets is recommended (Fig 8-1). Failure to obtain a clinically significant platelet increment in a sample of blood obtained 10-60 minutes following the infusion of random-donor platelets is suggestive of neonatal alloimmune thrombocytopenia due to HPA-1a incompatibility; this is because 98% of random-donor platelets are HPA-1a positive and thus incompatible in this clinical situation. It should be recognized, however, that a response to a random-donor platelet concentrate occasionally occurs in infants with alloimmune thrombocyto- penia, reflecting low levels of pathological alloantibodies in the blood of the affected infant or the chance selection of antigen-negative, random-donor platelets.[37] This latter explanation is more likely in cases of alloimmunization caused by relatively low-incidence alloantigens such as HPA-5b.

In marked contrast to the recommended treatment of neonatal autoimmune thrombocytopenia, IVIgG and corticosteroids are, at best, adjunctive therapies in infants with neonatal alloimmune thrombocytopenia. Although responses to IVIgG have been reported, neonates with alloimmune thrombocytopenia and very low platelet counts generally respond poorly, or not at all, to high-dose IVIgG. In such infants, the provision of compatible antigen-negative platelets should not be delayed while awaiting the unpredictable response to high-dose IVIgG. Even in a life-threatening situation, IVIgG therapy should be considered adjunctive and may, for example, be started in infants with severe thrombocytopenia or clinical bleeding while random-donor platelets are being transfused and arrangements are being made to harvest platelets from an antigen-negative compatible donor.

The case for corticosteroid therapy in neonatal alloimmune thrombocytopenia is even weaker. There is, at this time, no convincing evidence to support the use of this therapy for infants with neonatal alloimmune thrombocytopenia. Exchange transfusion may remove pathological maternal alloantibodies, but it is an involved procedure that is generally not con-

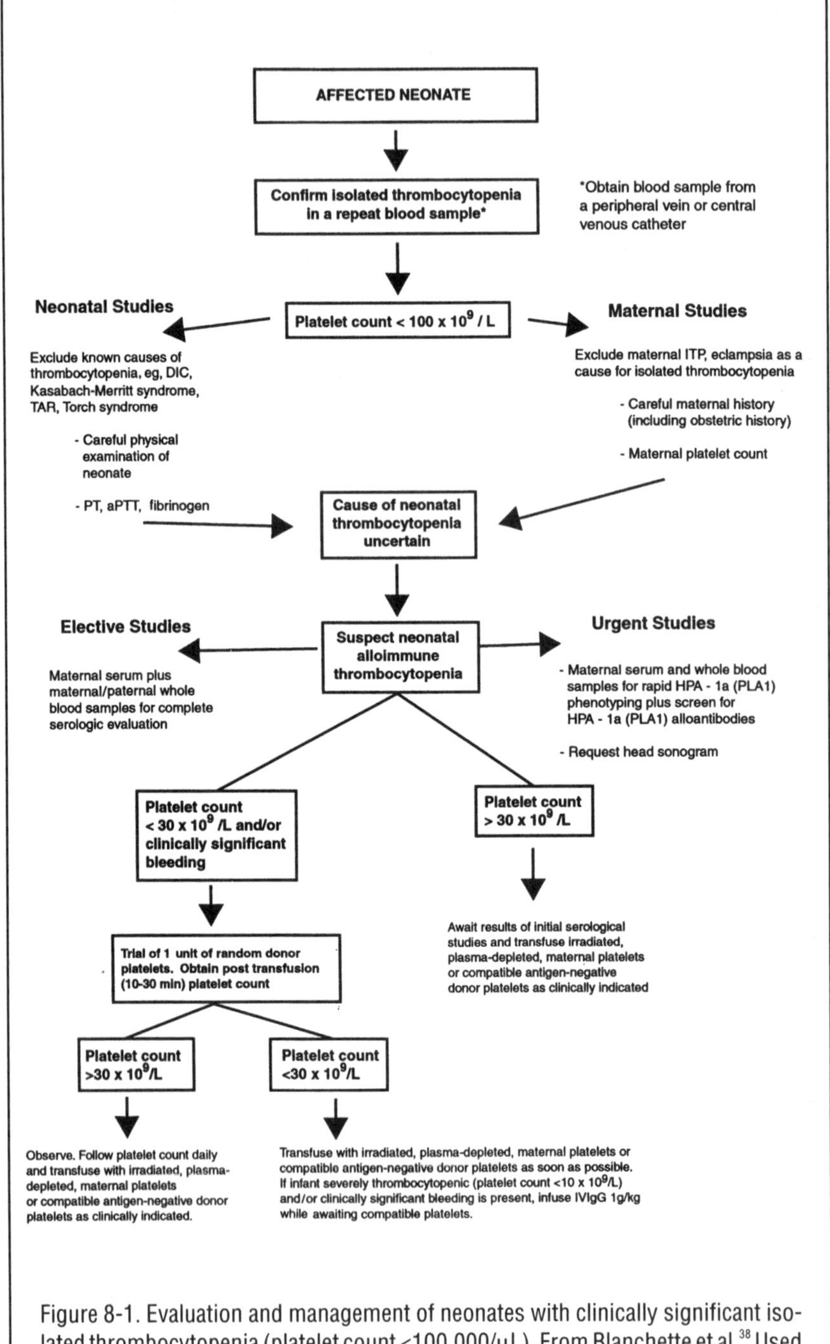

Figure 8-1. Evaluation and management of neonates with clinically significant isolated thrombocytopenia (platelet count <100,000/μL). From Blanchette et al.[38] Used with permission.

sidered except when dealing with an affected infant with severe thrombocytopenia and evidence of clinical bleeding and for whom compatible antigen-negative platelets cannot be obtained.

Antenatal management. Antenatal management of women alloimmunized to the HPA-1a antigen is a challenge because of the real risk of intracranial hemorrhage in the fetus before delivery.[32,39] Management options include elective early cesarean section, weekly intrauterine platelet transfusions, and IVIgG administered to the mother. Early cesarean section alone will not prevent antenatal hemorrhage because there are limits to how early this procedure can safely be performed, and in-utero hemorrhage has been reported prior to 34-36 weeks of gestation.[40] Weekly in-utero platelet transfusions appear to be too invasive and probably should be reserved for cases in which medical therapy for the mother has failed.[32] Antigen-negative compatible platelets should, however, be administered to the fetus 1) whenever cordocentesis is performed to determine the fetal platelet count, and 2) immediately before the elective delivery of any fetus with suspected thrombocytopenia. The therapeutic approach that is generally recommended for an alloimmunized mother is IVIgG at a dose of 1g/kg body weight per week, with or without concomitant corticosteroids.[32]

For intrauterine transfusion, platelets from group O Rh-negative donors are recommended.[41] Since the ABO group of the fetus is usually unknown, some experts suggest using only donors with low titers of anti-A and anti-B; however, there is no consensus on the need for this precaution.[42] The volume of platelets for an intrauterine transfusion must take into consideration the placental volume as well as the estimated fetal weight. Waters et al[43] have suggested the following formula to determine the volume of the platelet concentrate for intrauterine transfusion:

$$\frac{\text{Volume} = 2 \times \text{desired increment} \times \text{fetoplacental blood volume}}{\text{Platelet count of concentrate}}$$

The usual goal is to obtain a posttransfusion platelet count of 300-500,000/µL. Estimated blood volumes according to gestational age have been published[44]: at 18 weeks of gestation, the fetoplacental blood volume is approximately 117 mL/kg, and this falls gradually to 93 mL/kg at 31 weeks of gestation.

Extracorporeal Membrane Oxygenation

Extracorporeal membrane oxygenation (ECMO) is a technique for the short-term treatment of severe respiratory and cardiorespiratory failure. ECMO provides oxygenated blood to patients and thus functions as the "lung" for the patient. When a venoarterial circuit is used rather than a venovenous circuit, blood is artificially pumped through the body, and ECMO functions as the "heart" for the patient. ECMO is especially useful in selected neonates with reversible respiratory failure and in infants with cardiac failure following the repair of congenital heart defects. Behind success in all applications of ECMO is the belief that the underlying disease process is reversible; the patient can recover to normal cardiopulmonary function if supported for a limited period.

Bleeding during ECMO can be substantial, and significant bleeding (ie, that which requires multiple transfusions) occurs in up to one-third of all cases.[45] Postoperative patients, especially those who have undergone cardiac surgery, are at high risk for excessive bleeding. The cause of bleeding is multifactorial and includes both quantitative and qualitative platelet abnormalities, depletion of coagulation factors, and activation of the fibrinolytic pathways. In a review of blood component support for patients placed on ECMO, Meliones and Hanscolls[45] quoted a 13% risk of intracranial hemorrhage in patients placed on ECMO and recommended that prophylactic platelet transfusions be given to maintain a platelet count of at least 100,000/µL. This recommendation, although clinically reasonable, is not yet supported by results of a controlled study. Platelet products used during ECMO should be as fresh as possible, ABO matched, and irradiated.

Guidelines for Platelet Transfusion in Older Children

Decreased Platelet Production

Decreased platelet production occurs in children with congenital or acquired aplastic anemia or with marrow infiltration with leukemic or other malignant cells, and/or following myeloablative chemotherapy. The majority of studies addressing the indications for platelet transfusions for patients with decreased platelet production have been performed in patients with acute leukemia. It is reasonable, however, to use results of these studies to guide platelet transfusion therapy for the majority of patients with hypoproliferative thrombocytopenia.

Before platelets were available for transfusion, hemorrhage in patients with leukemia and severe thrombocytopenia was often fatal. In a report from the National Cancer Institute,[46] hemorrhage was considered to have been the major cause of death in 52% of 414 patients with acute leukemia studied from 1954 to 1963. With the introduction of plastic blood collection systems in the late 1960s, platelets became available for the treatment of patients with thrombocytopenic bleeding. By the 1980s, deaths due to hemorrhage gradually decreased to the point where only 3% of adults with acute nonlymphoblastic leukemia (ANLL) had lethal hemorrhagic complications.[47]

In the 1970s and 1980s, several studies addressed the issue of prophylactic vs therapeutic platelet transfusions for thrombocytopenic patients with acute leukemia.[48-54] These studies demonstrated that platelets given prophylactically do decrease the incidence of significant bleeding episodes in patients with leukemia; however, they did not demonstrate a longer survival in patients transfused prophylactically compared with those transfused only in the presence of active bleeding. Despite this, several experts began to recommend the use of prophylactic platelet transfusions.[55-58] The debate over prophylactic vs therapeutic platelet transfusion therapy continues to be active.[59,60] In a survey conducted in 1993 by the AABB, approximately 70% of 126 member institutions responding to the survey and treating pediatric hematology/oncology patients reported that the major use of platelets was for prophylaxis, whereas 20% transfused platelets primarily therapeutically and 10% followed a policy combining both approaches.[61]

For those physicians and institutions who choose to use prophylactic platelet transfusions, the current debate centers around the choice of platelet count at which to routinely administer platelet concentrates. In the reviews cited, published in the late 1970s and early 1980s and advocating the use of prophylactic platelet transfusions for leukemic patients, it was often suggested that the platelet count be maintained above 20,000/µL. This figure appears to have been derived from a much-quoted study by Gaydos et al[62] published in 1962, in which the authors tried to determine if there was a threshold platelet level above which bleeding rarely occurred and below which it commonly occurred. They conducted a retrospective review of 92 patients (40 of whom were 21 years or older and 52 of whom were under 21) with acute leukemia and determined the percentage of days with bleeding manifestations at various platelet levels. Gross hemorrhage was documented for less than 1% of days at all platelet levels above 20,000/µL, for 4% of days in which platelet counts were 10-20,000/µL, for 6% of days in which platelet counts were 5-10,000/µL, and for 31% of days in which platelet counts were less than 1000/µL. Sixteen of the 92 patients suffered fatal intracranial hemorrhages: 8 were in "blastic crisis" (not further defined by the authors) and had a median platelet count of 10,000/µL; and the remaining 8 were not in blastic crisis (7 had a platelet count below 5000/µL, and one had a platelet count of 5-10,000/µL). It should also be recognized that when this study was performed, the platelet inhibitory effects of aspirin were not appreciated, and some patients may have been receiving aspirin for control of fever. Although the authors concluded that no clear "threshold" platelet count could be identified, this study has nonetheless been often cited in support of the choice of a platelet threshold of 20,000/µL for prophylactic transfusion.

Recently, the necessity of maintaining a minimum platelet count of 20,000/µL in all patients with malignancies has been questioned. At a Consensus Development Conference sponsored by the National Institutes of Health in 1986 and addressing platelet transfusion therapy, the panel concluded that patients with severe thrombocytopenia may benefit from prophylactic transfusion but that the commonly used threshold value of 20,000/µL may sometimes be safely lowered.[1] Even more conservative recommendations have been published since then. In a review published in 1991, Slichter[63] recommended that only patients with platelet counts of less than 5000/µL should routinely be given prophylactic platelet transfusions, and for those with platelet counts above 5000/µL, clinical judgment should be used to assess the need for platelet therapy. Beutler[64] likewise suggested abandoning the practice of routinely transfusing patients whenever the platelet count drops below 20,000/µL; he, too, suggested that if any threshold is to be chosen for prophylactic transfusions in a stable patient, it should be 5000/µL, with transfusions at higher platelet counts being reserved for patients in whom additional risk factors exist. Finally, the members of the panel of a consensus conference on platelet transfusion conducted by the Royal College of Physicians of Edinburgh in November 1997 concluded that a platelet threshold of 10,000/µL is as safe as higher levels for treating most patients without additional risk factors.[65,66]

The rationale for these more conservative recommendations is based on results of older studies as well as on more recent ones addressing the safety of lowering threshold levels for prophylactic platelet transfusions. Among the studies cited addressing the issue of prophylactic versus therapeutic platelet transfusions, one was a retrospective review of 70 children with acute lymphoblastic leukemia (ALL) studied during induction and first remission.[52] Platelets were given only for significant bleeding associated with a platelet count below 20,000/µL. In this study there were no deaths due to hemorrhage, and 84% of patients achieved complete remission without a single platelet transfusion despite the fact that 49% had platelet counts below 20,000/µL at some time during the induction phase. Unfortunately, the actual platelet nadirs were not specified. This is the only study (to these authors' knowledge) that specifically addresses the issue in pediatric patients, although most of the studies that are discussed in this chapter included adolescent patients.

Over the last 13 years, 6 groups of investigators have reported the results of the use of relatively stringent indications for prophylactic platelet transfusions.[67-72] In a retrospective study published in 1986, the safety of using prophylactic platelet transfusion only for platelet counts below 10,000/µL in patients with ALL and ANLL was evaluated by analyzing all episodes of thrombocytopenia in which platelet counts were less than 20,000/µL.[67] In all, 117 episodes of thrombocytopenia were studied. There were 67 episodes of bleeding, of which 85% were minor and 15% were major (severe hematuria, hematemesis, melena). There were no intracranial hemorrhages, and there was only one death due to hemorrhage in a patient with a platelet count of less than 5000/µL. All the severe bleeding episodes occurred in patients with decreasing platelet counts and concomitant fever. At platelet counts of 10-20,000/µL vs platelet counts of less than 10,000/µL, patients with ALL had more bleeding episodes than patients with ANLL. In both groups, there were more episodes of bleeding with platelet counts of 10-20,000/µL in leukemia-related thrombocytopenia than in chemotherapy-related thrombocytopenia. Patients less than 18 years old also had a significantly greater number of bleeding episodes than adults, this was observed both with ALL and ANLL at platelet counts below 10,000/µL and with ANLL (but not ALL) at platelet counts of 10-20,000/µL. No further details or possible explanations for these observations concerning age were discussed by the authors.

In a prospective study published in 1991 involving 104 patients (mean age of 42 years with a range of 15-71 years) with newly diagnosed acute leukemia, investigators reported results for the routine use of prophylactic platelet transfusions at a threshold platelet count of 5000/µL or less. In the presence of fresh minor hemorrhagic manifestations or fever, prophylactic platelet transfusions were administered at platelet counts of 6-10,000/µL and in the presence of coagulation disorders and/or heparin therapy at platelet counts of 11-20,000/µL. In accordance with this prospective protocol, a platelet transfusion was withheld on 69% of days when a morning platelet count was 6-20,000/µL. Thirty-one major bleeding episodes occurred in the 104 patients, 3 patients died of complications related to bleeding (one thrombocytopenic patient with platelet refractoriness, one nonthrombocytopenic patient with DIC and heparin therapy, and one thrombocytopenic patient with acute promyelocytic leukemia and an unrecognized spinal cord hematoma). These authors made no mention of an influence of age on the frequency or severity of bleeding episodes.

Table 8-3. Studies Comparing Standard vs Restrictive Protocols for Administering Prophylactic Platelet Transfusions

Investigator	Study Design	Patients	Transfusion Protocol		Major Bleeding Episodes		Total Number of PTs or RDPCs Administered	
			Standard Group	Restrictive Group	Standard Group	Restrictive Group	Standard Group	Restrictive Group
Gil-Fernandez[69] (1996)	Single institution, retrospective, nonrandomized	Patients aged 13 to 59 years undergoing marrow transplantation	N = 87 PC <20,000/μL Patients treated in 1990-91; (41 auto, 46 allo)	N = 103 PC <10,000/μL or <20,000/μL and factors associated with increased consumption; patients treated in 1993-94 (50 auto, 53 allo)	14 episodes/ 12 patients*; 4 deaths due to hemorrhage: PC >20,000/μL in 3/4 at start of bleeding, 2/4 had platelet refractoriness	13 episodes 12 patients*; 3 deaths due to hemorrhage: PC >10,000/μL in all 3 at start of bleeding; 1/3 had platelet refractoriness	Median (range): RDPC: 73 (3-943) (1 RDPC/10 kg, no maximum number RDPC per PT)	Median (range): RDPC: 54 (0-647) (1 RDPC/ 10 kg, maximum of 6 RDPC per PT)
Heckman[70] (1997)	Single institution, prospective, randomized	Patients aged 19 to 32 years with de novo or relapsed ALL or ANLL; excluded if ANLL-M3, DIC, or fulminant sepsis during induction chemotherapy	N = 41 PC ≤20,000/μL	N = 37 PC ≤10,000/μL	Reported total bleeding episodes (ie, did not separate minor vs major): median (25th, 75th percentile) 2 (1,5)*	4 (2,7)*	Mean (range): PT: 11(6-5)	Mean (range): PT: 7 (5-11)

Table 8-3. Studies Comparing Standard vs Restrictive Protocols for Administering Prophylactic Platelet Transfusions (Continued)

			Transfusion Protocol		Major Bleeding Episodes		Total Number of PTs or RDPCs Administered	
Investigator	Study Design	Patients	Standard Group	Restrictive Group	Standard Group	Restrictive Group	Standard Group	Restrictive Group
Rebulla[71] (1997)	Multicenter, prospective, randomized	Patients aged 16 to 70 years with de novo ANLL (excluding ANLL-M3) during induction chemotherapy	N = 120 PC <20,000/μL	N = 135 PC <10,000/μL or 10-20,000/μL and fever, or invasive procedure, or any bleeding (minor or major)	33 episodes/ 24 patients*; no deaths due to bleeding	39 episodes/ 29 patients*; one death due to hemorrhage: an intracerebral hemorrhage in a patient with a PC of 32,000/μL at start of bleeding	Mean (range): PT: 6 (1-22)	Mean (range): PT: 8 (2-27)
Wandt[72] (1998)	Multicenter, prospective, nonrandomized	Patients aged 17 to 73 years with de novo ANLL (excluding ANLL-M3)	N = 58 Protocol in 9 centers; PC <20,000/μL	N = 47 Protocol in 8 centers; PC <10,000/μL or <15,000/μL with fever, DIC, or white blood count >50,000/uL	7 episodes/ 7 patients; 2/7 died; PC at start of bleeding 36 and 50,000/μL; deaths not due to bleeding	No major bleeding episodes*	Mean (range): Apheresis units: 4.8 (0-33) RDPC: 25.4 (0–188)	Mean (range): Apheresis units: 3.0 (0-16) RDPC: 15.4 (0–152)

ANLL = Acute nonlymphoblastic leukemia; ALL = acute lymphoblastic leukemia; DIC = disseminated intravascular coagulation
PC = platelet count; PT = platelet transfusions; RDPC = randon-donor platelet concentrates
*No statistically significant differences between the two groups.
Only one study (Rebulla et al[71]) reported pretransfusion platelet levels: 14,000 and 9000/μL for the standard and restrictive groups, respectively.
In none of the studies were there any statistically significant differences between the two groups of patients with respect to attainment of complete remission or mortality.

Between 1996 and 1998, 4 studies (one retrospective, 3 prospective) were published comparing the standard practice of administering a prophylactic platelet transfusion at a platelet count of 20,000/µL against a more stringent or restrictive policy.[69-72] These studies are summarized in Table 8-3. Each study used somewhat different criteria for prophylactic platelet transfusions in the group for whom a more restrictive policy was used, and it is not possible to clearly determine from these reports the extent to which the 2 groups in each study were in fact different (ie, how many and how often patients in the restrictive groups were considered to have "additional risk factors for bleeding" and therefore received transfusions at platelet levels of 10-20,000/µL). This is particularly true for the 2 nonrandomized studies. In addition, pretransfusion platelet counts were reported only in one of the studies. Nevertheless, in the four studies the investigators concluded that the use of more restrictive prophylactic platelet transfusion criteria resulted in a decrease in the number of platelet transfusions administered without any decrease in the complete remission rate or any increase in serious morbidity or mortality.

While more stringent prophylactic platelet transfusion policies may be appropriate for many patients, two groups of leukemic patients appear to be at particularly high risk of fatal hemorrhage during induction chemotherapy—namely, those with hyperleukocytosis and/or acute promyelocytic leukemia (ANLL, FAB M3). The German BFM study group reported the causes of early death in 294 children with ANLL.[73] Thirty (10%) died prior to or in the first 12 days of therapy, and of these deaths, 12 were due to hemorrhage alone. Eight patients had hyperleukocytosis (ie, leukocyte counts >100,000/µL); 2 had platelet counts of 50-100,000/µL, and only 2 had platelet counts of less than 20,000/µL. These 8 patients had platelet counts of 20-50,000/µL. The authors noted that several of the hemorrhagic deaths occurred during the period of rapid blast reduction. In patients with acute promyelocytic leukemia, rates of early fatal hemorrhage of 9-26% have been reported.[66,74] This bleeding tendency is associated with the presence of DIC and fibrinolysis, thought to be related to the release of procoagulant substances from the promyelocytic granules.

The incidence of hemorrhage in patients with solid tumors and thrombocytopenia has been addressed in at least 2 reports, although neither specifically studied pediatric patients.[75,76] These studies have revealed that the risk factors for hemorrhage in patients with solid tumors are similar to those in leukemic patients, although an additional consideration is the predisposition to hemorrhage associated with local tumor invasion.

In summary, given currently available data, the use of either therapeutic or prophylactic platelet transfusions for children with thrombocytopenia due to malignant disease and/or chemotherapy can be justified. However, the exclusive use of therapeutic transfusions should be considered only in settings where frequent evaluations by an experienced team of physicians can be carried out and where platelet concentrates, if necessary, can be quickly obtained and administered. Alternatively, for physicians at institutions electing to transfuse platelets prophylactically, consideration should be given to using a threshold platelet count at which platelets are routinely administered and to setting that threshold below 20,000/µL. Just as the indication for a red cell transfusion should not be determined solely on the basis of a hemoglobin level, the decision to administer a platelet transfusion should also be individualized, taking into account the clinical situation as well as the platelet count.

Prophylactic platelet transfusions are indicated for thrombocytopenic patients undergoing invasive procedures. At least one study suggests that major surgical procedures can be safely performed in leukemic patients at platelet counts of 50,000/µL or greater.[77] However, there are virtually no published studies addressing the issue of hemostatic platelet counts for 2 of the most common invasive procedures that patients with hematologic or other malignancies undergo—namely, lumbar puncture and the insertion of permanent, indwelling central venous catheters. The previously mentioned AABB survey showed that 62.6% of respondents required a count of 50,000/µL to perform such procedures. Marrow aspiration and biopsy can be safely performed (with respect to local bleeding) at any platelet level.

Studies addressing the indications for prophylactic platelet transfusions similar to those described for patients with acute leukemia or undergoing marrow transplantation have not been performed in children with congenital marrow failure syndromes (likely because of the small number of patients available for study). For the most part, however, it would seem reasonable to approach these children in the same way as children with thrombocytopenia due to malignant disease and/or chemotherapy. Yet it may also be appropriate to use a slightly lower threshold for prophylactic platelet transfusion (eg, 5000/µL) in children with congenital marrow failure syndromes if they are clinically stable with no bleeding manifestations; this is so particularly because their thrombocytopenia is chronic (therefore requiring prolonged treatment), a factor that may place these patients at increased risk of developing platelet alloimmunization and refractoriness.

Suggested guidelines for prophylactic platelet transfusions in pediatric patients with thrombocytopenia due to decreased platelet production are summarized in Table 8-4.

Table 8-4. Suggested Guidelines for Prophylactic Platelet Transfusions in Pediatric Patients with Thrombocytopenia Due to Decreased Platelet Production

- Platelet count £ 10,000/mL*
- Platelet count < 20,000/mL and disseminated intravascular coagulation, severe mucositis, anticoagulation therapy, extreme hyperleukocytosis, a platelet count likely to fall below 10,000/mL prior to next possible evaluation, or risk of bleeding due to local tumor invasion
- Platelet count < 50,000/mL during induction therapy for promyelocytic leukemia
- Platelet count < 50,000/mL and minor invasive procedure (eg, bronchoscopy, central line placement, biopsy, spinal tap)
- Platelet count < 50-100,000/mL and major surgical intervention (threshold level to depend on the nature of the procedure and the presence or absence of additional risk factors for bleeding)

*Some physicians may use a lower platelet count (eg, 5000/mL) in stable patients with congenital marrow failure syndromes.

Platelet Transfusion Support for Selected Disorders

The indications for platelet transfusions in children with thrombocytopenia due to factors other than decreased platelet production have not been well-studied. Guidelines are primarily based on studies performed in adult patients and/or on expert opinion.

Increased Platelet Destruction

Patients with thrombocytopenia due to ITP should be treated with platelet transfusions only in the presence of central nervous system or other life-threatening bleeding.[78] Prior to surgical procedures (eg, splenectomy), the platelet count can usually be raised to levels sufficient to ensure adequate hemostasis through the use of corticosteroids or IVIgG. A variety of conditions other than ITP (eg, septicemia, trauma, obstetric complications) may result in platelet consumption that is sufficiently severe to require platelet transfusion. In these conditions, the platelet increment and survival are usually decreased, and a larger number of units, administered at more frequent intervals, may be necessary.

Massive Transfusion

Thrombocytopenia is often associated with massive transfusion. Depending on the underlying cause(s) of bleeding, the thrombocytopenia may be dilutional owing to platelet loss through hemorrhage and/or to platelet consumption. Platelet transfusion therapy should be based on a consideration of several factors, including the platelet count, an assessment of the role of thrombocytopenia as a cause of bleeding, and the estimated platelet count necessary for hemostasis given the patient's clinical situation.

Platelet Dysfunction

Platelet dysfunction possibly requiring platelet transfusion is most commonly encountered in patients in two situations: when taking platelet inhibitory drugs and following cardiopulmonary bypass. Platelet dysfunction due to platelet inhibitory drugs is unlikely to contribute to bleeding if the platelet count is above 50,000/µL. Treatment with desmopressin acetate has been shown to prevent bleeding complications in patients who have taken aspirin within 7 days of a surgical intervention.[79,80]

Platelet dysfunction lasting 4-6 hours after cardiopulmonary bypass has been well documented.[81,82]These patients are also usually thrombocytopenic. Nevertheless, studies have not shown a benefit for the use of prophylactic platelet transfusions for patients undergoing cardiopulmonary bypass.[83] Platelet transfusions should be reserved for those patients who, following cardiopulmonary bypass, have excessive bleeding thought to be due to platelet function abnormalities and/or thrombocytopenia.[1,84]

Congenital Platelet Function Disorders

Congenital abnormalities of platelet function form a heterogenous group of disorders, some of which are associated with mild to moderate thrombocytopenia. Abnormalities may be quantitative or qualitative, and the severity of bleeding is variable. Affected patients should be instructed to avoid the use of aspirin and other platelet-inhibiting drugs. Platelet transfusions may be indicated for the prevention or treatment of bleeding in these patients. The decision to recommend platelet transfusions prophylactically should involve consideration of the severity of the congenital defect; a careful review of the child's personal bleeding history and that of similarly affected family members; the severity of the hemostatic challenge; and the potential role of alternate therapies, especially desmopressin acetate and/or antifibrinolytic agents (tranexamic acid and epsilon aminocaproic acid). Topical therapy (eg, fibrin sealants) should be considered for the prevention and/or treatment of bleeding from the oral cavity such as may occur following dental extractions.[85]

Repeated platelet transfusion in patients with Glanzmann's thrombasthenia and Bernard-Soulier syndrome may lead to the development of alloantibodies against glycoproteins (IIb/IIIa and Ib/IX) and to a state of nonresponsiveness to random-donor platelets. To lessen the risk of this relatively rare but clinically significant complication, these patients, wherever possible, should receive blood group and HLA-compatible single-donor platelets that are leukocyte-reduced. A conservative or stringent platelet transfusion protocol is also recommended.

Platelet Products

Volume-Reduced Platelet Concentrates

Standard or apheresis platelet concentrates from which the majority of plasma has been removed following centrifugation are referred to as volume-reduced platelet concentrates. This practice is prevalent in blood banks that serve neonatal intensive care units. In the aforementioned survey of neonatal transfusion practices that was conducted by the AABB Pediatric Hemotherapy Committee in 1989-1990, 46% of 407 responding US hospitals indicated that they routinely centrifuged platelet concentrates to reduce their volume before transfusion to neonates.[4] The comparable statistic for Canadian hospitals, based on an identical survey, was 48%.[86]

Although the removal of plasma from platelet concentrates is an acceptable practice in selected clinical situations (ie, when preparing antigen-negative maternal platelets for transfusion to newborns with neonatal alloimmune thrombocytopenia), the decision to request a volume-reduced platelet product is often based on a practical consideration: the fact that the transfusion of such a product can be completed more quickly than that of a standard platelet product. However, this does not take into account the significant amount of time (minimum of 2 hours) required to prepare a volume-reduced platelet product.[34] Accordingly, it should be recognized that the platelet product generally available for immediate transfusion to a thrombocytopenic patient who is actively bleeding or at high risk for significant hemorrhage is an unmodified platelet concentrate or pool of such concentrates.

In addition, transfusion medicine specialists are reasonably concerned that the extra manipulation (ie, centrifugation and resuspension) involved in preparing a volume-reduced platelet product might be expected to have a detrimental effect on platelet quality. To study this question, the effect of volume reduction (centrifugation at 2000 × *g* for 6 minutes followed by plasma removal) of standard platelet concentrates that have been stored for 2-5 days was examined.[87] In-vitro platelet recovery after the volume reduction step was 88.8% ± 2.2 (mean ± SEM); it did not differ among platelet concentrates stored for different times. The loss of platelets was not due to lysis during centrifugation, as the release of lactate dehydrogenase was only 0.1% ± 0.1 (basal level = 4.2% ± 0.3 in the plasma of the pooled standard platelet concentrates). The pH of the concentrates before volume reduction was 7.1 ± 1.7 (ie, within the range considered to be associated with platelet effectiveness upon transfusion),[88-90] and it was not altered by manipulation. Platelets recovered from the hypotonic stress of added water[91] to the same extent both before and after volume reduction (67.9% ± 1.7 vs 65.2% ± 2.3, respectively). Aggregation and secretion of [^{14}C]serotonin from prelabeled platelets stimulated with 10 µM adenosine diphosphate, 1.5 µg/mL collagen, 1 µM A23187, or pairs of these agonists were determined; responses tended to decrease with increasing time of storage but were not affected by volume reduction.

These findings are in keeping with those of Moroff et al[92] who reported that in-vitro platelet recovery after volume reduction (centrifugation at 580 × *g* for 20 minutes) was at least 85%, that volume reduction did not cause enhanced discharge of lactate dehydrogenase from platelets, and that platelet morphology, mean platelet volume, hypotonic stress response, synergistic aggregation, and platelet factor 3 activity (ie, procoagulant surface exposure) were not affected by the processing steps. In addition, Gollehon et al[93] found that volume reduction did not increase the platelet surface exposure of P-selectin, an indicator of granule release. Thus, the extra manipulation of standard platelet concentrates is not detrimental as judged by in-vitro responses, and platelet losses are acceptable.

More important than the in-vitro function of volume-reduced platelets is their in-vivo recovery. Moroff et al[92] showed that volume reduction of platelets stored for 1-5 days resulted in acceptable platelet increments in critically ill neonates with thrombocytopenia transfused with these hyperconcentrated products. Simon and Sierra[94] reported that platelets stored for 5 days and volume reduced by centrifugation at 2000 × *g* for 10 minutes or at 5000 × *g* for 6 minutes, when infused into normal (adult) volunteers, showed normal viability.

These findings notwithstanding, others are cautious about the use of volume-reduced products.[95] In the report of the 1989-1990 survey of US neonatal centers, the AABB Pediatric Hemotherapy Committee states that "because of the potential for harm, institutions transfusing volume-reduced platelets should monitor both the quality of the final product (ie, number of platelets, degree of clumping, and function) and in-vivo effects such as posttransfusion increment in platelet count and adverse reactions, including altered vital signs and pulmonary distress."[4(p534)] The committee noted that the final desired volumes of 10-15 mL for 61% of respondents and of 18-25 mL for an additional 30% of respondents are within the range of an unmodified platelet concentrate likely to give the desired increase in platelet count,[4] and they concluded that "nothing is gained by *routine* volume reduction of platelet concentrates. This technique should be reserved for special infants for whom marked volume reduction of all intravenous fluids is truly needed."[4(p534)]

Routine volume reduction of platelet concentrates for neonates is not warranted. This is also true for platelet transfusion support of older children. Several points support this recommendation. First and most important, volume reduction is generally not indicated because clinically significant platelet increments can be achieved after transfusion of an adequate volume of standard or apheresis platelet concentrates. Thus, volume reduction of platelets for transfusion to neonates or older children should be considered only in selected clinical situations in which repeated platelet transfusions may be necessary over a short interval and volume considerations are clinically important. Additional reasons for not advocating routine volume reduction of platelet concentrates include 1) loss of platelets during the additional preparation,[87,96] 2) risk of bacterial contamination associated with the additional manipulation, and 3) delayed availability of the final product.

Selection for Donor-Recipient Compatibility

Platelets possess intrinsic ABH antigens and extrinsically absorbed A and B antigens.[97,98] Nevertheless, ABO-incompatible platelets (ie, platelets with A and/or B antigens given to a recipient with a corresponding antibody) are usually clinically effective. However, in some patients, particularly those receiving multiple platelet transfusions, there may be a poorer posttransfusion response than that obtained with ABO-compatible platelets, and some studies have suggested that the transfusion of ABO-incompatible platelets is associated with the development of platelet refractoriness.[99-101] Also, there are reports of acute intravascular hemolysis following the transfusion of platelet concentrates containing ABO antibodies incompatible with the recipient's red cells.[102-104] Therefore, it would seem prudent, particularly in small children where the volume of plasma may be relatively large with respect to the patient's total blood volume, to use ABO-matched platelets whenever possible (Table 8-5). If ABO- matched platelets are not available, units that are plasma compatible with the recipient's red cells should be chosen. If this is also not possible, units with low titers of anti-A or anti-B should be selected, or platelets may be volume-reduced. Testing of platelet concentrates for red cell compatibility is not necessary unless red cells are detected by visual inspection.

Platelets do not carry Rh antigens.[105] However, the quantity of RBCs in platelet concentrates is sufficient to induce Rh sensitization even in immunosuppressed cancer patients.[106-108] Rh sensitization caused by platelet transfusions in Rh-negative patients can be prevented by the administration of Rh Immune Globulin (RhIG).[109,110] Thus, if platelets from an Rh-positive donor or from a donor of unknown Rh phenotype are given to an Rh-negative recipient, administration of RhIG should be considered, especially for female patients. The amount of RhIG necessary to prevent sensitization depends on the number of red cells in the platelet concentrate. A dose of 25 µg (125 IU) of RhIG will protect against 1 mL of red

Table 8-5. Possible Choices of ABO Blood Groups for Platelet Transfusions

Recipient Blood Group	Acceptable ABO Group of Donor Platelets
O	O, A, B, AB
A	A, AB
B	B, AB
AB	AB, A

In emergency situations, platelets in plasma with antibodies against recipient A and/or B antigens may be transfused in older children. However, in younger children and infants, platelet concentrates containing antibodies against recipient A and/or B antigens should not be used unless the anti-A/B is of low titer and/or the majority of plasma has been removed. Adapted with permission from Hume.[111]

cells.[110,112] If available, it is preferable to use a preparation of RhIG that can be administered intravenously.

Adverse Effects Following Platelet Transfusions

Adverse effects following platelet transfusions include transfusion-transmitted infections and noninfectious complications, such as allergic reactions, febrile nonhemolytic transfusion reactions (FNHTRs), alloimmunization, immunomodulation, and transfusion-associated graft-vs-host disease (TA-GVHD). Several of these complications are reviewed in detail elsewhere in this volume. However, additional commentary, with a pediatric bias, is provided about cytomegalovirus (CMV) infection, GVHD, and FNHTRs.

Cytomegalovirus Infection

CMV infection ranges from a mild or even asymptomatic infection in healthy immunocompetent individuals to a much more serious, and sometimes fatal, illness in immunocompromised patients. These populations include very low birthweight (<1250 g) neonates, fetuses who require intrauterine transfusions, marrow and solid organ transplant recipients, and other severely immunocompromised individuals. Features of CMV infection in these patient groups include fever, cytopenias, pneumonia, hepatitis, graft rejection, and increased risk of bacterial and fungal infection.

Three types of transfusion-associated CMV infection may occur: primary infection and 2 kinds of secondary infection; reactivation and reinfection. Primary infection occurs in a seronegative recipient of blood from a donor who is actively or latently infected. Reactivation occurs when a CMV-seropositive patient is transfused with blood from either a CMV-seropositive or a CMV-seronegative donor. The leukocytes in the transfused product trigger an allograft reaction that reactivates the recipient's latent CMV.[113] Re- or coinfection occurs in a CMV-seropositive recipient of blood with a strain of CMV that differs from the strain that initially infected the recipient. The only way to distinguish reinfection or coinfection from reactivation is to use molecular markers whereby multiple strains of CMV may be identified in the recipient.

Prevention of transfusion-transmitted primary CMV infection is of paramount importance in the risk groups defined and relies on the use of IgG seronegative blood components or, reflecting the fact that CMV is harbored in white cells, the use of blood components that have been leukocyte-reduced.[114] The use of IgG seronegative blood (or blood components) is considered by many to be the gold standard with regard to the prevention of transfusion-transmitted CMV, notwithstanding the fact that several publications support the efficacy of leukocyte-reduced blood components as a strategy to prevent transfusion-associated CMV.[115-119] In light of this, the study by Bowden et al is important.[120] The investigators conducted a clinical trial in which 502 seronegative recipients of autologous or seronegative allogeneic marrow transplants were randomly selected to receive either CMV-seronegative or filtered leukocyte-reduced red cells and platelets. Out of 250 patients who received filtered blood and blood products, 6 developed CMV disease, including 5 cases of fatal pneumonia. Of the 252 patients receiving seronegative blood, 4 developed CMV disease but none of the cases was fatal. Although the investigators concluded, on the basis of an "intention to treat" analysis, that seronegative and filtered units were equal with respect to the risk of transfusion-transmitted CMV infection and disease, the explanation for the difference in mortality between the two groups remains unclear. If leukocyte-reduced blood products are used either as an equivalent to seronegative products or because such products are not available, it is important that they contain less than 5×10^6 white blood cells. It should be emphasized that bedside filters are unreliable in this context and that filtration should occur in the setting of blood centers or hospital blood banks that have stringent quality control measures in place.

The AABB has published recommendations regarding the use of CMV-reduced-risk blood (Table 8-6). In a recent review of the hazards of transfusion, Luban et al[121] described the practice at Children's National Medical Center in Washington, DC, where the CMV status of all newly diagnosed oncology patients is determined on their first pretransfusion specimen. Children who are CMV-seronegative and who are placed on a protocol that may result in either transplantation or stem cell rescue are given CMV-seronegative blood products. CMV-seropositive patients are provided with leukocyte-reduced products to reduce febrile reactions and as a surrogate for CMV-negative products. Other patients who have a low likelihood of transplantation, regardless of CMV serostatus, receive untested, non-leukocyte-reduced, irradiated products unless their clinical circumstances change or they develop FNHTRs. Each institution should define its own approach, which should be reviewed regularly and modified as required on the basis of available literature and discussion with appropriate health-care groups (eg, hematologists/oncologists, neonatologists, and transplant physicians).

Table 8-6. AABB Recommendations on Use of CMV-Reduced-Risk Blood

Category*	Clinical Circumstance	CMV-Seronegative Blood (Unmodified)	LR Blood (CMV-Unscreened)
I	CMV+ patient	Not indicated	Not indicated
	CMV– patient	Not indicated	Not indicated
II	CMV+ patient	Not indicated	Use of LR blood to prevent viral reactivation awaits further research
	CMV– patient	Either CMV-seronegative blood or LR blood is indicated	Either CMV-seronegative blood or LR blood is indicated
III	CMV+ recipient	Not indicated	Not indicated
	CMV– recipient of CMV- organ donor	Either CMV-seronegative blood or LR blood is indicated	Either CMV-seronegative blood or LR blood is indicated
IV	CMV+ recipient	Not indicated	Use of LR blood to prevent viral reactivation awaits further research
	CMV– recipient of CMV+ donor	Either CMV-seronegative blood or LR blood is indicated	Either CMV-seronegative blood or LR blood is indicated
V	CMV+ recipient	Either CMV-seronegative blood or LR blood is indicated	Either CMV-seronegative blood or LR blood is indicated
	CMV– recipient	Either CMV-seronegative blood or LR blood is indicated	LR blood may be slightly preferred to CMV-seronegative blood (passive CMV immunoglobulin)

*Category I patients: General hospital patients and general surgery patients (including cardiac surgery); patients receiving chemotherapy that is not intended to produce severe neutropenia (adjuvant therapy for breast cancer, treatment of chronic lymphocytic leukemia, etc); patients receiving corticosteroids (patients with immune thrombocytopenia purpura, collagen vascular diseases, etc); full-term infants.
Category II patients: Patients receiving chemotherapy that is intended to produce severe neutropenia (leukemia, lymphoma, etc); pregnant patients; HIV-infected individuals.
Category III patients: Solid-organ allograft patients who do not require massive transfusion support.
Category IV patients: Patients receiving allogeneic and autologous hematopoietic progenitor cell transplants.
Category V patients: Low birthweight (<1200 g) premature infants.
CMV = cytomegalovirus; LR = leukokcyte-reduced
Source: American Association of Blood Banks. *Association Bulletin* 97-2.

Transfusion-Associated Graft-vs-Host Disease

TA-GVHD is caused by engraftment of donor T lymphocytes into a host unable to reject them.[122] Studies of leukocyte clearance after transfusion have shown that, in immunocompetent subjects, donor leukocytes are rapidly eliminated within the first 2-3 days following transfusion.[123] For GVHD to occur following transfusion, two conditions need to exist: 1) the donor and host must be antigenically dissimilar enough to stimulate proliferation of infused donor T cells; and 2) the host must be incapable of rejecting the alloreactive T cells because of an underlying congenital or acquired cellular immune deficiency or, more rarely, because of tolerance to the infused donor T cells. This latter scenario may occur following a transfusion from a donor who is homozygous for an HLA haplotype for which the host is haploidentical. In this setting, host leukocytes fail to eliminate compatible donor T cells, which then proliferate after exposure to foreign host cell antigens, engraft, and cause GVHD.[124]

Children at risk for TA-GVHD include the following groups: extremely premature neonates; infants who received intrauterine transfusions and who require exchange transfusion postnatally; children with congenital deficiencies involving the cellular immune system (eg, severe combined immune deficiency, DiGeorge syndrome, reticular dysgenesis, and purine nucleoside phosphorylase deficiency); and children with hematologic malignancies or solid tumors who are immune-suppressed following chemotherapy, radiation treatment, or both. The association between Hodgkin's disease and the development of TA-GVHD is related to intrinsic T-cell defects known to occur with this disorder.

TA-GVHD is an acute illness that occurs from a few days to up to 4 weeks following a transfusion of a cellular blood component, such as platelets containing a sufficient number of immunocompetent T lymphocytes. The threshold dose of lymphocytes required to cause TA GVHD is uncertain; however, there have been reports of fatal TA-GVHD in children with severe combined immunodeficiency in which a dose of only 8×10^4 lymphocytes/kg body weight appeared to be transfused.[125] Characteristic features of TA-GVHD include fever, a central maculopapular rash that spreads to involve the extremities, diarrhea, liver dysfunction, and pancytopenia. The disorder is nearly always fatal, with the majority of patients dying within a few days to a few weeks, usually as a complication of marrow failure.[126] The diagnosis of TA-GVHD is usually based on the clinical presentation in conjunction with histologic findings on skin biopsy. However, in ill, multitransfused patients, it is possible that some cases of TA-GVHD may go undiagnosed and that abnormalities may be attributed to other causes (eg, viral infections, drug reactions) that may present with similar clinical features. In questionable cases, documentation of the persistence of donor lymphocytes by cytogenetic, HLA, or DNA analyses provides supportive evidence for a diagnosis of TA-GVHD.

Since the treatment of TA-GVHD is ineffective and this disorder is fatal in more than 90% of cases, it is important that this devastating complication of transfusion be prevented in at-risk patients. The only validated strategy for preventing TA-GVHD is gamma-irradiation of blood components before transfusion. The recommended dose is 2500 cGy to the midplane of the component, with a minimum of 1500 cGy to the other regions of the product.[121] Washing and filtration can substantially reduce the burden of donor leukocytes in transfused blood products but should *never* be regarded as an acceptable substitute for gamma irradiation in patients at risk for GVHD following transfusion. Indications for the use of irradiated blood components in pediatric subjects are listed in Table 8-7. Some institutions elect to irradiate all blood components transfused to newborns and older children in order to avoid missing a child with an undiagnosed or unrecognized cellular immunodeficiency state.

Febrile Nonhemolytic Transfusion Reactions

FNHTRs are a common complication following platelet transfusions. Typical features include chills and/or rigors and an elevation in temperature that generally appears approximately 1 hour after the start of the transfusion.[127] An acceptable definition of an FNHTR is a rise in temperature of more than 1 C over the baseline level (minimum temperature 38 C) during or within 4 hours following the transfusion and for which there is no other explanation.

In 1957, Brittingham and Chaplin[127] performed careful transfusion studies in 5 patients with a history of recurrent severe febrile transfusion reactions. White cell agglutinins were present in all cases. The investigators clearly demonstrated that reactions could be prevented by removing the buffy coat before administering the transfusion and suggested that isoantibodies against white cells and possibly against platelets are a common cause of repeated febrile transfusion reactions. Subsequent studies documented white cell antibodies in approximately two-thirds of patients with FNHTRs.[128,129] More recently, the importance of proinflammatory cytokines as a cause of FHNTRs has been appreciated.[130,131] These cytokines (interleukin [IL]-1β, tumor necrosis factor [TNF]-α, IL-6, and IL-8) are synthesized and released from white cells during storage of platelet concen-

Table 8-7. Guidelines for Use of Irradiated Blood Components in Children and Infants

Fetus/newborn infants less than 4 months of age

- Fetus requiring in-utero transfusion
- Newborn undergoing exchange transfusion following an in-utero transfusion
- Premature infant < 1200 g birthweight
- Congenital leukemia or other malignancy undergoing chemotherapy
- Recipient of familial blood or HLA-matched cellular blood component(s)
- Known or suspected congenital cellular immunodeficiency

Children older than 4 months of age

- Known or suspected congenital cellular immunodeficiency
- Malignancy (hematological/solid tumor) undergoing chemotherapy/radiotherapy
- Recipient of solid organ or hematopoietic transplantation
- Recipient of familial blood or HLA-matched cellular blood component(s)

Children for whom risk of GVHD is not well enough established to support recommendation of irradiation*

- Infants < 4 months of age and birthweight > 1200 g in a neonatal intensive care setting but without a history as described above
- All children undergoing open-heart procedures, including extracorporeal membrane oxygenation
- Any child with a conal-truncal heart defect until congenital T-cell immunodeficiency is ruled out
- Human immunodeficiency virus infection

*Local facts, such as the degree of ethnic homogenicity between the donor-recipient groups, influence the decision to irradiate blood products for these groups. Adapted with permission from Luban et al.[121]

trates at 22 C; concentrations of cytokines increase significantly after 3 days of storage and beyond.[132-134] Strategies that are effective in reducing the frequency of FNHTRs include leukocyte reduction of the platelet concentrate before storage (prestorage leukocyte reduction) or before transfusion (by centrifugation or filtration). Prestorage leukocyte reduction by either filtration or removal of the buffy coat ensures a platelet product with low levels of both white cells and cytokines.[135]

FNHTRs should be treated with antipyretics such as acetaminophen; corticosteroids are of value in severe cases. Antihistamines are not indicated unless the patient simultaneously experiences an immediate allergic reaction to plasma components in the platelet concentrates. Children who

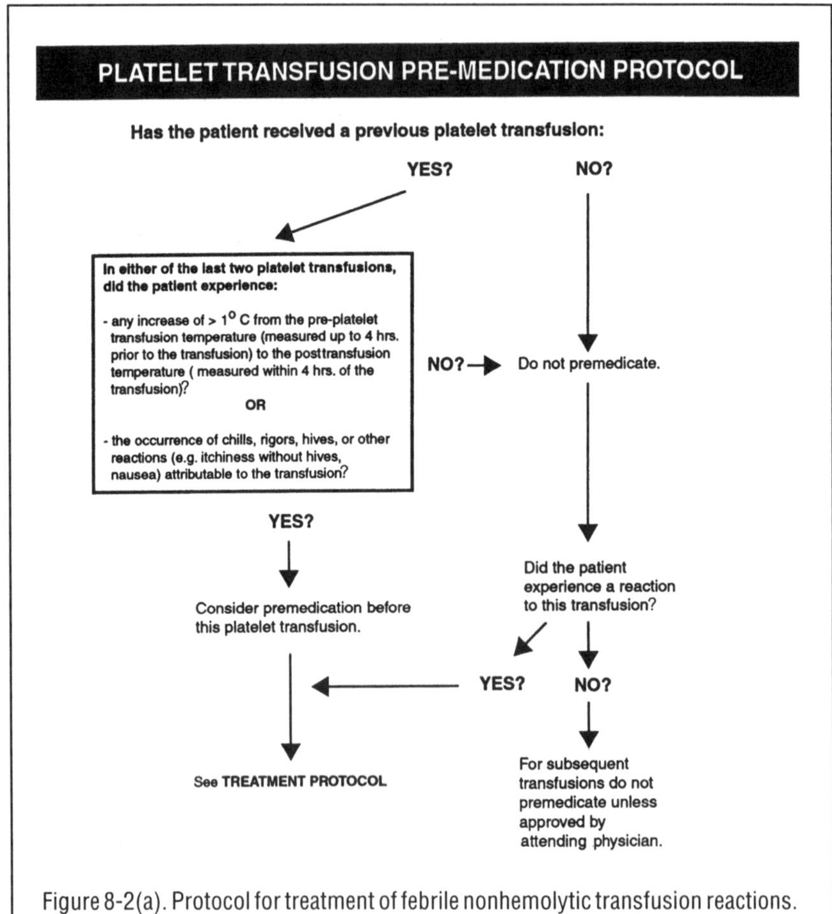

Figure 8-2(a). Protocol for treatment of febrile nonhemolytic transfusion reactions.

experience an initial FNHTR do not invariably experience a similar reaction at the next transfusion. It is important, therefore, that such children not be labeled as "allergic to platelets" and started on a program of prophylactic premedication before all subsequent transfusions. This is a frequent approach in pediatric hematology/oncology units and one that leads to unnecessary medication and often a shift to expensive alternate platelet products such as matched single-donor apheresis platelet concentrates. A stepwise approach to the management of this common clinical problem is preferred [Figs 8-2(a) and (b)].

Summary

Platelets are an essential component of the supportive care of selected children with thrombocytopenia. Although much is known about platelet

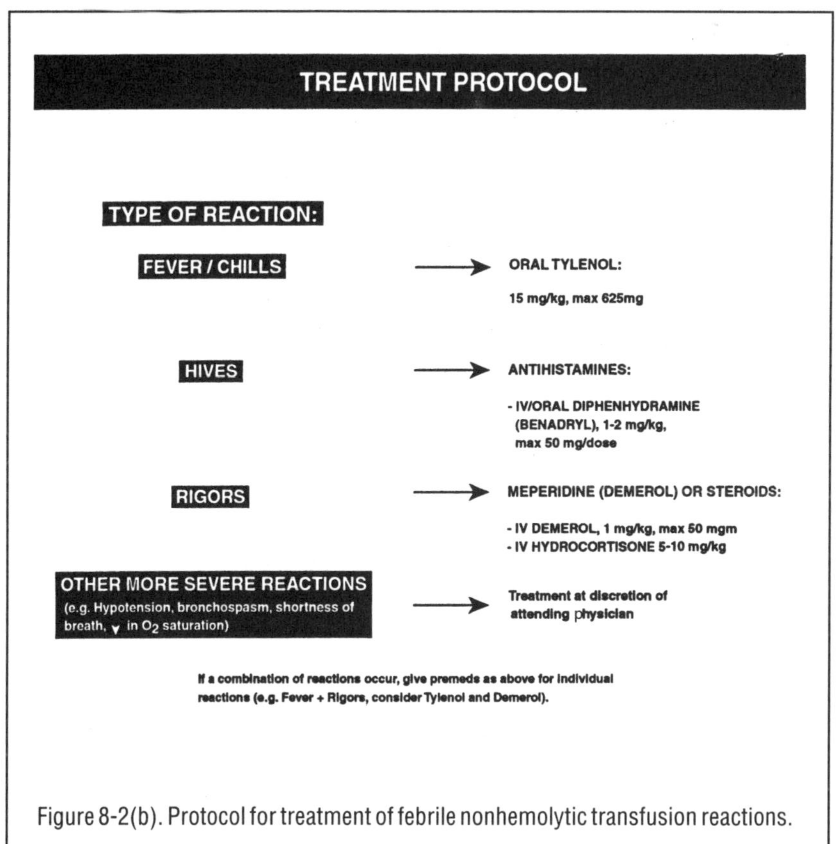

Figure 8-2(b). Protocol for treatment of febrile nonhemolytic transfusion reactions.

transfusion therapy in children, much remains to be learned. Future studies will define better ways to store platelets without a loss of function, as well as more sensitive techniques both to identify and to inactivate and/or remove contaminating infectious agents in platelet concentrates. The major clinical challenge will be to define better strategies to prevent platelet alloimmunization and to select appropriate thresholds for platelet transfusion in subgroups of patients (eg, neonates placed on ECMO and children with central nervous system tumors undergoing radiation therapy and/or chemotherapy). A number of these questions will be satisfactorily answered only after properly designed, prospective, controlled clinical trials have been completed with adequate numbers of pediatric subjects.

References

1. National Institutes of Health, Consensus Development Conference. Platelet transfusion therapy. JAMA 1987;257:1777-80.
2. Blanchette VS, Hume HA, Levy GJ, et al. Guidelines for auditing pediatric blood transfusion practices. Am J Dis Child 1991;145:787-96.
3. Fresh-Frozen Plasma, Cryoprecipitate and Platelets Administration Practice Guidelines Development Task Force of the College of American Pathologists. Practice parameter for the use of fresh-frozen plasma, cryoprecipitate, and platelets. JAMA 1994;271:777-81.
4. Strauss RG, Levy GJ, Sotelo-Avila C, et al. National survey of neonatal transfusion practices; II: Blood component therapy. Pediatrics 1993;91:530-6.
5. Castle V, Andrew M, Kelton J, et al. Frequency and mechanism of neonatal thrombocytopenia. J Pediatr 1986;108:749-55.
6. Andrew M, Castle V, Saigal S, et al. Clinical impact of neonatal thrombocytopenia. J Pediatr 1987;110:457-64.
7. Andrew M, Vegh P, Caco C, et al. A randomized, controlled trial of platelet transfusions in thrombocytopenic premature infants. J Pediatr 1993;123:285-91.
8. Lupton BA, Hill A, Whitfield MF, et al. Reduced platelet count as a risk factor for intraventricular hemorrhage. Am J Dis Child 1988; 142:1222-4.
9. Zipursky A, Palko J, Milner R, et al. The hematology of bacterial infections in premature infants. Pediatrics 1976;57:839-53.

10. Zipursky A, deSa D, Hsu E, et al. Clinical and laboratory diagnosis of hemostatic disorders in newborn infants. Am J Pediatr Hematol Oncol 1979;1:217-26.
11. Hutter JJ Jr, Hathaway WE, Wayne ER. Hematologic abnormalities in severe neonatal necrotizing enterocolitis. J Pediatr 1976;88:1026-31.
12. Kasabach HH, Merritt KK. Capillary hemangioma with extensive purpura: Report of a case. Am J Dis Child 1940;59:1063-70.
13. Larson EC, Zinkham WH, Eggleston JC, et al. Kasabach-Merritt syndrome: Therapeutic considerations. Pediatrics 1987;79:971-80.
14. McCrae KR, Samuels P, Schreiber AD. Pregnancy-associated thrombocytopenia: Pathogenesis and management. Blood 1992;80:2697-714.
15. Scott JR, Cruikshank DP, Kochenour NK, et al. Fetal platelet counts in the obstetric management of immunologic thrombocytopenic purpura. Am J Obstet Gynecol 1980;136:495-9.
16. Karpatkin M, Porges RF, Karpatkin S. Platelet counts in infants of women with autoimmune thrombocytopenia. Effect of steroid administration to the mother. N Engl J Med 1981;305:936-9.
17. Kelton JG, Inwood MJ, Barr RM, et al. The prenatal prediction of thrombocytopenia in infants of mothers with clinically diagnosed immune thrombocytopenia. Am J Obstet Gynecol 1982;144: 449-54.
18. Samuels P, Bussel JB, Braitman LE, et al. Estimation of the risk of thrombocytopenia in the offspring of pregnant women with presumed immune thrombocytopenic purpura. N Engl J Med 1990; 323:229-35.
19. Kelton JG. Management of the pregnant patient with idiopathic thrombocytopenic purpura. Ann Intern Med 1983;99:796-800.
20. Blanchette VS, Turner C. Treatment of acute idiopathic thrombocytopenic purpura (letter). J Pediatr 1986;108:326-7.
21. Woerner SJ, Abildgaard CF, French BN. Intracranial hemorrhage in children with idiopathic thrombocytopenic purpura. Pediatrics 1981;67:453-60.
22. Ballin A, Andrew M, Ling E, et al. High-dose intravenous gammaglobulin therapy for neonatal autoimmune thrombocytopenia. J Pediatr 1988;112:789-92.
23. Blanchette V, Andrew M, Perlman M, et al. Neonatal autoimmune thrombocytopenia: Role of high-dose intravenous immunoglobulin G therapy. Blut 1989;59:139 44.

24. Blanchette VS, Luke B, Andrew M, et al. A prospective, randomized trial of high-dose intravenous immunoglobulin G therapy, oral prednisone therapy, and no therapy in childhood acute immune thrombocytopenic purpura. J Pediatr 1993;123:989-95.
25. Blanchette V, Imbach P, Andrew M, et al. Randomised trial of intravenous immunoglobulin G, intravenous anti-D, and oral prednisone in childhood acute immune thrombocytopenic purpura. Lancet 1994;344:703-7.
26. Carcao MD, Zipursky A, Butchart S, et al. Short-course oral prednisone therapy in children presenting with acute immune thrombocytopenic purpura (ITP). Acta Paediatr 1998;424(suppl):71-4.
27. Baumann MA, Menitove JE, Aster RH, et al. Urgent treatment of idiopathic thrombocytopenic purpura with single-dose gammaglobulin infusion followed by platelet transfusion. Ann Intern Med 1986; 104:808-9.
28. Pearson HA, Shulman NR, Marder VJ, Cone TE Jr. Isoimmune neonatal thrombocytopenic purpura. Clinical and therapeutic considerations. Blood 1964;23:154-77.
29. Blanchette VS, Chen L, de Friedberg ZS, et al. Alloimmunization to the Pl^{A1} platelet antigen: Results of a prospective study. Br J Haematol 1990;74:209-15.
30. Mueller-Eckhardt G, Kiefel V, Grubert A, et al. 348 cases of suspected neonatal alloimmune thrombocytopenia. Lancet 1989;1: 363-6.
31. Skacel PO, Stacey TE, Tidmarsh CEF, Contreras M. Maternal alloimmunization to HLA, platelet and granulocyte-specific antigens during pregnancy: Its influence on cord blood granulocyte and platelet counts. Br J Haematol 1989;71:119-23.
32. Bussel J, Kaplan C, McFarland J, and the Working Party on Neonatal Immune Thrombocytopenia on the Neonatal Hemostasis Subcommittee of the Scientific and Standardization Committee of the ISTH. Recommendations for the evaluation and treatment of neonatal autoimmune and alloimmune thrombocytopenia. Thromb Haemost 1991;65:631-4.
33. Andrew M, Kelton J. Neonatal thrombocytopenia. Clin Perinatol 1984;11:359-71.
34. Vengelen-Tyler V, ed. Technical manual. 12th ed. Bethesda, MD: American Association of Blood Banks, 1996:700-3.

35. Tchernia G, Morel-Kopp MC, Yvart J, Kaplan C. Neonatal thrombocytopenia and hidden maternal autoimmunity. Br J Haematol 1993; 84:457-63.
36. McGill M, Mayhaus C, Hoff R, Carey P. Frozen maternal platelets for neonatal thrombocytopenia. Transfusion 1987;27:347-9.
37. O'Brien T, O'Brien B, Cosgrove JF, Counahan R. Isoimmune thrombocytopenia treated with random donor platelets. Ir Med J 1981;74: 81-2.
38. Blanchette VS, Kühne T, Hume H, Hellmann J. Platelet transfusion therapy in newborn infants. Trans Med Rev 1995;9:215-30.
39. Johnson J-AM, Ryan G, Al-Musa A, et al. Prenatal diagnosis and management of neonatal alloimmune thrombocytopenia. Semin Perinatol 1997;21:45-52.
40. Herman JH, Jumbelic MI, Arcona RJ, Kickler TS. In utero cerebral hemorrhage in alloimmune thrombocytopenia. Am J Pediatr Hematol Oncol 1986;8:312-7.
41. Hume HA. Fetal and neonatal transfusion. In: Pamphilon DH, ed. Modern transfusion medicine. Boca Raton, FL: CRC Press, 1995: 193-215.
42. Prenatal management of fetal alloimmune thrombocytopenia (editorial). Vox Sang 1993;65:180-9.
43. Waters A, Murphy M, Hambley N, Nicolandes K. Management of alloimmune thrombocytopenia in the fetus and neonate. In: Nance SJ, ed. Clinical and basic science aspects of immunohematology. Arlington, VA: American Association of Blood Banks, 1991:155-77.
44. Murphy MF, Metcalfe P, Hambley H, et al. Successful antenatal management of severe neonatal alloimmune thrombocytopenia (NAIT) using fetal intraperitoneal IgG and serial platelet transfusion (abstract). Blood 1992;80(suppl 1):217a.
45. Meliones JN, Hanscolls DR. Extracorporeal membrane oxygenation: The role of blood components. In: Chambers LA, Issitt LA, eds. Supporting the pediatric transfusion recipient. Bethesda, MD: American Association of Blood Banks, 1994:87-109.
46. Hersh EM, Bodey GP, Nies BA, Freireich EJ. Causes of death in acute leukemia. A ten-year study of 414 patients from 1954-1963. JAMA 1965;193:99-103.
47. Schiffer CA. Prophylactic platelet transfusion. Transfusion 1992;32: 295-8.

48. Roy AJ, Jaffe N, Djerassi I. Prophylactic platelet transfusions in children with acute leukemia: A dose response study. Transfusion 1973;13:283-90.
49. Higby DJ, Cohen E, Holland JF, Sinks L. The prophylactic treatment of thrombocytopenic leukemic patients with platelets: A double blind study. Transfusion 1974;14:440-6.
50. Soloman J, Bofenkamp T, Fahey J, et al. Platelet prophylaxis in acute non-lymphoblastic leukaemia (letter). Lancet 1978;1:267.
51. Gockerman JP, Davis J. Platelet transfusion in acute leukemic patients (abstract). Blood 1979;54:122A.
52. Ilett SJ, Lilleyman JS. Platelet transfusion requirements of children with newly diagnosed lymphoblastic leukemia. Acta Haematol 1979;62:86-9.
53. Murphy S, Litwin S, Herring LM, et al. Indications for platelet transfusion in children with acute leukemia. Am J Hematol 1982;12: 347-56.
54. Feusner J. Supportive care for children with cancer. Guidelines of the Childrens Cancer Study Group. The use of platelet transfusions. Am J Pediatr Hematol Oncol 1984;6:255-60.
55. Aisner J. Clinical use of platelet transfusion for patients with cancer. In: Platelet physiology and transfusion. Arlington, VA: American Association of Blood Banks, 1978:39-50.
56. Schiffer CA. Some aspects of recent advances in the use of blood cell components. Br J Haematol 1978;39:289-94.
57. Kelton JG, Blajchman MA. Platelet transfusions. Can Med Assoc J 1979;121:1353-8.
58. Tomasulo PA, Lenes BA. Platelet transfusion therapy. In: Menitove JE, McCarthy LJ, eds. Hemostatic disorders and the blood bank. Arlington, VA: American Association of Blood Banks, 1984:63-89.
59. Baer MR, Bloomfield CD. Controversies in transfusion medicine. Prophylactic platelet transfusion therapy: Pro. Transfusion 1992; 32:377-80.
60. Patten E. Controversies in transfusion medicine. Prophylactic platelet transfusion revisited after 25 years: Con. Transfusion 1992;32:381-5.
61. Pisciotto PT, Benson K, Hume H, et al. Prophylactic versus therapeutic platelet transfusion practices in hematology and/or oncology patients. Transfusion 1995;35:498-502.

62. Gaydos LA, Freireich EJ, Mantel N. The quantitative relation between platelet count and hemorrhage in patients with acute leukemia. N Engl J Med 1962;266:905-9.
63. Slichter SJ. Platelet transfusions—a constantly evolving therapy. Thromb Haemost 1991;66:178-88.
64. Beutler E. Platelet transfusions: The 20,000/µL trigger. Blood 1993; 81:1411-3.
65. Norfolk DR, Ancliffe PJ, Contreras M, et al. Consensus Conference on Platelet Transfusion, Royal College of Physicians of Edinburgh, 27-28 November 1997. Br J Haematol 1998;101:609-17.
66. Contreras M. Final statement from the Consensus Conference on Platelet Transfusion. Transfusion 1998;38:796-7.
67. Aderka D, Praff G, Santo M, et al. Bleeding due to thrombocytopenia in acute leukemias and reevaluation of the prophylactic platelet transfusion policy. Am J Med Sci 1986;291:147-51.
68. Gmür J, Burger J, Schanz U, et al. Safety of stringent prophylactic platelet transfusion policy for patients with acute leukaemia. Lancet 1991;338:1223-6.
69. Gil-Fernandez JJ, Alegre A, Fernandez-Villalta MJ, et al. Clinical results of a stringent policy on prophylactic platelet transfusion: Non-randomized comparative analysis in 190 bone marrow transplant patients from a single institution. Bone Marrow Transplant 1996;18:931-5.
70. Heckman KD, Weiner GJ, Davis CS, et al. Randomized study of prophylactic platelet transfusion threshold during induction therapy for adult acute leukemia: 10,000/µL versus 20,000/µL. J Clin Oncol 1997;15:1143-9.
71. Rebulla P, Finazzi G, Marangoni F, et al. A multicenter randomized study of the threshold for prophylactic platelet transfusions in adults with acute myeloid leukemia. Gruppo Italiano Malattie Ematologiche Maligne dell'Adulto. N Engl J Med 1997;337:1870-5.
72. Wandt H, Frank M, Ehninger G, et al. Safety and cost effectiveness of a 10×10^9/L trigger for prophylactic platelet transfusions compared with the traditional 20×10^9/L trigger: A prospective comparative trial of 105 patients with acute myeloid leukemia. Blood 1998;91: 3601-6.
73. Creutzig U, Ritter J, Budde M, et al. Early deaths due to hemorrhage and leukostasis in childhood acute myelogenous leukemia. Cancer 1987;60:3071-9.

74. Rodeghiero F, Avvisati G, Castaman G, et al. Early deaths and anti-hemorrhagic treatments in acute promyelocytic leukemia. A GIMEMA retrospective study in 268 consecutive patients. Blood 1990;75:2112-7.
75. Belt RJ, Leite C, Haas CD, Stephens RL. Incidence of hemorrhagic complications in patients with cancer. JAMA 1978;239:2571-4.
76. Dutcher JP, Schiffer CA, Aisner J, et al. Incidence of thrombocytopenia and serious hemorrhage among patients with solid tumors. Cancer 1984;53:557-62.
77. Bishop JF, Schiffer CA, Aisner J, et al. Surgery in leukemia: A review of 167 operations on thrombocytopenia patients. Am J Hematol 1987;26:147-55.
78. George JN, Woolf SH, Raskob GE, et al. Idiopathic thrombocytopenic purpura: A practice guideline developed by explicit methods for the American Society of Hematology. Blood 1996;88:3-40.
79. Flordal PA, Sahlin S. Use of desmopressin to prevent bleeding complications in patients treated with aspirin. Br J Surg 1993;80:723-4.
80. Sheridan DP, Card RT, Pinilla JC, et al. Use of desmopressin acetate to reduce blood transfusion requirements during cardiac surgery in patients with acetylsalicylic-acid-induced platelet dysfunction. Can J Surg 1994;37:33-6.
81. Beurling-Harbury C, Galvan CA. Acquired decrease in platelet secretory ADP associated with increased postoperative bleeding in post-cardiopulmonary bypass patients and in patients with severe valvular heart disease. Blood 1978;52:13-23.
82. Harker LA, Malpass TW, Branson HE, et al. Mechanism of abnormal bleeding in patients undergoing cardiopulmonary bypass: Acquired transient platelet dysfunction associated with selective α-granule release. Blood 1980;56:824-34.
83. Simon TL, Akl BF, Murphy W. Controlled trial of routine administration of platelet concentrates in cardiopulmonary bypass surgery. Ann Thorac Surg 1984;37:359-64.
84. American Society of Anesthesiologists Task Force on Blood Component Therapy. Practice guidelines for blood component therapy. Anesthesiology 1996;84:732-47.
85. Martinowitz U, Schulman S. Fibrin sealant in surgery of patients with a hemorrhagic diathesis. Thromb Haemost 1995;74:486-92.
86. Hume H, Blanchette V, Strauss RG, Levy GJ. A survey of Canadian neonatal blood transfusion practices. Transfus Sci 1997;18:71-80.

87. Rand ML, He L, Al-Musa A, et al. Volume reduction of stored platelet concentrates does not affect in vitro platelet responses. Blood 1997; 90(suppl 1, pt 2):138b.
88. Machin SJ, Kelsey H, Seghatchian J, et al. Platelet transfusion. Thromb Haemost 1995;74:246-52.
89. Klinger MHF. The storage lesion of platelets: Ultrastructural and functional aspects. Ann Hematol 1996;73:103-12.
90. Seghatchian J, Krailadsiri P. The platelet storage lesion. Transfus Med Rev 1997;11:130-44.
91. Holme S, Heaton WA, Courtright M. Improved *in vivo* and *in vitro* viability of platelet concentrates stored for seven days in a platelet additive solution. Br J Haematol 1987;66:233-8.
92. Moroff G, Friedman A, Robkin-Kline L, et al. Reduction of the volume of stored platelet concentrates for use in neonatal patients. Transfusion 1984;24:144-6.
93. Gollehon TJ, King DE, Craig FE. Does hyperconcentration result in platelet activation? A flow-cytometric study of hyperconcentrated random donor platelets. Vox Sang 1998;75:124-7.
94. Simon TL, Sierra ER. Concentration of platelet units into small volumes. Transfusion 1984;24:173-5.
95. Strauss RG. Transfusion therapy in neonates. Am J Dis Child 1991; 145:904-11.
96. Bredehoeft SJ, Campbell ML. Impact of modification sequence on platelet yield in preparation of small volume platelet products. Transfusion 1993;33(suppl):6S.
97. Dunstan RA, Simpson MB, Knowles RE, Rosse WF. The origin of ABH antigens on human platelets. Blood 1985;65:615-9.
98. Kelton JG, Hamid C, Aker S, Blajchman MA. The amount of blood group A substance on platelets is proportional to the amount in the plasma. Blood 1982;59:980-5.
99. Brand A, Sintnicolaas K, Claas FHJ, Eernisse JG. ABH antibodies causing platelet transfusion refractoriness. Transfusion 1986;26:463-6.
100. Lee EJ, Schiffer CA. ABO incompatibility can influence the results of platelet transfusion. Results of a randomized trial. Transfusion 1989; 29:384-9.
101. Carr R, Hutton JL, Jenkins JA, et al. Transfusion of ABO-mismatched platelets leads to early platelet refractoriness. Br J Haematol 1990; 75:408-13.

102. Pierce RN, Reich LM, Mayer K. Hemolysis following platelet transfusions from ABO-incompatible donors. Transfusion 1985;25:60-2.
103. Ferguson DJ. Acute intravascular hemolysis after a platelet transfusion. Can Med Assoc J 1988;138:523-4.
104. Reis MD, Coovadia AS. Transfusion of ABO-incompatible platelets causing severe haemolytic reaction. Clin Lab Haematol 1989;11: 237-40.
105. Dunstan RA, Simpson MB, Rosse WF. Erythrocyte antigens on human platelets. Absence of Rh, Duffy, Kell, Kidd, and Lutheran antigens. Transfusion 1984;24:243-6.
106. Goldfinger D, McGinnis MH. RH incompatible platelet transfusions—risks and consequences of sensitizing immunosuppressed patients. N Engl J Med 1971;284:942-4.
107. McLeod BC, Piehl MR, Sassetti RJ. Alloimmunization to RhD by platelet transfusions in autologous bone marrow transplant recipients. Vox Sang 1990;59:185-9.
108. Baldwin ML, Ness PM, Scott D, et al. Alloimmunization to D antigen and HLA in D-negative immunosuppressed oncology patients. Transfusion 1988;28:330-3.
109. Heim MU, Bock M, Kolb HJ, et al. Intravenous anti-D gammaglobulin for the prevention of rhesus isoimmunization caused by platelet transfusions in patients with malignant disease. Vox Sang 1992;62:165-8.
110. Zeiler T, Wittmann G, Zingsem J, et al. A dose of 100 IU intravenous anti-D gammaglobulin is effective for the prevention of RhD immunisation after RhD-incompatible single donor platelet transfusion (letter). Vox Sang 1994;66:243.
111. Hume HA. Blood components: Preparation, indications, and administration. In: Lilleyman J, Hann I, Blanchette V, eds. Pediatric hematology. London: Churchill-Livingstone, 1999:709-39.
112. National Blood Transfusion Service Immunoglobulin Working Party. Recommendations for the use of anti-D immunoglobulin. Prescribers J 1991;31:137-45.
113. Soderberg-Naucler C, Fish KN, Nelson JA. Reactivation of latent human cytomegalovirus by allogeneic stimulation of blood cells from healthy donors. Cell 1997;91:119-26.
114. Przepiorka D, LeParc GF, Werch J, Lichtiger B. Prevention of transfusion-associated cytomegalovirus infection. Practice parameter.

American Society of Clinical Pathologists. Am J Clin Pathol 1996; 106:163-9.

115. Verdonck LF, de Graan-Hentzen YC, Dekker AW, et al. Cytomegalovirus seronegative platelets and leukocyte-poor red blood cells from random donors can prevent primary cytomegalovirus infection after bone marrow transplantation. Bone Marrow Transplant 1987;2:73-8.
116. Gilbert GL, Hayes K, Hudson IL, James J. Prevention of transfusion-acquired cytomegalovirus infection in infants by blood filtration to remove leucocytes. Neonatal Cytomegalovirus Infection Study Group. Lancet 1989;1:1228-31.
117. de Graan-Hentzen YC, Gratama JW, Mudde GC, et al. Prevention of primary cytomegalovirus infection in patients with hematologic malignancies by intensive white cell depletion of blood products. Transfusion 1989;29:757-60.
118. De Witte T, Schattenberg A, Van Dijk BA, et al. Prevention of primary cytomegalovirus infection after allogeneic bone marrow transplantation by using leukocyte-poor random blood products from cytomegalovirus-unscreened blood-bank donors. Transplantation 1990;50:964-8.
119. Bowden RA, Slichter SJ, Sayers MH, et al. Use of leukocyte-depleted platelets and cytomegalovirus-seronegative red blood cells for prevention of primary cytomegalovirus infection after marrow transplant. Blood 1991;78:246-50.
120. Bowden RA, Slichter SJ, Sayers M, et al. A comparison of filtered leukocyte-reduced and cytomegalovirus (CMV) seronegative blood products for the prevention of transfusion-associated CMV infection after marrow transplant. Blood 1995;86:3598-603.
121. Luban NLC, Pisciotto P, Manno C. Hazards of transfusion. In: Lilleyman JS, Hann IM, Blanchette VS, eds. Pediatric hematology. London: Churchill Livingstone, 1999:741-57.
122. Anderson KC, Weinstein HJ. Transfusion-associated graft-versus-host disease. N Engl J Med 1990;323:315-21.
123. Lee T-H, Donegan E, Slichter S, Busch MP. Transient increase in circulating donor leukocytes after allogeneic transfusions in immunocompetent recipients compatible with donor cell proliferation. Blood 1995;85:1207-14.
124. Shivdasani RA, Haluska FG, Dock NL, et al. Brief report: Graft-versus-host disease associated with transfusion of blood from unrelated HLA-homozygous donors. N Engl J Med 1993;328:766-70.

125. Rubenstein A, Radl J, Cottier H, et al. Unusual combined immunodeficiency syndrome exhibiting kappa-IgD paraproteinemia, residual gut immunity and graft-versus-host reaction after plasma infusion. Acta Paediatr Scand 1973;62:365-72.
126. Linden JV, Pisciotto PT. Transfusion-associated graft-versus-host disease and blood irradiation. Transfus Med Rev 1992;6:116-23.
127. Brittingham TE, Chaplin H Jr. Febrile transfusion reactions caused by sensitivity to donor leukocytes and platelets. JAMA 1957;165: 819-25.
128. Brubaker DB. Clinical significance of white cell antibodies in febrile nonhemolytic transfusion reactions. Transfusion 1990;30:733-7.
129. Decary F, Ferner P, Giavedoni L, et al. An investigation of nonhemolytic transfusion reactions. Vox Sang 1984;46:277-85.
130. Brand A. Passenger leukocytes, cytokines, and transfusion reactions. N Engl J Med 1994;331:670-1.
131. Ferrara JLM. The febrile platelet transfusion reaction: A cytokine shower. Transfusion 1995;35:89-90.
132. Muylle L, Joos M, Wouters E, et al. Increased tumor necrosis factor α (TNFα), interleukin 1, and interleukin 6 (IL-6) levels in the plasma of stored platelet concentrates: Relationship between TNFα and IL-6 levels and febrile transfusion reactions. Transfusion 1993;33:195-9.
133. Stack G, Snyder EL. Cytokine generation in stored platelet concentrates. Transfusion 1994;34:20-25.
134. Aye MT, Palmer DS, Giulivi A, Hashemi S. Effect of filtration of platelet concentrates on the accumulation of cytokines and platelet release factors during storage. Transfusion 1995;35:117-24.
135. Muylle L, Peetermans ME. Effect of prestorage leukocyte removal on the cytokine levels in stored platelet concentrates. Vox Sang 1994;66:14-7.

In: Kickler TS, and Herman JH, eds.
Current Issues in Platelet Transfusion Therapy and Platelet Alloimmunity
Bethesda, MD: AABB Press, 1999

9

The Laboratory Approach to Suspected Immune Thrombocytopenia

MARYANN KEASHEN-SCHNELL AND
SCOTT MURPHY, MD

ANTIBODIES AGAINST PLATELETS PLAY A MAJOR ROLE in a variety of pathological processes. While clinical evaluation remains of utmost importance, serologic investigation of platelet antibodies in the laboratory is often crucial to diagnosis. This chapter describes the platelet antigen systems, the diseases that commonly result in the referral of patients, and the laboratory methods that are available for the study of these patients. These evaluations stress the approaches used in the authors' laboratory; other approaches are in use and will be discussed.

Maryann Keashen-Schnell, Supervisor, Platelet/Neutrophil Serology Laboratory, and Scott Murphy, MD, Chief Medical Officer, American Red Cross Blood Services, Penn-Jersey Region, Philadelphia, Pennsylvania

Platelet Surface Antigens

As in other areas of immunology, platelet antigens were first named for the proband or first antibody producer to bring the antigen under study.[1] The historical nomenclature for these antigens can be confusing. Most platelet-specific antigen systems are two allele systems with one high-incidence and one low-incidence antigen/allele. Glycoprotein locations have been assigned for each allele pair.[2,3] The differences in the alleles result from single amino acid differences at specific locations in the amino acid sequences of the glycoproteins. In turn, the amino acid differences are determined by specific changes in the nucleotide sequences at the DNA level.

A standardized nomenclature for platelet antigens was proposed by the Working Party on Platelet Serology and adopted by the International Society of Blood Transfusion.[1] In this new and more orderly numeric system, platelet antigens are designated as HPA (human platelet antigen) and numbered (with Arabic numbers) according to their discovery date; this number is then followed by a lowercase “a” or “b,” which denotes the high (a) or low (b) frequency of each member of the antigen pair. For example, the first and best-known antigen was referred to as Zw^a in Europe and Pl^{A1} in the United States; under the new nomenclature, it is now called HPA-1a, and the lower-frequency allele (Pl^{A2} or Zw^b) is now HPA-1b. To date, there are nine antigen systems that have defined alleles.

Table 9-1 provides a list of the HPA antigens, indicating the new and old systems of nomenclature and their glycoprotein locations.[4] The phenotypic frequencies stated are based on Caucasian population data from the United States and Europe. The precise amino acid and base pair substitutions that differentiate one platelet antigen from another have now been determined through DNA technology. The designation of these antigens as “human” platelet antigens may be misleading, however, as identical epitopes are present on the platelets of other mammalian species, including pigs, mules, and horses. Thrombocytopenia of newborns in these species as a result of placental transfer of maternal platelet antibodies has been reported.[5] These antigens also appear on cells other than platelets. HPA-1 and HPA-4 have been detected on endothelial cells, fibroblasts, and smooth muscle cells. HPA-5 is expressed on T lymphocytes and endothelial cells.

The antigen Nak is not the result of an amino acid substitution. Its positive or negative status correlates with the presence or absence of glycoprotein IV on the platelet surface.[6] Individuals lacking glycoprotein IV can produce antibodies to it after transfusion or pregnancy.[7] These antibodies can result in refractoriness to platelet transfusion. Racial differences have been reported in the frequency with which this glycoprotein is deleted.[7]

Table 9-1. Human Platelet-Specific Antigens

New Nomenclature	Old Nomenclature	Molecular Name	Phenotype Frequency (approx. %)	
			Caucasians	Asians
HPA-1a	Pl^{A1} (Zw^{a})	GPIIIa-Leu33	98	>99
HPA-1b	Pl^{A2} (Zw^{b})	GPIIIa-Pro33	27	3.7 (Japanese)
HPA-2a	Ko^{b}	GPIb-Thr145	99	?
HPA-2b	Ko^{a} (Sib^{a})	GPIb-Met145	14-17	25
HPA-3a	Bak^{a}	GPIIb-Ile843	85-90	80 (Japanese)
HPA-3b	Bak^{b}	GPIIb-Ser843	64-66	71 (Japanese)
HPA-4a	Yuk^{b} (Pen^{a})	GPIIIa-Arg143	99.9	>99.9
HPA-4b	Yuk^{a} (Pen^{b})	GPIIIa-Gln143	<0.1	0.2 (Chinese) 1.7 (Japanese)
HPA-5a	Br^{b} (Zav^{b})	GPIa-Glu505	99	99
HPA-5b	Br^{a} (Zav^{a},Hc^{a})	GPIa-Lys505	21	8.7 (Chinese) 18 (Japanese)
HPA-6W*	Ca,Tu	GPIIIa-Arg489Gln		
HPA-7W	Mo	GPIIIa-Pro407Ala		
HPA-8W	Sr	GPIIIa-Arg636Cys		
HPA-9W	Max	GPIIb-Val837Met		

*W "workshop" (both alleles not defined yet). Reproduced with permission from Garratty.[4]

In addition to HPA antigens, HLA Class I and ABH antigens are expressed in varying densities on the platelet surface.[8] Production of antibodies directed against HLA Class I antigens is the major immunologic cause of platelet transfusion failure. Therefore, the detection of antibodies against HLA antigens expressed on the platelet surface is often crucial in optimizing the efficacy of platelet transfusion therapy. The amount of ABH antigen expressed on platelets varies greatly from one individual to another.[9] Antibodies directed against ABH antigens can complicate platelet transfusion therapy[10] and may play a larger role than previously believed in thrombocytopenia of the newborn.

Clinical Indications for Serologic Investigation

Most commonly, the clinical problem caused by platelet antibodies is thrombocytopenia, but occasionally antibodies can impair the function of platelet glycoproteins, thereby causing a variety of functional defects.[11,12] Nonetheless, the investigative efforts of most platelet serology laboratories focus on thrombocytopenic states and are directed to the following categories.

Alloimmunity

Alloantibodies directed against platelet-specific HLA and ABH antigens are responsible for three distinct syndromes: neonatal alloimmune thrombocytopenia (NAIT), posttransfusion purpura (PTP), and refractoriness to platelet transfusion.

Neonatal Alloimmune Thrombocytopenia

Fetal thrombocytopenia is the result of the transfer of maternal alloantibody across the placental barrier. It is often compared with its red cell equivalent, hemolytic disease of the newborn (HDN). As with HDN, NAIT can occur as early as 20 weeks of gestation. Unlike HDN, however, NAIT is often seen in the first pregnancy. It can result in fetal death or retardation due to intracranial hemorrhage in utero. The incidence of this disease is approximately 1:2000-5000 births, with intracranial hemorrhage reported in approximately 10-15% of NAIT cases.[13] The most commonly reported fetomaternal incompatibility has been in the HPA-1 system followed by the HPA-5 system.[14,15] There is considerable controversy in this regard, but this syndrome may also result from HLA[16] and ABH antibodies as well as from antibody to platelet-specific antigens.[17]

Posttransfusion Purpura

In contrast to NAIT, in which the antibody producer does not become thrombocytopenic, PTP is associated with severe thrombocytopenia in a patient who has produced platelet-specific alloantibody(ies) shortly after blood transfusion, usually with red cell components. This rare but well-described syndrome is characterized by an abrupt drop in platelet count occurring 7-10 days after transfusion.[18] The usual patient is an older multiparous female, but many reports include both male patients with a history of prior transfusion and young female patients.[19] In the acute phase of PTP, autologous antigen-negative platelets as well as transfused platelets are destroyed. After recovery, the patient's platelets circulate normally despite the continuing presence of alloantibody. Similarities have been noted between PTP and hemolysis of autologous red cells during delayed hemolytic transfusion reactions caused by some red cell antibodies.[4] There is no definitive explanation for the destruction of autologous cells in either situation.

Refractoriness to Platelet Transfusion

Many multitransfused thrombocytopenic patients fail to have increments in the platelet count after transfusion. This can result from immune or nonimmune causes.[20] The usual cause of immune refractoriness is formation of platelet-reactive HLA Class I antibodies by the recipient. More rarely, immune refractoriness can be attributed to the production of alloantibodies directed against platelet-specific[21] and/or ABH antigens.[10]

Autoimmunity

Autoimmune Thrombocytopenic Purpura

In practice, the diagnosis of autoimmune thrombocytopenic purpura (AITP) is made by the exclusion of all other clinical causes for thrombocytopenia.[22] However, serologic evaluation may be helpful in some situations. Patients with AITP generally produce autoantibody against one or more platelet glycoproteins or portions of glycoproteins rather than against the specific antigens listed in Table 9-1. In many cases, antibody may be present only on the patient's platelets and not in the serum. Unlike red cell autoimmunity, in which direct testing of cell-bound antibody is possible even when there is severe anemia, a minimum platelet concentration in the patient's blood (generally >20,000/μL) is required to obtain sufficient cells for testing. This makes laboratory investigation of AITP difficult in the severely thrombocytopenic patient.

Drug-Induced Thrombocytopenia

Patients become thrombocytopenic during or soon after therapy with some drugs. Although many drugs have been cited as inducing thrombocytopenia, quinine (quinidine), sulfa drugs, and heparin are the most frequently incriminated. Quinine (quinidine) and sulfa drugs appear to produce conformational changes in surface glycoproteins, creating a neoantigen to which autoantibody is formed.[23] Typically, the drug must be present for antibody to react. In heparin-induced thrombocytopenia (HIT), the target of the antibody is a macromolecular complex formed by heparin (or other highly sulfated oligosaccharides) and platelet factor 4 (PF4).[24,25] This complex is bound to the surface of the patient's platelets by attachment of the Fc portion of the antibody to the platelet Fc receptor.[26] Paradoxically, heparin therapy to prevent in-vivo clotting carries the risk of thrombotic complications via activation of platelets by HIT antibodies and the subsequent formation of procoagulant, platelet-derived microparticles.[27]

Investigative Techniques Employed

As in the study of red cell serology, serologic methods used in the investigation of platelet antibodies fall into two categories: direct testing to assess the presence of antibodies bound to the surface of the patient's platelets, and indirect testing to measure antibodies present in the patient's serum. The authors' laboratory uses a combination of whole-cell and glycoprotein-based enzyme-linked immunosorbent assay (ELISA) techniques for the routine investigation of platelet allo- and autoantibodies. A function-based serotonin release assay (^{14}SREIA) adapted for ELISA testing and a PF4-ELISA assay are used for the detection of heparin-induced antibodies.

Platelet Suspension Immunofluorescence Test

The platelet suspension immunofluorescence test (PSIFT) was described by von dem Borne et al in 1978.[28] In it, platelets for panel and patient testing are isolated from EDTA-anticoagulated blood by differential centrifugation and stored at 4 C in a modified Hanks balanced salt buffer.[29] For indirect testing, serum or plasma and platelets are incubated together. Platelets are then washed, and fluorescence-tagged antihuman IgG (fluorescein isothiocyanate) is added. After another incubation, platelets are washed and examined by fluorescent microscopy. Antibodies bound to platelets are detected by the presence of cell-bound fluorescence. This assay remains in use in the authors' laboratory and is performed as originally published with minor modifications for use in microplates.

PSIFT detects antibody to platelet-specific (HPA), HLA, and ABO antigens. HLA antigens can be eluted from target platelets to aid in the distinction.[30,31] Platelets are incubated with 0.4 M chloroquine diphosphate for 2 hours at room temperature. They are then washed and used in parallel with untreated platelets in the PSIFT. The expression of HLA Class I antigens should be removed or greatly reduced, while platelet-specific antigens remain on the platelet surface. This technique is useful when a mixture of platelet-specific and HLA antibodies is suspected. However, results must be interpreted with caution. From time to time, a strong HLA antibody will continue to react with chloroquine-treated platelets.

Solid-Phase Red Cell Adherence Assay

The solid-phase red cell adherence (SPRCA) assay was first reported by Rachel et al in 1985[32] and is widely used today in its commercial form (Immucor Inc, Atlanta, GA). In the SPRCA assay (Fig 9-1), antibody is detected through the use of red cells, which are coated with antihuman globulin (AHG). Target platelets can be derived from platelet concentrates, platelet-rich plasma, or suspensions of washed and stored platelets. They are immobilized as monolayers on the surface of plastic, U-bottom microwells. Serum or plasma is added to the wells and allowed to incubate with the platelet monolayers in the presence of low-ionic-strength saline and washed. After washing of the platelet monolayers, AHG-coated indicator red cells are added and the microplates are centrifuged. If platelet antibody is present in the serum, the red cells attach to the platelet monolayer, adhering to the bottom of the microwell and forming a thin film. If there is no antibody, the red cells pellet in a bullet-type fashion. As with the PSIFT, this method also detects antibody to platelet-specific (HPA), HLA, and ABH an-

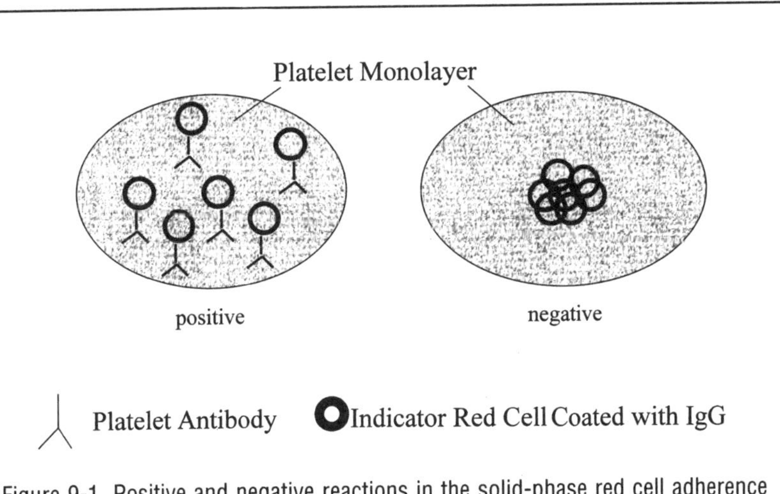

Figure 9-1. Positive and negative reactions in the solid-phase red cell adherence (SPRCA) assay. In positive reactions, antihuman globulin-coated indicator red cells form a thin film on the platelet monolayer because they are bound to it by antibody. In negative reactions, the red cells pellet in the well because they are not bound to the monolayer.

tigens. In the authors' experience, techniques for eluting HLA antigen have been even less reliable in this assay than in the PSIFT.

Microlymphocytotoxicity

This is the classical method for demonstrating the presence of HLA antibodies in serum. Since the target cell is the lymphocyte, HPA and ABH antibodies are not detected. In the Amos modification of the National Institutes of Health lymphocytotoxicity protocol,[33] serum is incubated with one of several commercially available panels of lymphocytes for 30 minutes at room temperature (22 C ± 2 C) in wells of microtiter trays under a coating of mineral oil. The panel of lymphocytes is chosen to obtain appropriate diversity of HLA Class I antigens. The trays are washed one time, complement is added, and the trays are then incubated at room temperature for 60 minutes. This is followed by staining with a mixture of acridine orange and ethidium bromide (Fluoroquench, One Lambda Inc, Canoga Park, CA). Lymphocytes in the microtiter wells are then examined under a fluorescence microscope. The acridine orange portion of the staining mixture indicates live cells by crossing intact cell membranes, intercalating with DNA, and generating green fluorescence. Dead cells emit ethidium bromide, causing red fluorescence. Reactivity for each well is scored on the basis of the percentage of cell death, according to the American Society of Histocompatibility and Immunogenetics scoring system.[34] Panel-reactive antibody (PRA) is determined by the number of positive reactions divided by the panel size.[35] Analysis of the wells that do and do not demonstrate cell death also permits the identification of those HLA antigens to which the patient has and has not formed antibody. Precise identification sometimes requires the use of an additional cross-reactive group cell panel containing additional specific cells.[36]

The Centers for Disease Control and Prevention protocol (Fig 9-2) for determining PRA follows the principle of the Amos-modified protocol with the following additional steps. After the initial incubation of lymphocytes with patient serum, the microtiter trays are washed 3 times and AHG is added to each well. After a 2-minute incubation at room temperature, complement is added and testing proceeds as in the Amos-modified protocol. This variation of the original method allows the detection of some low-titer (cytotoxicity-negative, absorption-positive) antibodies.

Monoclonal Antibody Immobilization of Platelet Antigens

An individual positive reaction in the PSIFT or the SPRCA assay does not identify the glycoprotein target of the antibody. However, the monoclonal

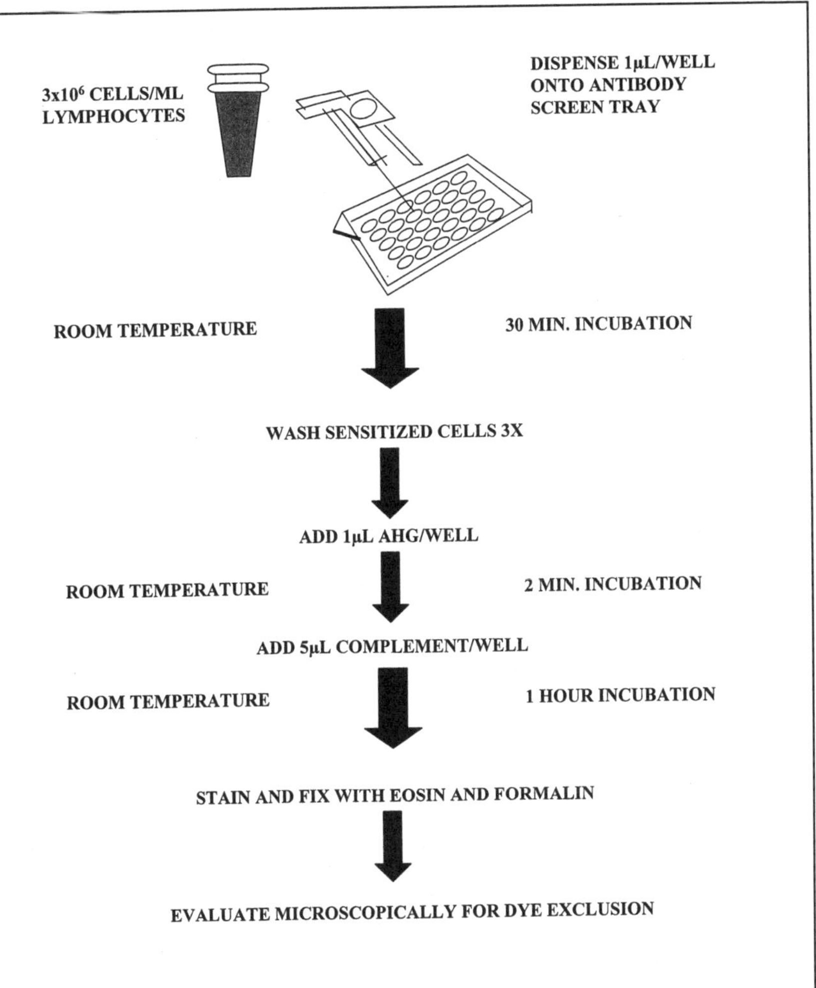

Figure 9-2. Antihuman globulin (AHG) augmented microlymphocytotoxicity assay. One microliter of the patient's serum, AHG, and complement are added sequentially to a panel of lymphocytes in wells of microtiter trays. Antibody to HLA Class I antigens causes cell lysis, which is detected microscopically.

antibody immobilization of platelet antigens (MAIPA) assay and the GTI assays (described in the next section) do provide glycoprotein specificity. Figure 9-3 outlines the MAIPA assay, which was first described by Kiefel et al in 1987.[37,38] In indirect testing, platelets are incubated with serum that may contain auto- or alloantibody and glycoprotein-specific murine monoclonal antibody. In direct testing, the patient's washed platelets are incu-

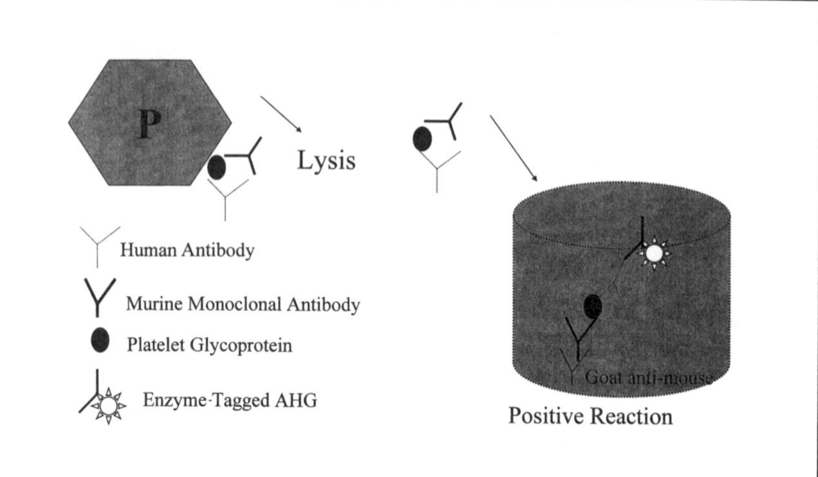

Figure 9-3. Monoclonal antibody immobilization of platelet antigens (MAIPA) assay. In an indirect test, platelets (P) are incubated with the patient's serum, a murine monoclonal antibody, and a platelet membrane glycoprotein. After cell lysis, the supernatant is added to a microwell coated with a goat antimouse antibody, which binds the monoclonal antibody. The presence of the attached human antibody is identified by an enzyme-conjugated antihuman globulin (AHG).

bated with monoclonal antibody only. The cells are lysed, and debris is cleared by centrifugation. If there is a human antibody directed against the glycoprotein identified by the monoclonal antibody, the supernatant (lysate) will contain a triplex of human antibody, murine monoclonal antibody, and platelet antigen/glycoprotein. This complex is immobilized to the wells of a flat-bottom microwell with a goat antimouse antibody, which attaches to the murine monoclonal antibody. The presence of the human antibody is detected by an enzyme-conjugated antihuman IgG. In addition to direct and indirect antibody detection, platelet antigen typing can be performed using a patient's platelets and specific human antiserum.

The advantage of this technique is that the patient's serum can be added to several wells, each containing a monoclonal antibody to a different glycoprotein. Monoclonals used are typically directed against glycoproteins IIb/IIIa, Ib/IX, Ia/IIa, and HLA Class I antigen. With varying phenotypes of the target platelets being used, the reactivity pattern can easily distinguish antibodies directed against different glycoproteins such as HLA and the various HPA antigens. However, there are problems with this assay that must be recognized. Some monoclonal antibodies interfere with the detection of human antibodies because they bind to the identical location on the glycoprotein as the patient's antibody.[39] Individual laboratories need to evaluate the monoclonal antibodies used with this in mind. Furthermore, some human sera contain antibody to murine immunoglobulin, which can result in a false-positive reaction in the standard assay. Two-stage assays that include a step to remove such antibody have been described.[39]

GTI Platelet Antibody Detection Systems

GTI-PAK™-12 and GTI-PAK™Plus (GTI Inc, Brookfield, WI) are ELISA test systems in which the patient's serum is added to microwell strips precoated with purified platelet glycoprotein from group O donors who have been selected to provide specific phenotypes expressed on glycoproteins IIb/IIIa and Ia/IIa. In addition, glycoprotein from a pool of donors provides glycoprotein Ib/IX, glycoprotein IV, and HLA Class I. Attachment of antibody to the glycoprotein is revealed by standard ELISA methodology (Fig 9-4). The GTI-PAK™-12 microwell strips contain wells with HPA-1a, -1b,-3a, -3b, -5a, and -5b. The PAK ™Plus system detects antibody directed against glycoprotein IV. These commercially available alternatives to the MAIPA assay allow glycoprotein-specific antibody detection with a very rapid turnaround time (2-3 hours). The GTI-PAK™-12 system reliably detects HLA antibody when the PRA is high. However, the authors have observed apparently false-positive reactions in the sera of patients treated with intravenous immunoglobulin and humanized mouse monoclonal antibodies as well as several false-negative results with sera containing monospecific HLA antibody.

Techniques for the Detection of Drug-Dependent Antibodies

Heparin-Induced Thrombocytopenia

The serotonin release assay (^{14}C-SRA) is a functional assay and is the most widely used to detect HIT antibody.[40] Normal platelets are radiolabeled with ^{14}C serotonin, which is concentrated within the dense granules of the platelets. The labeled platelets are washed and incubated with the patient's serum in the presence of two concentrations of heparin (low, 0.1-0.3 U/mL; and high, 10-100 U/mL). It is presumed that enough PF4 is present to bind to heparin and antibody and that this triplex binds to the Fc reception, leading to platelet activation and serotonin release. The percentage of serotonin released is quantified by liquid scintillation counting. The criterion for a positive result is the combination of serotonin release (>20% of

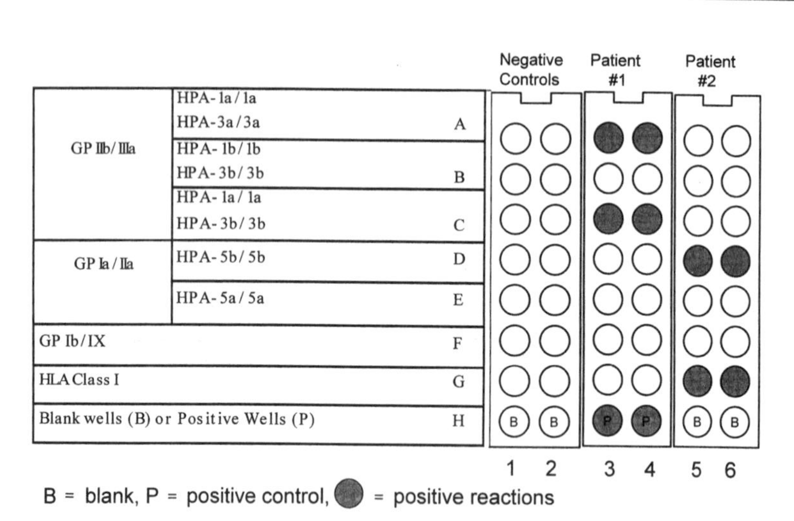

Figure 9-4. GTI-PAK™-12 system. Wells A-E contain glycoproteins with specific HPAs. Well F provides glycoprotein Ib/IX, and well G contains a mixture of HLA Class I antigens. Binding of antibody is revealed by standard ELISA technology. Patient #1 has anti-HPA-1a. One cannot exclude anti-HPA-3a being present as well. Patient #2 has anti-HPA-5b and HLA Class I antibody.

total incorporated) for patient serum and low heparin concentration and of background release (<20% of total incorporated) for both patient serum alone and for patient serum and high concentration of heparin. The presumed reason for the lower release at high concentrations of heparin is the disruption or dissociation of heparin/PF4 complexes from antibody because of antigen excess.

The authors' laboratory and most others do not have access to liquid scintillation counting. Therefore, the serotonin release enzyme immunoassay (SREIA) was developed in the authors' laboratory using an ELISA rather than a radioisotopic endpoint. The SREIA technique combines the traditional serotonin release principle (ability of HIT-IgG with heparin and PF4 to activate platelets, causing serotonin release) with a commercially available ELISA test system for the measurement of serotonin.[41] Patient and control sera are incubated with washed platelets in the presence of low and high concentrations of heparin. Maximum serotonin release is determined by the incubation of the platelets with thrombin, 4 U/mL. The resulting supernatants are assayed for serotonin content using the serotonin

ELISA immunoassay (Immunotech Inc, Westbrook, ME). A release of more than 20% of the serotonin released by thrombin at a low heparin concentration and a less than 20% release for patient serum alone and at the higher heparin concentration is considered a positive reaction. The authors are in the process of comparing results of this assay with those obtained with the classical ^{14}C-SRA technique.

Heparin/PF4 ELISA assays measure antibody directed against a complex of heparin and PF4 bound to the surface of microtiter wells.[24,42] Patient serum is added to coated microtiter wells, incubated, and washed. Antibody binding is detected with a standard ELISA technique. Assays of this type detect antibodies directed against heparin/PF4 and, more rarely, PF4 alone. These assays are technically simpler and less time-consuming than serotonin release assays. Others have already reported similar comparisons.[42] A study comparing a commercially available ELISA assay developed by GTI Inc with the SREIA and the ^{14}C-SRA is under way at the American Red Cross's Penn-Jersey Region laboratory. It has not yet been determined which of these assays will prove to have the best combination of accuracy and practicality.

Thrombocytopenia Due to Drugs Other Than Heparin

Platelet antibodies due to some drugs other than heparin can be detected using the PSIFT with the following modifications. A pool of target platelets from 3 or 4 group O donors is incubated with patient serum and negative and positive controls in both the presence and absence of drug solution. Drug solution is prepared by dissolving the suspected drug in phosphate-buffered saline/bovine serum albumin (0.2%) to a final drug concentration of 1 mg/mL.[43,44] Target platelets are also tested with drug solution alone to establish background reactivity. Next, the platelets are washed using the drug solution as the wash buffer for all reaction wells where the drug is present. The platelets are then examined microscopically for the presence of membrane fluorescence on platelets incubated with patient serum and drug and for the absence of fluorescence on platelets incubated with patient serum or drug alone. This combination is indicative of drug-dependent antibody.

A large number of drugs are suspected of causing drug-induced thrombocytopenia. However, positive control sera are not available for the vast majority. Therefore, testing for these drugs is difficult. Quinine (quinidine) and sulfa drugs react in this fluorescence test system, and well-characterized positive controls are available.

Other Techniques

Molecular techniques, such as polymerase chain reaction and flow cytometry, may also prove to be useful.

Molecular Techniques

Although advances in methodology have allowed more precise antibody identification, identification of the antigens on patients' platelets has been hampered by the limited availability of well-characterized antisera from immunized patients, the need for fresh platelets, and the minimum platelet concentration required for testing. New molecular techniques using the polymerase chain reaction[45-47] are not limited by these factors because platelets are replaced by any nucleated cell that provides DNA from the patient and antisera are replaced by sequence-specific primers and probes. Thus, these advances have allowed molecular genotyping for HPA-1 through HPA-6.

Flow Cytometry

Some investigators have found that the methods for antibody detection described are too insensitive to detect antibody in some situations. They have reported that flow cytometric methods can be used to enhance sensitivity.[48]

A Diagnostic Approach to Specific Conditions

With many techniques available, it is important for a platelet serology laboratory to choose the procedures that are most efficient in the diagnosis of immune thrombocytopenias. The approach will vary according to the potential diagnosis and will most often include a combination of assays from the categories mentioned previously. The approach used in the American Red Cross's Penn-Jersey Region laboratory follows.

Neonatal Alloimmune Thrombocytopenia

When this diagnosis is suspected, the hospital provides maternal serum and platelets from both the mother and the father. Little is added by asking for specimens from the newborn. On the day that the specimens arrive, the GTI-PAK™-12 is used to look for antibody in the mother's serum. This method has the advantage of clearly distinguishing between HPA antibody and the HLA antibody that is also commonly present. The SPRCA assay is also used to perform a crossmatch between the mother's serum and the father's platelets. Finally, the platelets of the mother and father are typed serologically for HPA-1a. All these methods are rapid enough to permit transmittal of a preliminary report to the referring hospital within 4-5 hours.

On a subsequent day, results are confirmed. The PSIFT is used for serologic antigen typing for HPA-1a and HPA-3a and for confirmation of the maternal antibody by screening against paternal platelets and a panel of platelets with known HPA types. If HPA-5 antibody has been detected with GTI-PAK™-12, confirmatory studies are carried out with the MAIPA assay using a monoclonal antibody to glycoprotein Ia-IIa. HPA-5 typing is also performed with the MAIPA assay. One needs to use this assay for studies of the HPA-5 system because of the low number of copies of glycoprotein Ia-IIa on each platelet—approximately 2000 relative to 25,000 for glycoprotein IIb-IIIa.[15] Whole cell assays such as the PSIFT and the SPRCA are too insensitive to detect such low levels of antibody binding.

The MAIPA assay can also be used to study the rare situation in which antibody in maternal serum reacts with paternal platelets in the SPRCA assay and/or the PSIFT, but the antigenic specificity of the antibody cannot be identified with GTI-PAK™-12. Using a series of monoclonal antibodies, researchers can determine the glycoprotein specificity in some cases.

Figure 9-5 shows the results of a study of 441 patients with the diagnosis of NAIT. In approximately one-third of the cases, no antibody was present. In another 29%, only HLA Class I antibody was found. In approximately 20%, HPA-1a antibody was found with a coexisting HLA Class I antibody in 34% of the cases. This combination emphasizes the value of GTI-PAK™-12, which immediately identifies anti-HPA-1a in the presence of HLA antibody (Fig 9-4). Antibody to HPA-3a and HPA-5b was much less common, with a total of 11 cases relative to the 91 HPA-1a cases. It may be that the percentage of patients with HPA-5 incompatibility will rise now that assay methods for these antibodies are more sensitive. Also, 15 patients had ABH antibody and 29 had autoantibody. Finally, in 22 patients, alloantibody was detected but the specificity could not be determined.

In approximately 10% of patients in whom no antibody was identified, a typical incompatibility existed: a father carrying HPA-1a and an HPA-1b homozygote mother. Such cases have been considered examples of NAIT due to HPA-1 incompatibility. It is assumed that the strength of the HPA-1a antibody is relatively weak, at least in vitro.

Posttransfusion Purpura

In contrast to some cases of NAIT, the authors have found that antibodies produced against HPA antigens in patients with PTP are uniformly quite

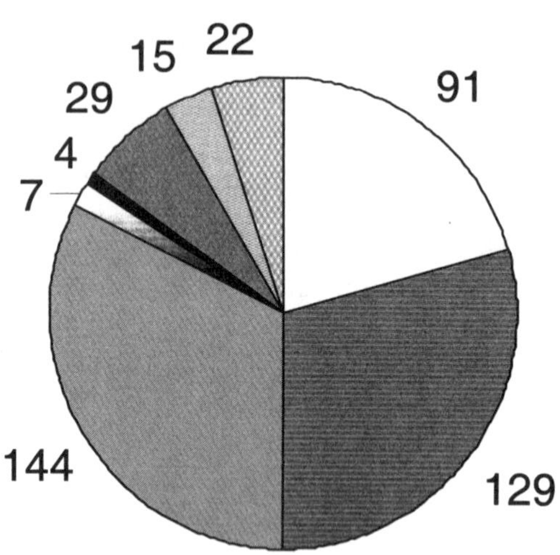

Figure 9-5. Antibodies identified in 441 patients referred for investigation of neonatal alloimmune thrombocytopenia (NAIT). Of these, 144 patients had no antibody, 129 had HLA Class I antibody only, 91 had anti-HPA-1a, 29 had autoantibody, 22 had alloantibody with no definable specificity, 15 had ABH antibody, seven had anti-HPA-5b, and four had anti-HPA-3a.

strong in the acute phase and detectable by all assay methods. Figure 9-6 shows the distribution of 25 patients referred for investigation of PTP in which antibody to HPA was found. Twenty of the 25 positive sera contained HPA-1a antibody, whereas examples of antibody to HPA-1b, HPA-3a, and HPA-5b were found in only a minority of cases. Fifteen of these 25 sera samples also contained antibody to HLA Class I antigen, emphasizing the need to use a glycoprotein-based assay such as GTI-PAK™-12 for the rapid identification of HPA antibodies when HLA antibodies are also present. With GTI-PAK™-12, a report can be sent to the referring hospital within a matter of hours. The result is always confirmed at a later date by PSIFT; the hospital is asked to provide platelets from the patient for typing when the platelet count has returned to normal.

The 25 samples cited were drawn from a total of 74 patients with a differential diagnosis of PTP. Figure 9-7 depicts the platelet count nadirs in the two patient groups with and without HPA antibodies. All but one of the sera with HPA antibody had nadir platelet counts below 20,000/μL, while those without HPA antibody commonly had nadir platelet counts above

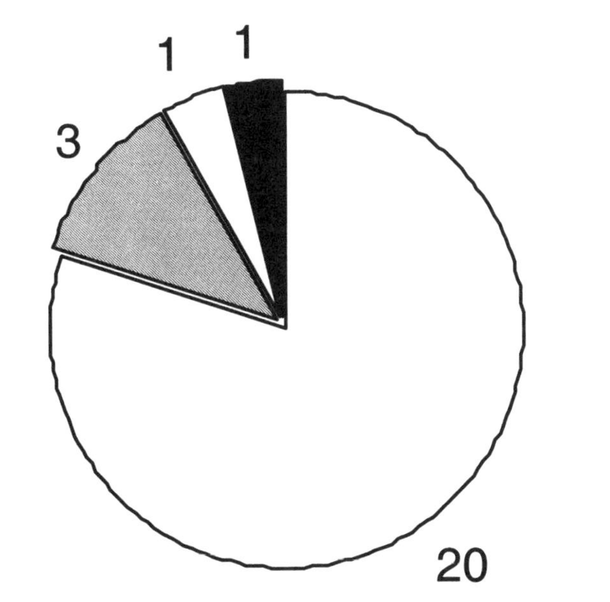

Figure 9-6. Antibodies identified in 25 patients referred for investigation of post-transfusion purpura (PTP). During the same time interval, no HPA antibodies were found in 49 referred patients. Among patients with HPA antibody, 20 had anti-HPA-1a, three had anti-HPA-1b, and one each had anti-HPA-3a and anti-HPA-5b.

20,000/mL. Medical histories suggest that many of the patients without HPA antibody were cardiac patients receiving heparin. It is common for the degree of thrombocytopenia in HIT to be relatively modest (30,000–80,000/µL). These results suggest that evaluation for PTP may commonly be requested in patients who, in fact, have HIT. Six of these HPA antibody-negative sera samples were assayed for HIT antibodies; 2 samples had positive results.

Management of Refractoriness to Platelet Transfusion

This approach is described in greater detail elsewhere.[49] Briefly, when refractoriness to platelet transfusion is suspected, the hospital provides not only lymphocytes for HLA typing but also a serum specimen so that antibody screening can be performed with microlymphocytotoxicity. Most true immunologic refractoriness is due to HLA antibodies, which can be

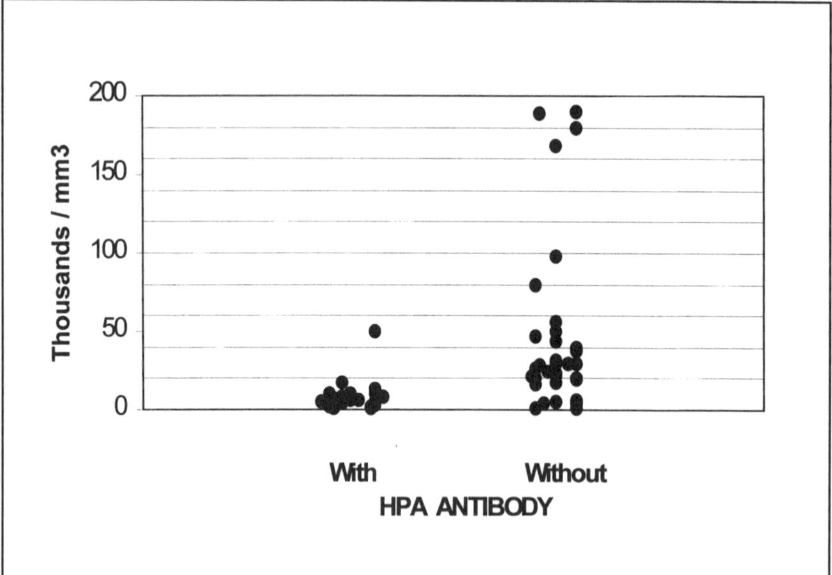

Figure 9-7. Nadir platelet counts in 74 patients evaluated for posttransfusion purpura (PTP). Of these, 25 patients had anti-HPA antibodies (left column). All but one had a nadir platelet count of less than 20,000/µL. In 49 patients without anti-HPA antibody (right column), platelet counts above 20,000/µL were common.

identified with this technique. If this screen is negative, the SPRCA assay is used to test the patient's serum against a panel of 10-20 randomly selected platelets. In 90% of cases with negative microlymphocytotoxicity, either this assessment is negative or the reactivity observed is compatible with IgG ABH antibody in a group O patient. If only ABH antibody is identified, the hospital uses only platelets from group O donors to treat the patient. In the less than 10% of cases in which other specificities appear to be possible in the SPRCA assay, the GTI-PAK™-12 and the MAIPA assay are used to look for HPA antibodies. If no antibody specificity is found, these patients can be managed by crossmatching randomly selected platelets with SPRCA.

In practice, approximately one-half of patients referred for matched platelet support have no evidence of HLA or HPA antibody in the laboratory. This reflects the fact that much refractoriness results from poorly understood clinical factors and not from alloimmunization.[20] However, if the microlymphocytotoxicity assay is negative, it is wise to ask for another specimen 3-4 weeks later to exclude the infrequent but important possibility that alloimmunization was just beginning at the time of the initial screen. If these 2 screens are both negative along with negative findings from an SPRCA investigation, matched platelets are rarely more beneficial than randomly selected products.

If antibody is found by microlymphocytotoxicity, the PRA is determined—that is, the percentage of wells in which cytotoxicity is observed. Also the results are analyzed to determine the HLA Class I antigens to which the patient has formed antibody. In general, if the PRA is less than 70%, one can successfully manage the patient by providing antigen-negative platelets (ie, platelets that lack the HLA antigens to which the patient has antibody).[50] If the PRA is greater than 70% and/or the hospital reports unsatisfactory platelet count increments to products being supplied, the SPRCA assay is used to crossmatch antigen-negative products. Finally, in these difficult cases, donors who are particularly good matches for the patient (ie, A or BU matches, platelets that have no antigens other than those that the patient has) are recruited.[51]

The success of this approach relies on the availability of a large (>2000) HLA-typed donor pool as well as on an HLA laboratory willing and able to determine the specificities of the antigens to which the patient has antibody. Other centers prefer to crossmatch using the SPRCA assay against a panel of randomly selected platelet products. Evidence in the literature[52] suggests that this approach is satisfactory for mild to moderately alloimmunized patients (ie, those with PRA less than 70%). However, for more highly immunized patients, it would be common to have nothing but incompatible components with random crossmatching. In such cases, identification of antibody specificities and the recruitment of A and BU matches can be most helpful.

Autoimmune Thrombocytopenic Purpura

A review by Kelton[53] traced the evolution of serologic methods for the study of AITP. Initially, indirect assays were used in which the patient's serum produced platelet lysis in the presence of complement or stimulated a platelet function such as aggregation or serotonin release. Except for the investigation of HIT, function-based assays are now used rarely in immunologic studies of platelets. Complement fixation and function-based assays were followed by the measurement of platelet-associated immunoglobulin (PAIgG), either that on the cell surface or the total contained in platelets following lysis. However, several investigators noted that, although elevated levels of PAIgG correlated with the severity of thrombocytopenia in AITP, equal degrees of elevation were observed in both immune and nonimmune thrombocytopenic disorders. For the most part, assays in this category are sensitive for the diagnosis of AITP but lack specificity. It is assumed that much of the increased PAIgG in immune and nonimmune thrombocytopenia represents "nonspecific" adherent IgG and not platelet antibody per se.

Knowledge of the structure of platelet glycoproteins and their epitopes and the production and commercial availability of monoclonal antibodies against individual platelet glycoproteins led to the development of glycoprotein-specific assays such as the MAIPA assay. These newer assays have the potential for distinguishing between nonspecific adherent IgG and true antibody against platelet membrane glycoprotein.

These approaches have potential but need greater refinement if they are to be widely applied. If the patient's platelet count is high enough to provide sufficient platelets for direct testing, the PSIFT can be used as a semiquantitative measure of the amount of surface immunoglobulin, and the MAIPA assay can be used to look for antibody specifically directed toward platelet glycoproteins. The problems with nonspecific increases in PAIgG have already been discussed. In typical cases of AITP, the MAIPA assay reveals evidence of glycoprotein-specific antibody in approximately 25% of cases.[54] On the other hand, positive results are rare in patients who clinically do not have AITP. Thus, MAIPA shows high specificity but low sensitivity.

Investigations are under way regarding the origins of this difficulty. The glycoprotein specificities of the monoclonal antibodies used include GPIIb/IIIa, GPIIIa/GPIX, GPIa, and HLA Class I. Those in routine use in the American Red Cross's Penn-Jersey Region laboratory are CD41 (Clone P2, GPIIb/IIIa), CD 49b (Clone Gi9, GPIa), and CD 42a (Clone S21, GPIX) (all from Immunotech); PL164 (GPIIIa, supplied by Dr. Cecile Kaplan, Paris, France); FMC25 (GPIX from Flinders Medical Centre, Bedford Park, Australia); and W6/32 (HLA Class I ABC locus from Harlan Sera Lab, Crawley Down, Sussex, England).

In studies of AITP, a monoclonal antibody to CD61 (Clone SZ21 GPIIIa) essentially never yields a positive result in the MAIPA assay, which suggests that it may bind to the same epitope to which autoantibody binds. Therefore, the authors no longer use it in AITP studies. More research needs to be done to identify the optimal monoclonal antibodies to use in this type of work.

References

1. von dem Borne AEGKr, DeCary F. ISCH/ISBT Working Party on Platelet Serology. Nomenclature of platelet-specific antigens (letter). Transfusion 1990;30:477.

2. von dem Borne AEGKr, Kaplan C, Minchinton R. Nomenclature of human platelet alloantigens. Blood 1995;85:1409-10.
3. Newman PJ. Nomenclature of human platelet-alloantigens: A problem with the HPA system? Blood 1994;83:1447-51.
4. Garratty G. Review: Platelet immunology similarities and differences with red cell immunology. Immunohematology 1995;11:112-24.
5. Buecher-Maxwell V, Scott MA, Godber L, Kristensen A. Neonatal alloimmune thrombocytopenia in a quarterhorse foal. J Vet Intern Med 1997;11:304-8.
6. Yamamoto N, Ikeda H, Tandon NN, et al. A platelet membrane glycoprotein (GP) deficiency in healthy blood donors: Nak[a-] platelets lack detectable GPIV (CD36). Blood 1990;76:1698-703.
7. Curtis BR, Aster RH. Incidence of the Nak-negative platelet phenotype in African Americans is similar to Asians. Transfusion 1996; 36:331-4.
8. Santoso S, Kiefel V, Mueller-Eckhardt C. Blood group A and B determinants are expressed on platelet glycoproteins IIa, IIIa, and Ib. Thromb Haemost 1991;65:196-201.
9. Ogasawara K, Ueki J, Takenaka M, Furihata K. Study on the expression of ABH antigens on platelets. Blood 1993;82:993-9.
10. Lee EJ, Schiffer CA. ABO compatibility can influence the results of platelet transfusion. Results of a randomized trial. Transfusion 1989; 29:384-9.
11. Keashen-Schnell M, Schuster SJ, Joiner K, et al. Clinical bleeding and thrombasthenic defect due to autoantibody directed against glycoprotein IIb/IIIa (abstract). Transfusion 1997;37(suppl):S158.
12. Yanabu M, Suzuki M, Soga T, et al. Influences of antiplatelet autoantibodies on platelet function in immune thrombocytopenic purpura. Eur J Haematol 1991;46:101-6.
13. Goldman M, Filion M, Prouiz C, et al. Neonatal alloimmune thrombocytopenia. Transfus Med Rev 1994;8:123-31.
14. Kiefel V, Santoso S, Katzmann B, Mueller-Eckhardt C. A new platelet-specific alloantigen Br[a]. Vox Sang 1988;54:101-6.
15. Kiefel V, Santoso S, Katzmann B, Mueller-Eckhardt C. The Br[a]/Br[b] alloantigen system on human platelets. Blood 1989:73:2219-23.
16. Lalezari P. HLA incompatibility is the most common cause of alloimmune neonatal thrombocytopenia (ANT) (abstract). Blood 1993;82:203a.
17. Kelton JG, Smith JW, Horsewood P, et al. ABH antigens on human platelets: Expression of the glycosyl phosphatidylinositol-anchored protein CD109. J Lab Clin Med 1998;132:142-8.

18. Shulman NR, Aster RH, Leitner A, et al. Immuno-reactions involving platelets. Post-transfusion purpura due to a complement-fixing antibody against a genetically controlled platelet antigen. A proposed mechanism for thrombocytopenia and its relevance in "autoimmunity." J Clin Invest 1961;40:1597.
19. Keashen-Schnell MA, Munizza M, Joiner K, et al. 53 cases of suspected post-transfusion purpura (abstract). Transfusion 1995;35 (suppl):S69.
20. Bishop JF, McGrath K, Wolf MM, et al. Clinical factors influencing the efficacy of pooled platelet transfusions. Blood 1988;71:383-7.
21. Herman JH, Kamel HT. Platelet transfusion. Current techniques, remaining problems, and future prospects. Am J Pediatr Hematol Oncol 1987;9:272-86.
22. George JN, Woolf SH, Raskob GE, et al. Idiopathic thrombocytopenic purpura: A practice guideline developed by explicit methods for the American Society of Hematology. Blood 1996;88:3-40.
23. Shulman NR, Reid DM. Mechanisms of drug-induced immunologically mediated cytopenias. Transfus Med Rev 1993;7:215-29.
24. Aminal J, Bridey F, Dreyfus M, et al. Platelet factor 4 complexed to heparin is the target for antibodies generated in heparin-induced thrombocytopenia. Thromb Haemost 1992;68:95-6.
25. Visentin GP, Ford SE, Scott JP, Aster RH. Antibodies from patients with heparin-induced thrombocytopenia/thrombosis are specific for platelet factor 4 complexed with heparin or bound to endothelial cells. J Clin Invest 1994;93:81-8.
26. Warkentin TE, Chong BH, Greinacher A. Heparin-induced thrombocytopenia: Towards consensus. Thromb Haemost 1998;79:1-7.
27. Warkentin TE. Heparin-induced thrombocytopenia, IgG-mediated platelet activation, platelet microparticle generation and altered procoagulant/anticoagulant balance in the pathogenesis of thrombosis and venous limb gangrene complicating heparin-induced thrombocytopenia. Transfus Med Rev 1996;10:249-58.
28. von dem Borne AEGKr, Verheught FWA, Oosterhuf F, et al. A simple fluorescence test for the detection of platelet antibodies. Br J Haematol 1978;39:195-207.
29. Kiss JE, Salamon DJ, Wilson J, et al. A method for platelet storage for use in platelet compatibility testing. Blood 1986;68(suppl):1074.
30. Nordhagen R, Flaathen S. Chloroquine removal of HLA antigens from platelets for the platelet immunofluorescence test. Vox Sang 1985;48: 156-9.

31. Blumberg N, Masel D, Mayert T, et al. Removal of HLA-A, B antigens from platelets. Blood 1984;63:448-50.
32. Rachel JM, Sinor LT, Tawlik OW, et al. A solid-phase red cell adherence test for platelet crossmatching. Med Lab Sci 1985;42:194-5.
33. Amos DB, Bashir H, Boyle W, et al. A simple micro cytotoxicity test. Transplantation 1969;7:220-3.
34. ASHI laboratory manual. 3rd ed. Lenexa, KS: American Society for Histocompatibility and Immunogenetics, 1994.
35. Tardif GN, MacQueen JM, eds. Tissue typing reference manual. 3rd ed. Richmond, VA: Southeastern Organ Procurement Foundation (SEOPF), 1993.
36. Fuller TC. Monitoring HLA alloimmunization. Analysis of HLA alloantibodies in the serum of prospective transplant recipients. J Clin Lab Med 1991;11:551-70.
37. Kiefel V, Santoso S, Weisheit M, Mueller-Eckhardt C. Monoclonal antibody-specific immobilization of platelet antigens (MAIPA): A new tool for the identification of platelet-reactive antibodies. Blood 1987;70:1722-6.
38. Kiefel V. The MAIPA assay and its applications in immunohematology. Transfus Med 1992;2:181-8.
39. Morel-Kopp MC, Daviet L, McGregor J, et al. Drawbacks of the MAIPA technique in characterizing human anti-platelet antibodies. Blood Coagul Fibrinolysis 1996;7:144-6.
40. Sheridan D, Carter C, Kelton JG. A diagnostic test for heparin-induced thrombocytopenia. Blood 1986;67:27-30.
41. Joiner K, Nance S, Keashen-Schnell MA, Murphy S. Heparin antibody detection. The first report of a novel enzyme immunoassay to measure serotonin release (abstract). Transfusion 1996;36(suppl):S238.
42. Arepally G, Reynolds C, Tomaski A, et al. Comparison of PF4/heparin ELISA assay with the ^{14}C-serotonin release assay in the diagnosis of heparin-induced thrombocytopenia. Am J Clin Pathol 1995;104: 648-54.
43. Petz LD, Branch DR. Drug-induced immune hemolytic anemia. In: Chaplin H, ed. Methods in hematology: Immune hemolytic anemias. New York: Churchill Livingstone 1985:47-94.
44. Walker RH, ed. Technical manual. 11th ed. Bethesda, MD: American Association of Blood Banks, 1993.
45. McFarland JG, Aster RH, Bussel JB, et al. Prenatal diagnosis of neonatal alloimmune thrombocytopenia using allele-specific oligonucleotide probes. Blood 1991;78:2276-82.

46. Skogen B, Bellissimo DB, Hessler MJ, et al. Rapid determination of platelet alloantigen genotypes by polymerase chain reaction using allele-specific primers. Transfusion 1994;34:955-60.
47. Kroll H, Kiefel V, Santoso S. Clinical aspects and typing of platelet alloantigens. Vox Sang 1998;74(suppl 2):345-54.
48. Kohler M, Dittmann J, Legler TJ, et al. Flow cytometric detection of platelet-reactive antibodies and application in platelet crossmatching. Transfusion 1996;36:250-5.
49. Murphy S, Varma M. Selecting platelets for transfusion of the alloimmunized patient: A review. Immunohematology 1998;14:117-23.
50. Petz LD, Garratty G, Clark BD, et al. The effectiveness of an antibody specificity prediction (ASP) method for selecting platelets for transfusion to alloimmunized patients (abstract). Blood 1995;86:546a.
51. Duquesnoy RJ, Filip DJ, Rodey GE, et al. Successful transfusion of platelets "mismatched" for HLA antigens to alloimmunized thrombocytopenic patients. Am J Hematol 1997;2:219-26.
52. Gelb AB, Leavitt AD. Crossmatch-compatible platelets improve corrected count increments in patients who are refractory to randomly selected platelets. Transfusion 1997;37:624-30.
53. Kelton JG. The serological investigation of patients with autoimmune thrombocytopenia. Thromb Haemost 1995;74;228-33.
54. Joiner K, Nance S, Keashen-Schnell MA, Murphy S. Detection of platelet autoantibodies using the monoclonal antibody immobilization of platelet antigens (MAIPA) assay (abstract). Transfusion 1995; 35(suppl):S68.

In: Kickler TS, and Herman JH, eds.
Current Issues in Platelet Transfusion Therapy and Platelet Alloimmunity
Bethesda, MD: AABB Press, 1999

10

Adverse Reactions to Platelet Transfusions

JOHN D. ROBACK, MD, PhD, AND
CHRISTOPHER D. HILLYER, MD

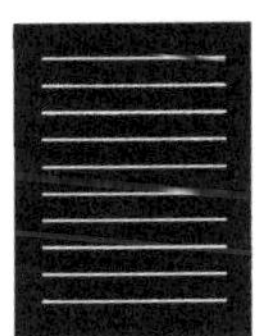

ADVERSE REACTIONS TO PLATELET TRANSFUSIONS ARE not uncommon. Their reported incidence is 5-30%, and in multitransfused patients, the rate may be significantly higher.[1-4] These reactions range from mild urticaria to life-threatening sepsis.[1,2] Because platelet recipients are often acutely ill, such as those who have just undergone marrow transplantation, these adverse reactions can lead to increased morbidity and mortality. Platelet transfusion reactions can be categorized as either *infectious* or *noninfectious*, as shown in Table 10-1. This chapter discusses these adverse sequelae with emphasis on recent insights into pathogenesis, ap-

John D. Roback, MD, PhD, Fellow, Transfusion Medicine Program, and Christopher D. Hillyer, MD, Associate Professor, Department of Pathology and Laboratory Medicine, and Director, Transfusion Medicine Program, Emory University School of Medicine, Atlanta, Georgia

Table 10-1. Adverse Reactions to Platelet Transfusions

Infectious	Noninfectious
Viral	Allergic
HIV-1 and -2	Urticarial
HBV, HCV	Anaphylactic
HTLV-I and -II	TRALI
CMV	Hypotensive
Other	Febrile nonhemolytic
Bacterial	Alloimmunization
	Immunomodulation
	TA-GVHD

HIV = human immunodeficiency virus; HBV = hepatitis B virus; HCV = hepatitis C virus; HTLV = human T-cell lymphotropic virus; CMV = cytomegalovirus; TRALI = transfusion-related acute lung injury; TA-GVHD = transfusion-associated graft-vs-host disease

proaches to treatment and prevention, and issues that remain to be resolved.

Infectious Complications—Viral

Human Immunodeficiency Virus-I and -II, Hepatitis B Virus, Hepatitis C Virus, and Human T-Cell Lymphotropic Virus-I and -II

Incidence and Significance

The risk of transfusion-transmitted virus infections has been estimated by examining the rates of seroconversion in repeat blood donors and calculating the probability that donations were made during the "window period."[5] By applying these incidence rates to the entire donor pool, researchers have been able to derive estimates for the risk of acquiring the following viruses via blood transfusion of screened units: Human immunodeficiency virus (HIV), 1 in 493,000 units (95% confidence interval [CI] = 202,000-2,778,000 [does not include HIV p24 antigen screening]); hepatitis B virus (HBV), 1 in 63,000 (95% CI = 31,000-147,000); hepatitis C virus (HCV), 1 in 103,000 (95% CI = 28,000-288,000); and human T-cell lymphotropic virus (HTLV), 1 in 641,000 (95% CI = 256,000-2,000,000).[5] With the recent implementation of HIV p24 antigen screening to detect infectious donations before the recipient has an antibody response, the incidence of HIV transmission by transfusion is likely to decline from the given estimate.[5] There is also increasing recognition that selected populations are at risk for the transfusion transmission of other viruses in addition to those cited above, including Epstein-Barr virus and cytomegalovirus (CMV) (the latter of which is discussed in more detail below).

When the transmitted viruses produce disease, the disease usually takes several years to develop. For HIV, the progression to acquired immunodeficiency syndrome (AIDS) appears inexorable, with a mean interval of approximately 10 years.[6,7] However, treatment of HIV-infected individuals with recently available antiviral therapies, including protease inhibitors, may alter this natural history. While the majority of HCV infections become chronic,[8,9] the long-term clinical significance of transfusion-transmitted HCV infections is not clear. In a retrospective study of 545 patients who harbored transfusion-transmitted "non-A, non-B hepatitis" for an average of 18 years, there was no increased risk of overall mortality and only a marginally significant increase in deaths due to liver disease as compared with matched controls.[10] Similarly, patients who contracted HBV via a contaminated yellow fever vaccine failed to show significant morbidity, including the development of hepatocellular carcinoma.[11] Transfusion-transmitted HBV may be reduced even further by widespread vaccination. Finally, whereas the frequency of HTLV-I/II transmission by transfusion of seropositive cellular components may vary from 12.8% to 44%[12,13] (or up to 80% with short-storage units and in some Japanese studies[12,14]), infected individuals have less than a 4% lifetime risk of developing adult T-cell leukemia-lymphoma or the progressive neurologic disease, tropical spastic paraparesis/HTLV-I-associated myelopathy.[15,16]

Prevention

Currently, the only means for preventing transfusion transmission of these viruses is through the screening of blood donors. However, recent studies indicate that inactivating viruses and other pathogens that contaminate blood components may become feasible. Derivatives of psoralen, when activated by long-wave ultraviolet light (UV-A), can crosslink DNA and thus block viral and bacterial replication. S-59, a proprietary, novel psoralen, can inactivate more than $10^{6.6}$ plaque-forming units per milliliter of HIV (free or cell-associated), more than $10^{6.8}$ infectious doses per milliliter of duck hepatitis B virus (HBV model), more than $10^{6.5}$ plaque-forming units per milliliter of bovine viral diarrhea virus (HCV model), more than $10^{6.6}$ colony-forming units (CFU)/mL *Staphylococcus epidermidis*, and more than $10^{5.6}$ CFU/mL *Klebsiella pneumonia*.[17] The treatment requires 3 to 4 minutes of UV-A exposure, and preliminary studies suggest that platelet function is not adversely affected. Other psoralen derivatives, such as aminomethyltrimethylpsoralen, also appear promising for blood component sterilization.[18]

Cytomegalovirus

Clinical Features of Transfusion-Transmitted Cytomegalovirus Infection

As compared with HIV, HBV, HCV, and HTLV, there are a number of fundamentally different issues associated with transfusion-transmitted CMV (TT-CMV) infections. First, the majority of the population (60-80%) is CMV seropositive[19,20]; thus, eliminating seropositive donors would significantly deplete the donor base. Second, recent studies suggest that some seronegative individuals harbor latent CMV infections that can be reactivated,[21] raising the possibility that some infectious units will not be detected by serology. Third, because CMV is highly cell-associated, the incidence of TT-CMV can be significantly reduced by leukocyte reduction.[22] However, it is still unclear what percentage of filtered seropositive units continue to harbor infectious CMV.[23-25] Finally, TT-CMV is of limited consequence in immunocompetent individuals since primary CMV infection in this population is often asymptomatic and rapidly controlled by the immune system.[26] In contrast, primary infection in immunocompromised patients is often clinically significant and can rapidly progress to retinal, gastrointestinal, and/or pulmonary disease, as well as to hematopoietic dysfunction.[19,20] Thus, it is critical that immunocompromised hosts (including patients with AIDS, immunosuppressed recipients of solid organ or marrow transplants, and fetuses of seronegative mothers[20,27]) receive "CMV-reduced-risk" blood. These issues are discussed in more detail below.

Central Role of Leukocytes

Leukocytes appear to play a pivotal role in CMV dissemination within an infected individual as well as between individuals.[22,28] In vitro, CMV can infect leukocytes at different points along the hematopoietic pathway, from early CD34+ hematopoietic progenitors to mature leukocytes, including lymphocytes and monocytes.[29-36] After primary CMV infection is suppressed, the virus is not completely eliminated but rather remains latent indefinitely in some of these cell populations.[37,38] Thus, many leukocyte subpopulations can support either latent or active CMV infection.

Seronegative Units as the "Gold Standard" to Prevent CMV Transmission

Historically, it has been recommended that immunocompromised seronegative patients receive blood components from CMV-seronegative donors.[22,28,39-41] Because the CMV antibodies that develop after infection were believed to persist indefinitely, seronegative donors were considered to have never been exposed to the virus.[20,38] However, the recent observation that latent CMV can be reactivated from leukocytes of healthy seronegative blood donors suggests that in some individuals, a significant CMV antibody response either was never present or diminished with time.[21] Alternatively, some seronegative donors may have recently been infected and not yet developed an antibody response. These possibilities could explain, at least in part, the 3-5% incidence of TT-CMV following the transfusion of seronegative units.

Production of Cytomegalovirus-Reduced-Risk Units by Leukocyte Reduction

An alternative approach to the use of seronegative units is to reduce the number of leukocytes in the components. Because CMV is a highly cell-associated virus,[32,42] removal of the cellular targets for CMV (ie, the leukocytes) from components should also remove CMV. In fact, the use of leukocyte-reduced units can markedly decrease the incidence of TT-CMV infection when compared with the use of non-leukocyte-reduced units.[43-47] In 1994, Hillyer et al[22] reviewed a number of clinical studies in which various leukocyte reduction methods were evaluated for their efficacy in reducing the incidence of TT-CMV. The authors concluded that components that were leukocyte reduced with 3-$\log_{10}$ leukocyte filters, or frozen-deglycerolized red cells, were equivalent to seronegative components for the purpose of reducing the incidence of TT-CMV. In contrast, washing components with saline removes some leukocytes but not to the same extent as does filtration. Thus, washed units cannot be considered equivalent to seronegative units although they too reduce the incidence of TT-CMV.[22,48] It is not yet clear which specific leukocyte subsets must be removed in order to prevent TT-CMV.

In 1995, Bowden et al[23] published results from a prospectively randomized clinical trial in which 502 seronegative recipients of autologous or seronegative allogeneic marrow transplants received either CMV seronegative or filter-leukocyte-reduced, unscreened red cells and platelets. The patients were longitudinally evaluated for evidence of CMV infection and the development of CMV disease. Using the predefined window for identifying TT-CMV (21-100 days posttransplantation, to exclude patients who acquired CMV prior to study enrollment), the authors found that the actuarial probabilities of developing CMV infection or disease were similar in patients receiving either filtered or seronegative components ($p>0.05$). On the basis of an intention-to-treat analysis, they concluded that seronegative and filtered units were equivalent in terms of the risks of TT-CMV infection and disease. However, when all data from days 0-100 were analyzed, the difference in the risk of progression to CMV disease between patients receiving filtered vs seronegative units reached accepted levels for statistical significance (2.4% vs 0%, respectively; $p = 0.03$). This finding has led other groups to question whether progression to CMV disease is in fact different in patients receiving filtered vs seronegative components.[24,25,49] It is also noteworthy that 5 of 6 patients who contracted CMV from filtered units developed CMV disease that progressed to fatal CMV pneumonia, whereas none of 4 patients infected with CMV from seronegative components developed CMV disease ($p = 0.005$ by Fisher's exact test[24]). The biologic basis for this difference remains unexplained.[23-25]

Other Viruses

Additional viruses may be transmitted by platelet transfusions, with subsequent clinical consequences. For example, parvovirus B19 transmission resulting in persistent B19 infection and chronic anemia has been reported.[50] Further, human herpesvirus 8, believed to be an etiologic agent of Kaposi's sarcoma and body cavity–based lymphoma, was identified in CD19+ cells from an apparently healthy blood donor and could infect CD19+ cells in vitro.[51] But, while this study raised the possibility of human herpes virus 8 transmission by transfusion, other studies suggest that transmission occurs predominantly, if not exclusively, through sexual activity.[52,53] It is also important to note that while some viruses, such as CMV, partition to the leukocyte compartment and can be largely removed by leukocyte reduction filtration, others cannot. Influenza virus,[54] vaccinia virus,[55] herpes simplex virus,[56] and HIV-I[57,58] either are platelet associated or exist as free virus, and cannot be quantitatively removed through either filtration or washing.

Infectious Complications—Bacterial

Incidence and Significance

The rate of bacterial contamination of platelet components is at least 10-100 times greater than the rate of contamination by many viruses (HIV-1/2, HBV, HCV, HTLV-I/II).[2,59-68] Yomtovian et al[2] determined that 6 of 3141 pooled platelet concentrates (PCs; 0.19%) were contaminated by bacteria while all 2476 single-donor apheresis platelet (SD-PLT) units examined were sterile. Blajchman,[67] as well as the Canadian Red Cross,[66,68] noted rates of PC bacterial contamination in the same range (0.04-0.3%). This incidence can be explained, at least in part, by room temperature storage of platelet components for up to 5 days, which is a sufficient interval for a small bacterial inoculum to proliferate extensively.[59-62]

Not all of these contaminated units produce signs and symptoms of sepsis upon transfusion. Morrow et al[65] identified 829 febrile reactions with 29,738 platelet transfusions (19,519 SD-PLT units; 10,219 pooled PCs) to patients with marrow failure; the PCs causing 7 of the reactions were contaminated with bacteria (0.8% incidence of contaminated units in patients with febrile reactions; 0.02% overall incidence of contaminated units). Components stored for 5 days were 5 times more likely to produce sepsis than those stored for 4 days or less. The incidence of septic reactions reported in this study was 2-15 times lower than the rate of platelet bacterial contamination.[2,66-68] This can be explained by the following factors. First, septic transfusion reactions may be overlooked in febrile neutropenic marrow recipients or mistaken for febrile nonhemolytic transfusion reactions (FNHTRs); in either case, the unit is not cultured for confirmation.[1,4,65] Second, some patients (3 of 4 in one study[2]) do not display the classic signs and symptoms of sepsis after having received bacterially contaminated units, possibly because the transfused bacterial load is not always clinically significant. Lastly, in cases where the culture of suspected platelet components grows skin flora, these isolates are often disregarded as culture artifacts.

Although 4-30 of 10,000 PCs harbor culturable bacteria, the clinical significance of this problem is unclear. On examination of transfusion-related deaths reported to the Food and Drug Administration (FDA) from 1976 to 1990, 19 deaths were attributed to the transfusion of platelet components contaminated by bacteria.[63] Culture results demonstrated a diverse array of contaminating species, including *Staphylococcus epidermidis*, *Staphylococcus aureus*, *Klebsiella* species, *Salmonella* species, *Streptococcus* species, *Enterobacter cloacae*, *Proteus mirabilis*, *Serratia* species, and *Bacillus* species. On the basis of an estimate of 500,000-1,000,000 annual platelet doses in the United States and without correcting for suspected underreporting,[63] sepsis-related mortality from contaminated platelets appears to be on the order of 1-2 per 1,000,000 platelet doses. This rate is comparable to the estimated mortality resulting from transfusion-transmitted HIV infections.

Pathogenesis

The isolation of skin flora from many of these components suggests that a common mechanism of component contamination is through "coring" of a small segment of incompletely sterilized skin by the venipuncture needle,[65,69] with the contaminated skin core drawn into the blood unit. Among the skin flora that can contaminate platelets, *Propionibacterium* species are of most significance in immunocompromised patients (many of whom receive platelet transfusions) and orthopedic surgery patients.[70] *Staphylococcus epidermidis* is also of importance in the immunocompromised patient, especially with the increasing rate of antibiotic resistance.[71] *Staphylococcus aureus* is another major pathogen.[72] When isolates are not derived from skin flora, the most probable mechanism is transient donor bacteremia.[68,73] For example, *Yersinia enterocolitica*, more commonly associated with bacterial contamination of red cell units,[74] was recently implicated in a septic reaction from a contaminated platelet unit.[75] Subsequent interviews revealed that the platelet donor had an episode of nausea and abdominal cramping near the time of donation, consistent with a transient *Yersinia enterocolitica* bacteremia.[75] While the bacteria that contaminate platelet units can produce sepsis in the transfusion recipient, the role of bacterial endotoxin in the "warm shock" response, which can develop shortly after the initiation of transfusion, is still unclear.

Prevention

Although many bacterial isolates from platelet units are derived from normal skin flora, these contaminants may be virtually unavoidable. About 20% of skin bacteria are found deep in the pilo-sebaceous unit and skin crevices, including antecubital fossa scars in repeat donors.[76] While these bacteria are inaccessible to sterilization, they can still be "cored" by the venipuncture needle.[69] Other potential causes of contamination, including transient donor bacteremia[68,73] and contamination during closed-system component processing,[77-79] appear to occur rarely. Finally, while the increased incidence of bacterial contamination with longer storage time suggests that limiting component storage to 3-4 days would decrease transfusion-associated sepsis,[2,65] this approach would also produce unacceptable component wastage and a reduced platelet supply. Thus, it is likely that the most effective interventions to prevent bacterial transmission by platelet transfusion will take place after component processing. Two general strategies have been proposed. The first approach is to identify and discard contaminated units prior to transfusion. The second is to sterilize all units to inactivate occasional contaminating bacteria.

Identification and Discard of Infected Units

Contaminating bacteria in platelet components can be detected with a number of techniques: bacterial culture (direct plating and rapid automated culture),[1,2,68,80,81] Gram's stain,[1,2,65,72,82-84] direct visualization of component "swirling,"[85,86] glucose and pH determinations,[86-88] bacterial nucleic acid detection (direct bacterial RNA hybridization[89,90] and polymerase chain reaction [PCR][91]), and blood gas determinations (pO_2 and pCO_2)[80,89,92] (see Table 10-2). Culture is the benchmark, with a theoretical sensitivity of 1 CFU and an experimental sensitivity 10^2 CFU/mL or less with automated culture technology.[1] However, bacterial culture frequently

Table 10-2. Techniques for Detecting Bacteria in Platelet Components

Detection Methodology	Detection Limit (CFU/mL)	Turnaround Time
Culture	1*/$<10^{2}$†	> 10 hours‡
Chemiluminescent rRNA probe	10^2 - 10^4	1-3 hours
Polymerase chain reaction	5×10^3	4-6 hours
Gram's stain (acridine orange)	10^5 - 10^6 (10^4 - 10^5)	≤ 30 minutes
Blood gas determinations	10^6 - 10^9	≤ 30 minutes
Platelet "swirling"	10^7 - 10^8	≤ 5 minutes
Dipstick pH, glucose	10^7 - 10^8	≤ 5 minutes

*Theoretical sensitivity
†Experimentally determined sensitivity with platelet units
‡Time to detection with automated culture system dependent on bacterial inoculum; large bacterial inocula can be detected in as little as 3 hours[80]
CFU = colony-forming unit; rRNA = ribosomal RNA

requires at least 10-12 hours for a result unless the unit is heavily contaminated.[68,80,81] It is also important to note that culturing the component segments is less sensitive than culturing the residual component in the bag, presumably because if the initial bacterial inoculum was small, it did not involve the limited volume in the segment. The other techniques yield results more rapidly but are also less sensitive. Gram's stain displays limited sensitivity, detecting 10^5-10^6 CFU/mL and identifying 50-100% of the platelet units that were positive by culture.[1,2,65,72,82-84] Direct bacterial identification with acridine orange stain and fluorescence microscopy is only slightly more sensitive (10^4-10^5 CFU/mL).[93-95] Visual assessment of platelet "swirling" and dipstick measurements of plasma pH and glucose both detect 10^7-10^8 CFU/mL,[85-88] which correlates with the stationary phase of bacterial growth. Plasma pCO_2, pO_2, and pH measured with blood gas analyzers were also insensitive, detecting bacteria at more than 10^6-10^9 CFU/mL.[80,89,92] Similar results were obtained using a pCO_2 indicator badge attached directly to the component bag.[80] Chemiluminescence detection of ribosomal RNA displayed a sensitivity of 10^2-10^4 CFU/mL,[89,90] and PCR, when used to detect *Yersinia enterocolitica* in red cell units, displayed a sensitivity of 5×10^3 CFU/mL.[91] However, chemiluminescence requires at least 1 hour to complete, while PCR often requires at least 4 hours. Thus, there is currently a trade-off between sensitivity and turnaround time, with no single technique clearly emerging as superior for the routine monitoring of bacterial contamination in platelet components.

Decontamination of Units

Leukocyte-reduction depletion filters can directly and indirectly remove bacteria from platelet units. Bacteria appear to adhere directly to the filter matrix during leukocyte-reduction filtration, with filters removing up to 10^6 CFU/mL in this manner.[1,68] The indirect mechanism, involving bacterial ingestion by, or adherence to, phagocytic leukocytes with subsequent removal of leukocytes by filtration, has been demonstrated by many groups.[74,95-102]

It has been argued that prestorage leukocyte reduction may be detrimental, allowing bacterial growth by the removal of phagocytes.[96] However, the concentration of bacteria in units immediately after filtration is actually lower than that in unmanipulated units, indicating indirect bacterial removal via leukocyte reduction.[98] Others have obtained similar results.[103] While these findings do not indicate that leukocyte-reduced units present a more favorable milieu for bacterial growth, the timing of leukocyte reduction appears to be important. To optimize phagocytosis prior to leukocyte reduction, the component should be left at room temperature for approximately 8 hours before filtering.[1]

Other approaches to decontaminating platelet units remain experimental. The psoralen derivative 8-methoxypsoralen can inactivate a spectrum of both gram-positive and gram-negative organisms (including *Staphylococcus aureus, Staphylococcus epidermidis, Escherichia coli, Yersinia enterocolitica, Salmonella choleraesuis, Serratia marcescens*, and *Pseudomonas aeruginosa*) that can contaminate platelet components.[104] Bacterial concentrations of 10^4-10^7 CFU/mL can be inactivated, which compares favorably with estimated bacterial concentrations of 10^1-10^3 CFU/mL in naturally infected units.[105] In-vitro platelet function was not adversely affected[104] by 8-methoxypsoralen treatment. Similar results were recently reported with another psoralen derivative, S-59.[17]

Noninfectious Complications

Allergic: Transfusion of Antigen or Antibody

The spectrum of allergic reactions ranges from relatively common and benign urticarial reactions to rare and life-threatening anaphylactic reactions. The incidence varies with the specific reaction.These reactions are believed to result from transfusion of plasma proteins, antigens, or antibodies. The formation of antigen-antibody complexes in the transfusion recipient initiates an inflammatory response of varying severity. Hypotensive reactions[106,107] represent an exception since they are likely not precipitated by antigen-antibody reactions. However, hypotensive reactions are discussed along with allergic reactions because they share common downstream inflammatory mediators, including bradykinin.[106,107]

Urticaria

Urticarial reactions (hives) are generally mild and benign, often occurring in the absence of other signs and symptoms. These reactions account for less than 25% of platelet transfusion reactions.[108,109] The proposed mechanism, interaction between recipient IgE and donor plasma constituents with subsequent histamine release from mast cells and basophils,[110] is supported by two observations. First, platelets washed free of plasma are associated with a lower incidence of urticarial reactions. Second, these reactions can be prevented or interrupted with antihistamines. However, the nature of the plasma antigens involved in these reactions has not been elucidated. When an urticarial reaction develops, the transfusion should be slowed or temporarily stopped until antihistamine administration interrupts the reaction. The transfusion may then resume at the initial rate.

Anaphylaxis

Life-threatening anaphylactic reactions generally manifest immediately after the onset of transfusion. They are characterized by marked hypertension followed by hypotension, shock, severe gastrointestinal symptoms, and dyspnea, usually in the absence of fever.[111] These reactions are rare, with only eight anaphylactic transfusion-related deaths reported to the FDA between 1976 and 1985.[70]

In a study of severe, unexplained, nonhemolytic transfusion reactions referred to a reference laboratory, 8% met the diagnostic criteria for anaphylactic reactions of the IgA-deficient type.[112] This well-characterized scenario occurs upon transfusion of an IgA-deficient patient who has previously formed IgA antibodies, often of the IgE class, in response to prior transfusion or pregnancy. IgA in transfused plasma crosslinks IgE on mast cells and basophils, initiating an inflammatory response with the release of histamine, serotonin, bradykinin, interleukin-1 (IL-1), and tumor necrosis factor-a (TNF-α).[113]

Anaphylactic reactions require immediate administration of epinephrine to prevent fatality. If further transfusions are required, the components should be obtained from IgA-deficient donors. Alternatively, washed cellular components could be substituted if IgA-deficient components are not available.[114]

Transfusion-Related Acute Lung Injury

Transfusion-related acute lung injury (TRALI) is characterized by signs and symptoms of noncardiogenic pulmonary edema appearing 1 to 6 hours after transfusion. It is accompanied by other manifestations, including chills, fever, dyspnea, and hypoxia, and may progress to resemble adult respiratory distress syndrome.[115,116] TRALI has been estimated to complicate 0.02% of transfusions, with a mortality rate approaching 5%.[115,116]

In contrast to urticarial and anaphylactic reactions, in which recipient antibodies react with substances in the transfused component, the pathogenesis of TRALI typically involves transfusion of donor antibodies that agglutinate recipient leukocytes.[115,116] The donor is usually a multiparous woman with HLA-specific antibodies formed through pregnancy. Antibodies against granulocyte-specific antigens may also be present.[113] Agglutinated antibody-leukocyte complexes in the pulmonary capillary bed can activate complement,[117] including C5a, a chemoattractant that can produce extensive neutrophil aggregation in the lungs. This mechanism may explain the observation that in some cases of TRALI, relatively small volumes of transfused blood can precipitate marked pulmonary edema.[118] In about 10% of cases, recipient antibodies can agglutinate transfused leukocytes; the downstream effects are as described.

Treatment of TRALI includes respiratory and hemodynamic support until pulmonary edema resolves, usually within 48-96 hours. High-dose bolus corticosteroids have been administered to decrease neutrophil aggregation; however, their efficacy has not been proven.[113]

Hypotensive Reactions

Hypotensive transfusion reactions are a relatively newly defined entity.[119] While hypotension may accompany hemolytic, anaphylactic, septic, and allergic transfusion reactions as well as TRALI, the unique feature of hypotensive reactions is that hypotension is the primary or only manifestation. A survey by the American Association of Blood Banks Transfusion Practices Committee identified 17 atypical platelet reactions characterized by hypotension.[119] These reactions displayed the following similarities: 75% of platelet components were filter leukocyte-reduced at the bedside; 88% of the reactions occurred within 1 hour of transfusion; 82% of the reactions were associated with respiratory distress, which was neither as severe nor as prolonged as in TRALI; and 82% of the reactions resolved rapidly after cessation of transfusion, without necessitating further intervention.

The role of bedside leukocyte reduction in the pathogenesis of hypotensive reactions is supported by a case report of a patient who on 3 consecutive days received Fresh Frozen Plasma (FFP) transfusions through a leukocyte reduction filter.[120] The patient was concurrently being treated with angiotensin-converting enzyme (ACE) inhibitors for hypertension. During each of the 3 transfusions, he rapidly developed symptoms consistent with a hypotensive reaction; each reaction resolved rapidly after the transfusion was discontinued. Over the subsequent 2 weeks, the patient received 24 units of FFP without the use of leukocyte-reduction filters. No adverse sequelae occurred. A more recent report further strengthens the linkage of the concurrent use of ACE inhibitors and negatively charged bedside leukocyte-reduction filters with the development of hypotensive reactions.[121]

Hypotensive reactions appear to be associated with bradykinin generation during leukocyte reduction using negatively charged (but not positively charged) filters.[106] The negatively charged filter surface appears to activate Hageman factor, which cleaves prekallikrein to kallikrein, which in turn converts high-molecular-weight kininogens to bradykinin. ACE inhibitors block the action of kininase II, one of the primary enzymes in bradykinin catabolism.[122-124] Thus, ACE inhibitors may potentiate bradykinin activation by the filter, and if patients treated with ACE inhibitors require leukocyte-reduced components, those components should be leukocyte-reduced, either prestorage or at bedside using positively charged filters.[121]

Febrile Nonhemolytic Transfusion Reactions

FNHTRs are the most common reactions associated with platelet transfusions.[3,4] Their primary manifestation is usually fever, sometimes accompanied by chills, rigors, nausea, or discomfort. These reactions generally occur toward the end of, or following, transfusion.

Pathogenesis: The Role of Cytokines

The pathogenic mechanisms underlying FNHTRs are not completely resolved. Current evidence suggests that there may be multiple distinct etiologies, each manifesting as a similar complex of signs and symptoms. An early proposal hypothesized a role for preformed recipient antibodies to donor leukocytes.[125-129] While supported by some experimental evidence, however, this hypothesis could not explain 3 well-characterized features of FNHTRs. First, these reactions more commonly occur following platelet transfusions than red cell transfusions even though red cell components contain 10-1000 times more leukocytes.[4] Second, they occur in males not previously transfused and thus unlikely to have generated leukocyte alloantibodies.[3] Third, the incidence and severity of FNHTRs increase in direct proportion to platelet storage time and leukocyte content.[130] These empirical observations suggest that additional mechanisms might contribute to FNHTRs in transfusion recipients.

To address this issue, Heddle et al[131] separated PCs into plasma and cellular fractions and randomly transfused both into recipients. When all resulting transfusion reactions were considered, the plasma fraction was significantly more likely than the cellular component to cause severe reactions. In addition, only the plasma fraction elicited febrile reactions (defined as at least a 1 C rise in body temperature). Quantitation of IL-1β and IL-6 by enzyme-linked immunosorbent assay demonstrated that elevated levels of these potent pyrogens[132,133] strongly correlated with increased incidence and severity of resulting transfusion reactions. Subsequent studies showed that, in addition to IL-1β and IL-6, PC plasma contains IL-8 and TNF-α. It is important to note that the levels of these cytokines increase progressively with PC storage and are correlated with component leukocyte counts.[131,134,135] These findings provide a possible explanation for the increased frequency of FNHTRs with PC units near outdate. Based on reverse transcriptase-PCR identification of cytokine messenger RNA from PC leukocytes, the cytokines are being actively synthesized and secreted during PC storage and not simply released by dying leukocytes.[136]

Additional studies further support the role of cytokines in FNHTRs. As discussed below, leukocyte-reduced PCs display lower cytokine levels and produce fewer adverse platelet reactions than do non-leukocyte-reduced components. In addition, when total PC plasma cytokine loads are calculated (on the basis of cytokine concentration and volume), the levels approach those previously shown to produce biologic effects with bolus injections.[134-137] While the cytokines may not be transfused individually at biologically active concentrations, synergistic effects of multiple plasma cytokines transfused simultaneously may produce the biologic effects that manifest as FNHTRs.

In addition to systemic effects in the transfusion recipient, cytokines may adversely affect platelet function.[138] Incubation of fresh platelets with IL-6 (<10 pg/mL) and IL-8 (<1500 pg/mL) at concentrations similar to those found in PCs stored for 1-2 days had no significant effect on platelet activation, as assessed by platelet P-selectin (CD 62) expression. However, there was marked platelet activation in response to concentrations of IL-6 (>125 pg/mL) and IL-8 (>3000 pg/mL) similar to that found in 3- to 4-day-old PCs. Platelet activation during storage may in turn correlate with poor transfusion outcome.

In contrast to cytokines released by leukocytes in PCs, other biologic response modifiers are released by platelets themselves during storage.[139] The chemokines platelet factor 4, β-thromboglobulin, and RANTES (regulated upon activation, normal T cell expressed and presumably secreted), which are normally stored in platelet organelles, all are released by platelets during storage, with their concentrations increasing as a function of storage time. These chemokines are inflammatory mediators and may synergize with cytokines released by leukocytes to cause FNHTRs in the transfusion recipient.

Prevention of Plasma Cytokine Elevation

Antipyretics can be used to treat the febrile component of FNHTRs, but the other side effects are usually not alleviated.[4] Thus, prevention of FNHTRs may prove more effective than treatment of ongoing reactions. Toward this end, investigators have attempted to decrease cytokine accumulation by lowering leukocyte content of platelet components. One approach is to alter fundamentally the platelet fractionation technique from the platelet-rich plasma (PRP) approach, used most frequently in the United States, to the buffy coat (BC) preparation technique, commonly used in Europe.[140,141] Due to differences in centrifugation and separation protocols, PRP-PC components contain significantly more leukocytes than BC-PC units (~5×10^8 vs ~5×10^7 leukocytes per platelet dose, respectively, in one study).[108] Alternatively, platelets can be prepared from SD-PLT procedures, resulting in process leukocyte-reduced components with ~10^4-10^6 leukocytes, depending on instrumentation and separation technique.[142] Direct comparisons have demonstrated significantly more adverse reactions with the transfusion of PRP-PCs (17% of transfusions) than with either BC-PCs or SD-PLTs (3-4% each).[108,143] Differences in transfusion reaction incidence were related to cytokine content of the component. BC-PCs displayed consistently lower levels of IL-1β, IL-6, IL-8, and TNF-α than did PRP-PCs,[141,144] while SD-PLT components contained the lowest levels of IL-1β, IL-6, and IL-8 over the entire storage period. However, SD-PLT components displayed elevated transforming growth factor-β (TGF-β) levels, possibly owing to leukocyte stimulation during the apheresis procedure.[137]

Leukocyte reduction by filtration is an alternative method to decrease white cells and thus cytokine and chemokine concentrations in component plasma. In experiments, filter leukocyte reduction attenuated the increase in IL-1β, IL-6, IL-8, and TNF-α normally seen with increasing storage time.[131,134,135,145] There is still debate in the literature regarding threshold leukocyte concentrations below which cytokines do not increase during storage. A range of target concentrations between 10^4 and 5×10^6 has been proposed,[134,135] which correlates with the levels seen in process leukocyte-reduced SD-PLT units but represents a 10^2 to 10^4-fold reduction in leukocyte content compared with that in standard PRP-PC units. It is important to note that leukocyte reduction decreases the incidence of FNHTRs but does not prevent all reactions.

Various experimental approaches have also been used to block cytokine generation during PC storage. For example, UV-B radiation (20,000 J/m^2) but not gamma radiation (30 Gy) prevents the production of IL-8 during platelet storage.[136] A fundamentally different approach is to store platelets at 4 C in a solution of second-messenger effectors to prevent the development of platelet storage lesion, typified by decreasing platelet numbers and the attenuation of agonist-activated aggregation and hypotonic shock response.[146-149] PCs stored in this manner do not display a dramatic increase in IL-6, IL-1β, or TNF-α immunoreactivity in the plasma fraction during storage and also do not support bacterial growth.[150]

Finally, it may be possible to deplete biological response modifiers from platelet component plasma prior to transfusion. The chemokines IL-8 and RANTES, as well as the complement anaphylatoxins C3a and C5a, all of which are cationic, directly bind to some commercially available, negatively charged leukocyte-reduction filters.[151-153] The cytokines IL-1β and IL-6 are not retained on the filters. Unfortunately, the binding of biologic response modifiers to the current generation of filters is saturable and effective only with small volumes of plasma (≤ 50 mL). Because leukocyte-reduction filters were not designed for this purpose, future modifications in filter composition with this application in mind may produce filters that efficiently bind not only chemokines and complement, but cytokines as well.

HLA and Red Cell Alloimmunization

Transfusion recipients exposed to allogeneic blood can generate specific immune responses to alloantigens in the component. With respect to platelet transfusions, alloimmunization to HLA and platelet-specific antigens is of greatest clinical concern because the resulting antibodies can lead to a platelet refractory state. Although estimates vary widely, up to 80% of multitransfused platelet recipients historically formed alloantibodies (primarily anti-HLA).[154,155] These rates were determined prior to widespread use of SD-PLTs and leukocyte-reduction filtration. More recently, Abou-Elella et al[156] reported that among 170 hematopoietic transplant patients without preexisting HLA antibodies, 8 (4.7%) developed persistent HLA antibodies and 9 (5.3%) were variably positive for antibodies, consistent with the 5-10% HLA alloimmunization rate currently accepted. Four of 193 hematopoietic transplant patients (2.1%) developed new red cell alloantibodies (anti-E, -M, -Jk^b, -Lu14), at a rate of 0.1% per red cell unit transfused. These patients received only leukocyte-reduced components, and transfused platelets were exclusively SD-PLT components.[156] The more extensively alloimmunized a patient becomes, the more difficult it may be to identify platelet units that produce a clinically significant effect, since the antibodies can result in rapid clearance of transfused platelets. The pathogenesis of alloimmunization, as well as clinical approaches to the alloimmunized patient, are discussed elsewhere in this volume.

Immunomodulation

The extent to which blood transfusion alters the host immune network, resulting in significant clinical sequelae, has been debated for years. There remains little doubt that transfused allogeneic leukocytes perturb the host immune system. However, the degree to which these perturbations, when propagated through the host immune network, affect the clinical progression of disease is still under active investigation.

Immunomodulatory Effects of Allogeneic Transfusion: Beneficial vs Adverse

In the mid-1970s, Opelz et al[157] and Opelz and Terasaki[158] reported that allogeneic red cell transfusion prior to transplantation improved renal graft survival. Graft survival increased in proportion to the number of transfusions, and the effect appeared dependent on the presence of viable leukocytes in the transfused component. Transfusion of platelet components alone also improved graft survival.[159] These beneficial effects of transfusion were confirmed in animal renal allograft models.[160,161]

Patients with recurrent spontaneous abortions also respond positively to transfusion. A growing fetus is a type of "allograft," whose major histocompatibility complex loci are usually only partially matched to the mother's. Under normal circumstances, the mother is tolerant to the graft and the pregnancy proceeds to term. However, immune suppression or derangements in tolerance can lead to fetal rejection, resulting in abortion. Consistent with the renal allograft studies, transfusion can also significantly reduce recurrent spontaneous abortion.[162-166] Interestingly, leukocytes from the father are more effective than those from random donors,[164] suggesting the specificity of transfusion-associated immunomodulation. In contrast, retrospective studies on the beneficial effects of transfusion in patients with immune-mediated chronic inflammatory bowel disease (eg, Crohn's disease) have not been conclusive. There are indications that transfusions delay the recurrence of Crohn's disease after surgery,[167,168] but other investigators have questioned the value of transfusion for immunomodulation in these patients.[169]

There also appear to be deleterious effects of transfusion-induced immunomodulation. Most data suggest that perisurgical transfusion increases the frequency of postoperative infections (recently reviewed in Blumberg and Heal[170]). Compared with patients who received unmanipulated components, those who received leukocyte-reduced components and thus were not exposed to the immunomodulatory effects of donor leukocytes experienced significantly fewer infections, shorter hospital stays, and reduced medical costs.[171-173] An increase in susceptibility to infection after transfusion has also been reported in animal studies.[174] These findings were supported by a retrospective study of 487 colorectal cancer surgery patients. After correcting for 20 confounding variables (including severity of illness, operative procedure, and historical risk of infection), those patients who received allogeneic blood transfusions had significantly more infections.[175] It is important to note that the difference in the incidence of infections between transfused and nontransfused groups was the primary factor contributing to an approximately 60% longer hospital stay (16.7 ± 0.81 vs 10.3 ± 0.26 days [p<.0001]) and approximately 75% greater hospital charges ($28,101 ± 1121 vs $15,978 ± 265 [p<.0001]) for patients who received allogeneic transfusions.

There are other adverse sequelae of transfusion that may result from immunomodulation. Viruses latent in host leukocytes, including CMV and HIV, can reactivate in vitro after stimulation by allogeneic donor leukocytes.[21,176] Viral reactivation in the transfusion recipient has also been suggested by studies of CMV-seropositive recipients of seronegative allogeneic blood,[177] as well as by the debated association between blood transfusion and shortened survival in AIDS patients.[178-180] There is also a lack of consensus regarding the role of immunomodulation in tumor growth and cancer recurrence after surgery. Experimental models have demonstrated that animals that received unmanipulated allogeneic transfusions had larger tumors than animals that received leukocyte-reduced transfusions.[181,182] Whether this same phenomenon occurs in cancer patients postoperatively is unclear.[183,184]

Mechanism

A number of potential mechanisms have been proposed to explain the immunomodulatory effects of allogeneic leukocytes. These include the generation of idiotype antibodies, the development of a suppressor cell network, and clonal deletion of alloreactive lymphocytes (reviewed in Blumberg and Heal[185] and in Klein[186]). Recent investigations show that allogeneic transfusions can shift the helper-T-1/helper-T-2 (Th1/Th2) cells steady state in favor of the Th2 response, thus dampening the cellular immune response.[185] Th1 cells, which secrete primarily IL-2 and interferon-γ, are believed to mediate immunologic rejection (eg, solid organ or marrow allografts, "fetal" allograft, tumors) as well as autoimmune phenomena (eg, Crohn's disease). In contrast, Th2 cells, which express IL-4, IL-10, and TGF-β, tend to downregulate the processes mediated by Th1 cells and thus suppress cell-mediated immunity.[187,188] It is currently unclear which of these proposed mechanisms is most important to transfusion-induced immunomodulation, or whether multiple mechanisms are active simultaneously. In addition, it appears that a simple shift in Th1 to Th2 cytokine profiles is a dramatic oversimplification of a complex process.[188] While this continues to be an area of active research, indications are that in the future, blood components may be engineered (through leukocyte reduction or modification) with the objective of specifically tailoring the immunomodulatory activity to the clinical situation.

Transfusion-Associated Graft-vs-Host Disease

It was first observed in the 1950s that some heavily transfused cardiac surgery patients developed fever, adenopathy, marked pancytopenia, diarrhea, liver function abnormalities, and a characteristic erythematous maculopapular rash between 2 and 30 days postoperatively.[189,190] This syndrome is now known as transfusion-associated graft-vs-host disease (TA-GVHD). A related syndrome, postoperative erythroderma, occurs in HLA-homogeneous populations and consists of a transient skin rash. This represents a mild and host-limited form of TA-GVHD.

Incidence

Examination of a number of published reports, as well as surveys of professional groups, suggests that while TA-GVHD is rare in the general United States population, the incidence rate is higher in some immunocompromised patient populations, including patients with malignancies and hematologic disorders.[191] These are probably underestimates because TA-GVHD may be difficult to diagnose in critically ill patients, appearing as a drug reaction or viral illness. The previous lack of recognition of TA-GVHD is evident from the observation that between 1976 and 1985, only a single TA-GVHD-related death was reported to the FDA.[70]

In Japan, in contrast, the incidence of postoperative erythroderma/TA-GVHD is 0.15% in immunocompetent patients undergoing cardiac surgery,[192] presumably because of the relative genetic homogeneity in Japan and increased directed donations by family members. Both of these factors may lead to an increased incidence of the one-way HLA match. Statistical considerations indicate that donations from parents/children, second-degree relatives, and siblings are 7.2-17.2, 4.1-9.1, and 3.9-8.8 times more likely, respectively, to have an HLA phenotype that could predispose to TA-GVHD than are donations from random donors.[193] Approximately 50%

of the reported cases of TA-GVHD in immunocompetent patients resulted from the use of directed donations from biologic relatives.[194]

Pathophysiology

TA-GVHD occurs from the transfusion of cellular blood components containing immunocompetent donor lymphocytes. If the donor and recipient are incompatible at major and/or minor histocompatibility loci, the donor lymphocytes recognize the transfusion recipient's cells as foreign and initiate an antirecipient graft-vs-host immune response.[195,196] In immunocompetent recipients, the donor lymphocytes are rapidly eliminated by the host allograft rejection response before TA-GVHD can develop.[197] However, the following immunocompromised patient populations cannot mount an effective immune response against the donor cells and are at risk

Table 10-3. Indications for Gamma Irradiation of Platelets to Prevent TA-GVHD

Accepted Indications	Potential Indications
Immunocompromised transplant recipients (solid organ or marrow) or patients prior to allogeneic marrow transplant	Patients on immunosuppressive therapy (including chemotherapy and irradiation)
Patients with Hodgkin's disease	Patients with AIDS
Recipients of blood donations from biologic relatives or (partially or completely) HLA-matched donors	Low-birthweight neonates
Intrauterine transfusions	Patients with hematologic malignancies other than Hodgkin's disease or solid tumors
Neonatal exchange transfusions or use of extracorporeal membrane oxygenation	
Patients with congenital, cell-mediated immunodeficiencies	

TA-GVHD = transfusion-associated graft-vs-host disease; AIDS = acquired immune deficiency syndrome

for developing TA-GVHD[191,198,199] (see Table 10-3): Fetuses and neonates, who have immature immune systems; patients with congenital cell-mediated immunodeficiencies; patients with hematologic malignancies such as Hodgkin's disease; and patients who are immunosuppressed with transplants (marrow or solid organ) or will soon undergo allogeneic marrow transplantation. In these patients, the donor lymphocytes can proliferate and rapidly eliminate the recipient's hematopoietic elements.

In a second scenario for the development of TA-GVHD, immunocompetent patients receiving HLA-matched platelet units or directed donations from biologic relatives may develop TA-GVHD secondary to a "one-way HLA match": The donor lymphocytes are homozygous for an HLA allele (eg, HLA-A9) for which the recipient is heterozygous (eg, HLA-A9, A28). In this situation, the recipient's immune system recognizes the donor cells as self (because HLA-A9 is self) and does not attack them. However, the donor lymphocytes recognize the recipient as foreign (because of the HLA-A28 allele), leading to TA-GVHD.

The primary difference between TA-GVHD and the GVHD seen in marrow recipients is the immune response to the host marrow. After transplantation, the host marrow is replaced by donor marrow and the GVHD effect is targeted primarily at peripheral tissues because the donor marrow is seen by the new (donor) immune system as self. In contrast, in TA-GVHD, the marrow is seen as foreign by the transfused lymphocytes and is targeted by the immune response leading to marrow aplasia, marked pancytopenia, and high mortality usually secondary to infectious complications.

Prevention

Therapy for TA-GVHD is largely unsuccessful, with overall mortality reported at 90-98%.[190,199] Thus, it becomes paramount to prevent the development of this disease. The only proven method to prevent TA-GVHD in common clinical use is gamma irradiation. Current standards dictate that in patients at risk for TA-GVHD (see Table 10-3), cellular blood components (whole blood, red cell units, platelet units, and granulocytes) as well as fresh plasma should be exposed to a minimum of 25 Gy of gamma irradiation prior to transfusion.[200,201] This dose is derived from experiments that demonstrate that 25-50 Gy can completely block proliferation of lymphocytes to mitogenic stimuli.[202,203] In addition, empirical observations have shown that while a single patient developed TA-GVHD after receiving 20 Gy-irradiated blood, no patients have developed TA-GVHD if their components were irradiated with at least 25 Gy.[191,204] Gamma irradiation of plate-

Table 10-4. Reduction of Adverse Reactions to Platelets

Reaction / Agent	Screening	Medication	Leukocyte Reduction	Gamma Irradiation	Washing
HIV, HBV, HCV, HTLV	+++	—	—	—	—
CMV	+++	—	+++	—	—
Bacterial	+	—	+	—	—
Allergic	—	+++		—	+++
FNHTR	—	+++	+++	—	+
HLA alloimmunization	—	—	+++	—	—
Immunomodulation	—	—	+++	—	—
TA-GVHD	—	—	—	+++	—

+++ = Effective and in common clinical use
+ = Possibly effective, but more investigation is necessary before use becomes widespread
— = Not recommended, not effective, or not yet shown to be effective
HIV = human immunodeficiency virus; HBV = hepatitis B virus; HCV = hepatitis C virus; HTLV = human T-cell lymphotopic virus; CMV = cytomegalovirus; FNHTR = febrile nonhemolytic transfusion reaction; TA-GVHD = transfusion-associated graft-vs-host disease

lets with 20-30 Gy does not decrease platelet function or platelet survival after transfusion.[205,206]

Conclusions

While platelet transfusions can provide life-saving support for thrombocytopenic bleeding patients, their administration can be complicated by a variety of adverse sequelae. The following procedures are currently used clinically to attenuate some platelet transfusion reactions (Table 10-4): Donor and donation screening, medication (antihistamines and antipyretics), leukocyte reduction, gamma irradiation, and component washing. Ongoing investigations are focused on further dissecting the biologic mechanisms that underlie these reactions, as well as on identifying new approaches to further "engineer" platelet products in order to maximize their clinical benefit while reducing the untoward side effects.

References

1. Blajchman MA, Ali AM, Richardson HL. Bacterial contamination of cellular blood components. Vox Sang 1994;67(suppl 3):25-33.
2. Yomtovian R, Lazarus HM, Goodnough LT, et al. A prospective microbiologic surveillance program to detect and prevent the transfusion of bacterially contaminated platelets. Transfusion 1993;33: 902-9.
3. Chambers LA, Kruskall MS, Pacini DG, Donovan LM. Febrile reactions after platelet transfusion: The effect of single versus multiple donors. Transfusion 1990;30:219-21.
4. Heddle NM, Klama LN, Griffith L, et al. A prospective study to identify the risk factors associated with acute reactions to platelet and red cell transfusions. Transfusion 1993;33:794-7.
5. Schreiber GB, Busch MP, Kleinman SH, et al. The risk of transfusion-transmitted viral infections. N Engl J Med 1996;334:1685-90.
6. Brookmeyer R. Reconstruction and future trends of the AIDS epidemic in the United States. Science 1991;253:37-42.
7. Donegan E, Stuart M, Niland JC, et al. Infection with human immunodeficiency virus type 1 (HIV-1) among recipients of antibody-positive blood donations. Ann Intern Med 1990;113:733-9.
8. Farci P, Alter HJ, Wong D, et al. A long-term study of hepatitis C virus replication in non-A, non-B hepatitis. N Engl J Med 1991;325: 98-104.
9. Iwarson S, Norkrans G, Wejstal R. Hepatitis C. Natural history of a unique infection. Clin Infect Dis 1995;20:1361-70.
10. Seeff LB, Buskell-Bales Z, Wright EC, et al. Long-term mortality after transfusion-associated non-A, non-B hepatitis. N Engl J Med 1992; 327:1906-11.
11. Seeff LB, Beebe GW, Hoofnagle JH, et al. A serologic follow-up of the 1942 epidemic of post-vaccination hepatitis in the United States Army. N Engl J Med 1987;316:965-70.
12. Sullivan MT, Williams AE, Fang CT, et al. Transmission of human T-lymphotropic virus types I and II by blood transfusion. A retrospec-

tive study of recipients of blood components (1983 through 1988). Arch Intern Med 1991;151:2043-8.
13. Manns A, Wilks RJ, Murphy EL, et al. A prospective study of transmission by transfusion of HTLV-I and risk factors associated with seroconversion. Int J Cancer 1992;51:886-91.
14. Inaba S, Sato H, Okochi K, et al. Prevention of transmission of human T-lymphotropic virus type I (HTLV-I) through transfusion, by donor screening with antibody to the virus: One year experience. Transfusion 1989;29:7-11.
15. Murphy EL, Hanchard B, Figueroa JP, et al. Modeling the risk of adult T-cell leukemia/lymphoma in persons infected with human T-lymphotropic virus type I. Int J Cancer 1989;43:250-3.
16. Kaplan JE, Osame M, Kubota H, et al. The risk of development of HTLV-I-associated myelopathy/tropical spastic paraparesis among persons infected with HTLV-I. J Acquir Immune Defic Syndr Hum Retrovirol 1990;3:1096-101.
17. Lin L, Cook DN, Wiesehahn GP, et al. Photochemical inactivation of viruses and bacteria in platelet concentrates by use of a novel psoralen and long-wavelength ultraviolet light. Transfusion 1997; 37:423-35.
18. Benade LE, Shumaker J, Xu Y, et al. Inactivation of free and cell-associated human immunodeficiency virus in platelet suspensions by aminomethyltrimethylpsoralen and ultraviolet light. Transfusion 1994;34:680-4.
19. Mocarski ES Jr. Cytomegaloviruses and their replication. In: Fields BN, Knipe DM, Howley PM, et al, eds. Fields virology. 3rd ed. Philadelphia: Lippincott-Raven, 1996:2447-92.
20. Britt WJ, Alford CA. Cytomegalovirus. In: Fields BN, Knipe DM, Howley PM, et al, eds. Fields virology. 3rd ed. Philadelphia: Lippincott-Raven, 1996:2493-523.
21. Soderberg-Naucler C, Fish KN, Nelson JA. Reactivation of latent human cytomegalovirus by allogeneic stimulation of blood cells from healthy donors. Cell 1997;91:119-26.
22. Hillyer CD, Emmens RK, Zago-Novaretti M, Berkman EM. Methods for the reduction of transfusion-transmitted cytomegalovirus infection: Filtration versus the use of seronegative donor units. Transfusion 1994;34:929-34.
23. Bowden RA, Slichter SJ, Sayers M, et al. A comparison of filtered leukocyte-reduced and cytomegalovirus (CMV) seronegative blood

products for the prevention of transfusion-associated CMV infection after marrow transplantation. Blood 1995;86:3598-603.

24. Landaw EM, Kanter M, Petz LD. Safety of filtered leukocyte-reduced blood products for prevention of transfusion-associated cytomegalovirus infection (letter). Blood 1996;87:4910.
25. Bowden RA, Slichter S, Sayers M, et al. Safety of filtered leukocyte-reduced blood products for prevention of transfusion-associated cytomegalovirus infection (response). Blood 1996;87:4910-1.
26. Koszinowski UH, Del Val M, Reddehase MJ. Cellular and molecular basis of the protective immune response to cytomegalovirus infection. Curr Top Microbiol Immunol 1990;154:189-220.
27. Tegtmeier GE. Transfusion-transmitted cytomegalovirus infections: Significance and control. Vox Sang 1986;51:22-30.
28. Hillyer CD, Syndman DR, Berkman E. The risk of cytomegalovirus infection in solid organ and bone marrow transplant recipients: Transfusion of blood products. Transfusion 1990;30:659-66.
29. von Laer D, Meyer-Koenig U, Serr A, et al. Detection of cytomegalovirus DNA in CD34+ cells from blood and bone marrow. Blood 1995;86:4086-90.
30. Zhuravskaya T, Maciejewski JP, Netski DM, et al. Spread of human cytomegalovirus (HCMV) after infection of human hematopoietic progenitor cells: Model of HCMV latency. Blood 1997;90:2482-91.
31. Braun RW, Reiser HC. Replication of human cytomegalovirus in human peripheral blood T cells. J Virol 1986;60:29-36.
32. Rice GPA, Schrier RD, Oldstone MBA. Cytomegalovirus infects human lymphocytes and monocytes: Virus expression is restricted to immediate-early gene products. Proc Natl Acad Sci U S A 1984;81:6134-8.
33. von Laer D, Serr A, Meyer-Koenig U, et al. Human cytomegalovirus immediate early and late transcripts are expressed in all major leukocyte populations *in vivo*. J Infect Dis 1995;172:365-70.
34. Maciejewski JP, Bruening EE, Donahue RE, et al. Infection of mononucleated phagocytes with human cytomegalovirus. Virology 1993;195:327-36.
35. Minton EJ, Tysoe C, Sinclair JH, Sissons JGP. Human cytomegalovirus infection of the monocyte/macrophage lineage in bone marrow. J Virol 1994;68:4017-21.
36. Lathey JL, Spector SA. Unrestricted replication of human cytomegalovirus in hydrocortisone-treated macrophages. J Virol 1991;65:6371-5.

37. Bruggeman CA. Cytomegalovirus and latency: An overview. Virchows Arch B 1993;64:325-33.
38. Rasmussen L. Immune response to human cytomegalovirus infection. Curr Top Microbiol Immunol 1990;154:221-54.
39. Bowden RA, Sayers M, Flournoy N, et al. Cytomegalovirus immune globulin and seronegative blood products to prevent primary cytomegalovirus infection after marrow transplantation. N Engl J Med 1986;314:1006-10.
40. Bowden RA, Sayers M, Gleaves CA, et al. Cytomegalovirus-seronegative blood components for the prevention of primary cytomegalovirus infection after marrow transplantation: Considerations for blood banks. Transfusion 1987;27:478-81.
41. Miller WJ, McCullough J, Balfour HH Jr, et al. Prevention of cytomegalovirus infection following bone marrow transplantation: A randomized trial of blood product screening. Bone Marrow Transplant 1991;7:227-34.
42. Einhorn L, Ost A. Cytomegalovirus infection of human blood cells. J Infect Dis 1984;149:207-14.
43. Verdonck LF, de Graan-Hentzen YC, Dekker AW, et al. Cytomegalovirus seronegative platelets and leukocyte-poor red blood cells from random donors can prevent primary cytomegalovirus infection after bone marrow transplantation. Bone Marrow Transplant 1987; 2:73-8.
44. Gilbert GL, Hayes K, Hudson IL, James J. Prevention of transfusion-acquired cytomegalovirus infection in infants by blood filtration to remove leucocytes. Lancet 1989;1:1228-31.
45. de Graan-Hentzen YCE, Gratama JW, Mudde GC, et al. Prevention of primary cytomegalovirus infection in patients with hematologic malignancies by intensive white cell depletion of blood products. Transfusion 1989;29:757-60.
46. DeWitte T, Schattenberg A, Van Dijk BA, et al. Prevention of primary cytomegalovirus infection after allogeneic bone marrow transplantation by using leukocyte-poor random blood products from cytomegalovirus-unscreened blood-bank donors. Transplantation 1990;50: 964-8.
47. Bowden RA, Slichter SJ, Sayers MH, et al. Use of leukocyte-depleted platelets and cytomegalovirus-seronegative red blood cells for prevention of primary cytomegalovirus infection after marrow transplant. Blood 1991;78:246-50.

48. Demmler GJ, Brady MT, Bijou H, et al. Posttransfusion cytomegalovirus infection in neonates: Role of saline-washed red blood cells. J Pediatr 1986;108:762-5.
49. Kanter MH, Petz L. The validity of statistical analyses in the transfusion medicine literature with specific comments concerning studies of the comparative safety of units donated by autologous, designated and allogeneic donors (editorial). Transfus Med 1995;5:91-5.
50. Cohen BJ, Beard S, Knowles WA, et al. Chronic anemia due to parvovirus B19 infection in a bone marrow transplant patient after platelet transfusion. Transfusion 1997;37:947-52.
51. Blackbourn DJ, Ambroziak J, Lennette E, et al. Infectious human herpesvirus 8 in a healthy North American blood donor. Lancet 1997;349:609-11.
52. Operskalski EA, Busch MP, Mosley JW, Kedes DH. Blood donations and viruses (letter). Lancet 1997;349:1327.
53. Lefrere J-J, Mariotti M, Girot R, et al. Transfusional risk of HHV-8 infection (letter). Lancet 1997;350:217.
54. Terada H, Baldini M, Ebbe S, Madoff MA. Interaction of influenza virus with blood platelets. Blood 1966;28:213-28.
55. Bik T, Sarov I, Livne A. Interaction between vaccinia virus and human blood platelets. Blood 1982;59:482-7.
56. Forghani B, Schmidt NJ. Association of herpes simplex virus with platelets of experimentally infected mice. Arch Virol 1983;76: 269-74.
57. Lee T-H, Stromberg RR, Henrard D, Busch MP. Effect of platelet-associated virus on assays of HIV-1 in plasma. Science 1993;262: 1585-6.
58. Lee T-H, Stromberg RR, Henrard DR, Busch MP. Detection of high levels of platelet-associated HIV-1: Implications for quantitation of plasma viremia (abstract). Transfusion 1993;33(suppl):37S.
59. Punsalang A, Heal JM, Murphy PJ. Growth of gram-positive and gram-negative bacteria in platelet concentrates. Transfusion 1989; 29:596-9.
60. Goddard D, Jacobs SI, Manohitharajah SM. The bacteriological screening of platelet concentrates stored at 22 C. Transfusion 1973; 13:103-6.
61. Buchholz DH, Young VM, Friedman NR, et al. Detection and quantitation of bacteria in platelet products stored at ambient temperature. Transfusion 1973;13:268-75.

62. Buchholz DH, Young VM, Friedman NR, et al. Bacterial proliferation in platelet products stored at room temperature: Transfusion-induced *Enterobacter* sepsis. N Engl J Med 1971;285:429-33.
63. Sazama K. Bacteria in blood for transfusion. A review. Arch Pathol Lab Med 1994;118:350-65.
64. Dodd RY. Adverse consequences of blood transfusion: Quantitative risk estimates. In: Nance ST, ed. Blood supply: Risks, perceptions and prospects for the future. Bethesda, MD: American Association of Blood Banks, 1994:1-24.
65. Morrow JF, Braine HG, Kickler TS, et al. Septic reactions to platelet transfusions. A persistent problem. JAMA 1991;266:555-8.
66. Goldman M, Blajchman MA. Blood product-associated bacterial sepsis. Transfus Med Rev 1991;5:73-83.
67. Blajchman MA. Bacterial contamination of blood products and the value of pre-transfusion testing. Immunol Invest 1995;24:163-70.
68. Blajchman MA, Ali AM. Bacteria in the blood supply: An overlooked issue in transfusion medicine. In: Nance ST, ed. Blood safety: Current challenges. Bethesda, MD: American Association of Blood Banks, 1992:213-28.
69. Gibson T, Norris W. Skin fragments removed by injection needles. Lancet 1958;2:983-5.
70. Sazama K. Reports of 355 transfusion-associated deaths: 1976 through 1985. Transfusion 1990;30:583-90.
71. Pfaller MA, Herwaldt LA. Laboratory, clinical, and epidemiological aspects of coagulase-negative staphylococci. Clin Microbiol Rev 1988;1:281-99.
72. Anderson KC, Lew MA, Gorgone BC, et al. Transfusion-related sepsis after prolonged platelet storage. Am J Med 1986;81:405-11.
73. Heal JM, Jones ME, Forey J, et al. Fatal *Salmonella* septicemia after platelet transfusion. Transfusion 1987;27:2-5.
74. Gong J, Hogman CF, Hambraeus A, et al. Transfusion-transmitted *Yersinia enterocolitica* infection. Vox Sang 1993;65:42-6.
75. Kuehnert MJ, Jarvis WR, Schaffer DA, Chaffin DJ. Platelet transfusion reaction due to *Yersinia enterocolitica* (letter). JAMA 1997;278:550.
76. Selwyn S, Ellis H. Skin bacteria and skin disinfection reconsidered. Br Med J 1972;1:136-40.

77. Heltberg O, Skov F, Gerner-Smidt P, et al. Nosocomial epidemic of *Serratia marcescens* septicemia ascribed to contaminated blood transfusion bags. Transfusion 1993;33:221-7.
78. Hogman CF, Fritz H, Sandberg L. Posttransfusion *Serratia marcescens* septicemia. Transfusion 1993;33:189-91.
79. Blajchman MA, Thornley JH, Richardson H, et al. Platelet transfusion induced *Serratia marcescens* sepsis due to vacuum tube contamination. Transfusion 1979;19:39-44.
80. Hogman CF, Gong J. Studies of one invasive and two noninvasive methods for detection of bacterial contamination of platelet concentrates. Vox Sang 1994;67:351-5.
81. Gong J, Hogman CF, Lundholm M, Gustafsson I. Novel automated microbial screening of platelet concentrates. APMIS 1994;102: 72-8.
82. Reik H, Rubin SJ. Evaluation of the buffy-coat smear for rapid detection of bacteremia. JAMA 1981;245:357-9.
83. Barrett BB, Andersen JW, Andersen KC. Strategies for the avoidance of bacterial contamination of blood components. Transfusion 1993; 33:228-33.
84. Chiu EKW, Yuen KY, Lie AKW, et al. A prospective study of symptomatic bacteremia following platelet transfusion and of its management. Transfusion 1994;34:950-4.
85. Bertolini F, Murphy S, for the Biomedical Excellence for Safer Transfusion (BEST) Working Party of the International Society of Blood Transfusion. A multicenter evaluation of reproducibility of swirling in platelet concentrates. Transfusion 1994;34:796-801.
86. Wagner SJ, Robinette D. Evaluation of swirling, pH, and glucose tests for the detection of bacterial contamination in platelet concentrates. Transfusion 1996;36:989-93.
87. Myhre BA, Demianew SH, Yoshimori RN, et al. pH changes caused by bacterial growth in contaminated platelet concentrates. Ann Clin Lab Sci 1985;15:509-14.
88. Burstain JM, Brecher ME, Workman K, et al. Rapid identification of bacterially contaminated platelets using reagent strips: Glucose and pH analysis as markers of bacterial metabolism. Transfusion 1997; 37:255-8.
89. Brecher ME, Boothe G, Kerr A. The use of a chemiluminescence-linked universal bacterial ribosomal RNA gene probe and blood gas

analysis for the rapid detection of bacterial contamination in white cell-reduced and nonreduced platelets. Transfusion 1993;33:450-7.

90. Brecher ME, Hogan JJ, Boothe G, et al. Platelet bacterial contamination and the use of a chemiluminescence-linked universal bacterial ribosomal RNA gene probe. Transfusion 1994;34:750-5.
91. Feng P, Keasler SP, Hill WE. Direct identification of *Yersinia enterocolitica* in blood by polymerase chain reaction amplification. Transfusion 1992;32:850-4.
92. Arpi M, Bremmelgaard A, Abel Y, et al. A novel screening method for the detection of microbial contamination of platelet concentrates. An experimental pilot study (letter). Vox Sang 1993;65:335-6.
93. McCarthy LR, Senne JE. Evaluation of acridine orange stain for detection of microorganisms in blood cultures. J Clin Microbiol 1980; 11:281-5.
94. Chongokolwatana V, Morgan M, Feagin JC, et al. Comparison of microscopy and bacterial DNA probe for detecting bacterially contaminated platelets (abstract). Transfusion 1993;33(suppl):50S.
95. Kim DM, Brecher ME, Bland LA, et al. Prestorage removal of *Yersinia enterocolitica* from red cells with white cell-reduction filters. Transfusion 1992;32:658-662.
96. Hogman CF, Gong J, Eriksson L, et al. White cells protect donor blood against bacterial contamination. Transfusion 1991;31:620-6.
97. Wenz B, Ciavarella D, Freundlich L. Effect of prestorage white cell reduction on bacterial growth in platelet concentrates. Transfusion 1993;33:520-3.
98. Hogman CF, Gong J, Hambraeus A, et al. The role of leukocytes in the transmission of *Yersinia enterocolitica* with blood components. Transfusion 1992;32:654-7.
99. Franzin L,Gioannini P. Growth of *Yersinia* species in artificially contaminated blood bags. Transfusion 1992;32:673-6.
100. Buchholz DH, AuBuchon JP, Snyder EL, et al. Removal of *Yersinia enterocolitica* from AS-1 red cells. Transfusion 1992;32:667-72.
101. Wenz B, Burns ER, Freundlich LF. Prevention of growth of *Yersinia enterocolitica* in blood by polyester fiber filtration. Transfusion 1992;32:663-6.
102. Pietersz RNI, Reesink HW, Pauw W, et al. Prevention of *Yersinia enterocolitica* growth in red-blood-cell concentrates. Lancet 1992; 340:755-6.

103. Wagner SJ, Moroff G, Katz AJ, Friedman LI. Comparison of bacteria growth in single and pooled platelet concentrates after deliberate inoculation and storage. Transfusion 1995;35:298-302.

104. Lin L, Londe H, Janda JM, et al. Photochemical inactivation of pathogenic bacteria in human platelet concentrates. Blood 1994;83: 2698-706.

105. Blajchman MA. Transfusion-associated bacterial sepsis: The phoenix rises yet again. Transfusion 1994;34:940-2.

106. Takahashi T, Abe H, Nakai K, Sekiguchi S. Bradykinin generation during filtration of platelet concentrates with a white cell-reduction filter (letter). Transfusion 1995;35:967.

107. Takahashi TA, Abe H, Sekiguchi S. More on kininogen measurements in platelet concentrates that are white cell (WBC) reduced with WBC-reduction filters (response). Transfusion 1996;36:940-1.

108. Muylle L, Wouters E, Peetermans ME. Febrile reactions to platelet transfusion: The effect of increased interleukin-6 levels in concentrates prepared by the platelet-rich plasma method. Transfusion 1996;36:886-90.

109. Riccardi D, Raspollini E, Rebulla P, et al. Relationship of the time of storage and transfusion reactions to platelet concentrates from buffy coats. Transfusion 1997;37:528-30.

110. Petranyi GG, Reti M, Harsanyi V, Szabo J. Immunologic consequences of blood transfusion and their clinical manifestations. Int Arch Allergy Immunol 1997;114:303-15.

111. Miller WV, Holland PV, Sugarbaker E, et al. Anaphylactic reaction to IgA: A difficult transfusion problem. Am J Clin Pathol 1970;54: 618-21.

112. Laschinger C, Shepherd FA, Naylor DH. Anti-IgA-mediated transfusion reactions in Canada. Can Med Assoc J 1984;130:141-4.

113. Ramsey G. The pathophysiology and organ-specific consequences of severe transfusion reactions. New Horiz 1994;2:575-81.

114. Baroti Toth C, Kramer J, Pinter J, et al. IgA content of washed red blood cells. Vox Sang 1998;74:13-4.

115. Popovsky MA, Moore SB. Diagnostic and pathogenetic considerations in transfusion-related acute lung injury. Transfusion 1985;25: 573-7.

116. Popovsky MA, Chaplin HC, Moore SB. Transfusion-related acute lung injury: A neglected, serious complication of hemotherapy. Transfusion 1992;32:589-92.

117. Seeger W, Schneider V, Kreusler B, et al. Reproduction of transfusion-related acute lung injury in an *ex vivo* lung model. Blood 1990;76:1438-44.
118. Wolf CFW, Canale VC. Fatal pulmonary hypersensitivity reaction to HLA incompatible blood transfusion: Report of a case and review of the literature. Transfusion 1976;16:135-40.
119. Hume HA, Popovsky MA, Benson K, et al. Hypotensive reactions: A previously uncharacterized complication of platelet transfusion? Transfusion 1996;36:904-9.
120. Fried MR, Eastlund T, Christie B, et al. Hypotensive reactions to white-cell reduced plasma in a patient undergoing angiotensin-converting enzyme inhibitor therapy. Transfusion 1996;36:900-3.
121. Mair B, LeParc GF. Hypotensive reactions associated with platelet transfusions and angiotensin-converting enzyme inhibitors. Vox Sang 1998;74:27-30.
122. Moore SB. Hypotensive reactions: Are they a new phenomenon? Are they related solely to transfusion of platelets? Does filtration of components play a role? Transfusion 1996;36:852-3.
123. Proud D, Kaplan AP. Kinin formation: Mechanisms and role of inflammatory disorders. Annu Rev Immunol 1988;6:49-83.
124. Colman RW, Scott CF, Brandwein H, Whitbread J. More on kininogen measurements in platelet concentrates that are white cell (WBC) reduced with WBC-reduction filter (letter). Transfusion 1996;36:939-40.
125. Payne R. The association of febrile transfusion reactions with leuko-agglutinins. Vox Sang 1957;2:233-41.
126. Payne R, Rolfs MR. Further observations on leukoagglutinin transfusion reactions, with special reference to leukoagglutinin transfusion reactions in women. Am J Med 1960;29:449-58.
127. Perkins HA, Payne R, Ferguson J, Wood M. Nonhemolytic febrile transfusion reactions: Quantitative effects of blood components with emphasis on isoantigenic incompatibility of leukocytes. Vox Sang 1966;11:578-600.
128. Brittingham TE, Chaplin H Jr. Febrile transfusion reactions caused by sensitivity to donor leukocytes and platelets. JAMA 1957;165: 819-25.
129. Andreu G, Dewailly J, Leberre C, et al. Prevention of HLA immunization with leukocyte-poor packed red cells and platelet concentrates obtained by filtration. Blood 1988;72:964-9.

130. Muylle L, Wouters E, De Bock R, Peetermans ME. Reactions to platelet transfusion: The effect of the storage time of the concentrate. Transfus Med 1992;2:289-93.
131. Heddle NM, Klama L, Singer J, et al. The role of the plasma from platelet concentrates in transfusion reactions. N Engl J Med 1994; 331:625-8.
132. Dinarello CA. Interleukin-1 and interleukin-1 antagonism. Blood 1991;77:1627-52.
133. Heinrich PC, Castell JV, Andus T. Interleukin-6 and the acute phase response. Biochem J 1990;265:621-36.
134. Stack G, Snyder EL. Cytokine generation in stored platelet concentrates. Transfusion 1994;34:20-5.
135. Aye MT, Palmer DS, Giulivi A, Hashemi S. Effect of filtration of platelet concentrates on the accumulation of cytokines and platelet release factors during storage. Transfusion 1995;35:117-24.
136. Fujihara M, Takahashi TA, Ogiso C, et al. Generation of interleukin-8 in stored apheresis platelet concentrates and the preventive effect of prestorage ultraviolet B radiation. Transfusion 1997;37:468-75.
137. Wadhwa M, Seghatchian MJ, Lubenko A, et al. Cytokine levels in platelet concentrates: Quantitation by bioassays and immunoassays. Br J Haematol 1996;93:225-34.
138. Lumadue JA, Lanzkron SM, Kennedy SD, et al. Cytokine induction of platelet activation. Am J Clin Pathol 1996;106:795-8.
139. Bubel S, Wilhelm D, Entelmann M, et al. Chemokines in stored platelet concentrates. Transfusion 1996;36:445-9.
140. Bertolini F, Rebulla P, Riccardi D, et al. Evaluation of platelet concentrates prepared from buffy coats and stored in a glucose-free crystalloid medium. Transfusion 1989;29:605-9.
141. Flegel WA, Wiesneth M, Stampe D, Koerner K. Low cytokine contamination in buffy coat-derived platelet concentrates without filtration. Transfusion 1995;35:917-20.
142. Sweeney JD, Holme S, Stromberg RR, Heaton WAL. In vitro and in vivo effects of prestorage filtration of apheresis platelets. Transfusion 1995;35:125-30.
143. Bishop D, Tandy N, Anderson N, et al. A clinical and laboratory study of platelet concentrates produced by pooled buffy coat and single donor apheresis technologies. Transfus Sci 1995;16:187-8.

144. Kluter H, Muller-Steinhardt M, Danzer S, et al. Cytokines in platelet concentrates prepared from pooled buffy coats. Vox Sang 1995; 69:38-43.

145. Muylle L, Joos M, Wouters E, et al. Increased tumor necrosis factor a (TNFα), interleukin 1, and interleukin 6 (IL-6) levels in the plasma of stored platelet concentrates: Relationship between TNFα and IL-6 levels and febrile transfusion reactions. Transfusion 1993;33:195-9.

146. Handin RI, Fortier NL, Valeri CR. Platelet response to hypotonic stress after storage at 4°C or 22°C. Transfusion 1970;10:305-9.

147. Watts SE, Tunbridge LJ, Smith K, Lloyd JV. Storage of platelets for tests of platelet function: Effects of temperature on platelet aggregation, platelet morphology and liberation of β-thromboglobulin. Thromb Res 1986;44:365-76.

148. Slichter SJ, Harker LA. Preparation and storage of platelet concentrates, II: Storage variables influencing platelet viability and function. Br J Haematol 1976;34:403-19.

149. Connor J, Currie LM, Allan H, Livesey SA. Recovery of *in vitro* functional activity of platelet concentrates stored at 4°C and treated with second-messenger effectors. Transfusion 1996;36:691-8.

150. Currie LM, Harper JR, Allan H, Connor J. Inhibition of cytokine accumulation and bacterial growth during storage of platelet concentrates at 4°C with retention of in vitro functional activity. Transfusion 1997;37:18-24.

151. Shimuzu T, Uchigiri C, Mizuno S, et al. Adsorption of anaphylatoxins and platelet-specific proteins by filtration of platelet concentrates with a polyester leukocyte reduction filter. Vox Sang 1994;66:161-5.

152. Snyder EL, Mechanic S, Baril L, Davenport R. Removal of soluble biologic response modifiers (complement and chemokines) by a bedside white cell-reduction filter. Transfusion 1996;36:707-13.

153. Geiger TL, Perrotta PL, Davenport R, et al. Removal of anaphylatoxins C3a and C5a and chemokines interleukin-8 and RANTES by polyester white cell-reduction and plasma filters. Transfusion 1997; 37:1156-62.

154. Howard JE, Perkins HA. The natural history of alloimmunization to platelets. Transfusion 1978;18:496-503.

155. Meryman HT. Transfusion-induced alloimmunization and immunosuppression and the effects of leukocyte depletion. Transfus Med Rev 1989;3:180-93.

156. Abou-Elella AA, Camarillo TA, Allen MB, et al. Low incidence of red cell and HLA antibody formation by bone marrow transplant patients. Transfusion 1995;35:931-5.
157. Opelz G, Sengar DPS, Mickey MR, et al. Effect of blood transfusions on subsequent kidney transplants. Transplant Proc 1973;5:253-9.
158. Opelz G, Terasaki PI. Improvement of kidney-graft survival with increased numbers of blood transfusions. N Engl J Med 1978;299: 799-803.
159. Betuel H, Cantarovitch D, Robert F, et al. Platelet transfusions preparative for kidney transplantation. Transplant Proc 1985;17: 2335-7.
160. Borleffs JCC, Marquat RL, Neuhaus P. Effect of matching for DR antigens and pretransplant blood transfusions on kidney graft survival in rhesus monkeys. Transplant Proc 1982;14:403-6.
161. Obertop H, Bijnen AB, Vriesendorp HM, Westbroek DL. Prolongation of renal allograft survival in DLA tissue-typed beagles after third-party blood transfusions and immunosuppressive treatment. Transplantation 1978;26:255-9.
162. Taylor C, Faulk WP. Prevention of recurrent abortion with leukocyte transfusions. Lancet 1981;2:68-70.
163. Mowbray JF. Autoantibodies, alloantibodies and reproductive success. Curr Opin Immunol 1989;2:761-4.
164. Mowbray JF, Gibbings C, Lidell H, et al. Controlled trial of treatment of recurrent spontaneous abortion by immunisation with paternal cells. Lancet 1985;1:941-3.
165. Unander AM. The role of immunization treatment in preventing recurrent abortion. Transfus Med Rev 1992;6:1-16.
166. Gatenby PA, Cameron K, Simes RJ, et al. Treatment of recurrent spontaneous abortion by immunization with paternal lymphocytes: Results of a controlled trial. Am J Reprod Immunol 1993;29:88-94.
167. Peters WR, Fry RD, Fleshman JW, Kodner IJ. Multiple blood transfusions reduce the recurrence rate of Crohn's disease. Dis Colon Rectum 1989;32:749-53.
168. Steup WH, Brand A, Weterman IT, et al. The effect of perioperative blood transfusion on recurrence after primary operation for Crohn's disease. Scand J Gastroenterol 1991;188(suppl):81-6.
169. Scott ADN, Ritchie JK, Phillips RKS. Blood transfusion and recurrent Crohn's disease. Br J Surg 1991;78:455-8.

170. Blumberg N, Heal JM. Blood transfusion immunomodulation. The silent epidemic. Arch Pathol Lab Med 1998;122:117-9.

171. Jensen LS, Andersen AJ, Christiansen PM, et al. Postoperative infection and natural killer cell function following blood transfusion in patients undergoing elective colorectal surgery. Br J Surg 1992;79: 513-6.

172. Jensen LS, Grunnet N, Hanberg-Sorensen F, Jorgensen J. Cost-effectiveness of blood transfusion and white cell reduction in elective colorectal surgery. Transfusion 1995;35:719-22.

173. Jensen LS, Kissmeyer-Nielsen P, Wolff B, Qvist N. Randomised comparison of leucocyte-depleted versus buffy-coat-poor blood transfusion and complications after colorectal surgery. Lancet 1996;348: 841-5.

174. Gianotti L, Pyles T, Alexander JW, et al. Identification of the blood component responsible for increased susceptibility to gut-derived infection. Transfusion 1993;33:458-65.

175. Vamvakas EC, Carven JH. Allogeneic blood transfusion, hospital charges, and length of hospitalization. A study of 487 consecutive patients undergoing colorectal cancer resection. Arch Pathol Lab Med 1998;122:145-51.

176. Busch MP, Lee TH, Heitman J. Allogeneic leukocytes but not therapeutic blood elements induce reactivation and dissemination of latent human immunodeficiency virus type 1 infection: Implications for transfusion support of infected patients. Blood 1992;80: 2128-35.

177. Adler SP, Baggett J, McVoy M. Transfusion-associated cytomegalovirus infections in seropositive cardiac surgery patients. Lancet 1985; 2:743-6.

178. Ward JW, Bush TJ, Perkins HA, et al. The natural history of transfusion-associated infection with human immunodeficiency virus: Factors influencing the rate of progression of disease. N Engl J Med 1989;321:947-52.

179. Groopman JE. Impact of transfusion on viral load in human immunodeficiency virus infection. Semin Hematol 1997;34:27-33.

180. Vamvakas E, Kaplan HS. Early transfusion and length of survival in acquired immune deficiency syndrome: Experience with a population receiving medical care at a public hospital. Transfusion 1993; 33:111-8.

181. Bordin JO, Blajchman MA. Transfusion-associated immunosuppression. In: Rossi EC, Simon TL, Moss GS, Gould SA, eds. Principles of transfusion medicine. 2nd ed. Baltimore, MD: Williams & Wilkins, 1996:803-12.
182. Lane TA. Leukocyte reduction of cellular blood components. Effectiveness, benefits, quality control, and costs. Arch Pathol Lab Med 1994;118:392-404.
183. Busch OR, Hop WC, Hoynck van Papendrecht MA, et al. Blood transfusions and prognosis in colorectal cancer. N Engl J Med 1993;328:1372-6.
184. Houbiers JG, Brand A, van de Watering LM, et al. Randomised controlled trial comparing transfusion of leucocyte-depleted or buffy-coat-depleted blood in surgery for colorectal cancer. Lancet 1994; 344:573-8.
185. Blumberg N, Heal JM. The transfusion immunomodulation theory: The Th1/Th2 paradigm and an analogy with pregnancy as a unifying mechanism. Semin Hematol 1996;33:329-40.
186. Klein HG. Immunomodulation caused by blood transfusion. In: Petz LD, Swisher SN, Kleinman S, Spence RK, et al, eds. Clinical practice of transfusion medicine. 3rd ed. New York: Churchill Livingstone, 1996:59-69.
187. Clerici M, Clerici E, Shearer GM. The tumor enhancement phenomenon: Reinterpretation from a Th1/Th2 perspective. J Natl Cancer Inst 1996;88:461-2.
188. Strom TB, Roy-Chaudhury P, Manfro R, et al. The Th1/Th2 paradigm and the allograft response. Curr Opin Immunol 1996;8: 688-93.
189. Shimodo T. On postoperative erythroderma. Geka 1955;17:487-92.
190. Brubaker DB. Human posttransfusion graft-versus-host disease. Vox Sang 1983;45:401-20.
191. Przepiorka D, Leparc GF, Stovall MA, et al. Use of irradiated blood components. Practice parameter. Am J Clin Pathol 1996;106:6-11.
192. Juji T, Takahashi K, Shibata Y, et al. Post-transfusion graft-versus-host disease in immunocompetent patients after cardiac surgery in Japan (letter). N Engl J Med 1989;321:56.
193. Kanter MH. Transfusion-associated graft-versus-host disease: Do transfusions from second-degree relatives pose a greater risk than those from first-degree relatives? Transfusion 1992;32:323-7.

194. Petz LD, Calhoun L, Yam P, et al. Transfusion-associated graft-versus-host disease in immunocompetent patients. Report of a fatal case associated with transfusion of blood from a second-degree relative, and a survey of predisposing factors. Transfusion 1993;33:742-50.
195. Terasaki PI. Identification of the type of blood cells responsible for the graft-versus-host reaction in chicks. J Exp Morphol 1959;7: 394-402.
196. Billingham RE. The biology of graft-versus-host reactions. Harvey Lect 1966;62:21-78.
197. Lee T-H, Donegan E, Slichter S, et al. Transient increase in circulating donor leukocytes after allogeneic transfusions in immunocompetent recipients compatible with donor cell proliferation. Blood 1995; 85:1207-14.
198. Anderson KC, Goodnough LT, Sayers M, et al. Variation in blood component irradiation practice: Implications for prevention of transfusion-associated graft-versus-host disease. Blood 1991;77: 2096-102.
199. Greenbaum BH. Transfusion-associated graft-versus-host disease: Historical perspectives, incidence and current use of irradiated blood products. J Clin Oncol 1991;9:1889-902.
200. Menitove JE, ed. Standards for blood banks and transfusion services. 19th ed. Bethesda, MD: American Association of Blood Banks, 1999:25.
201. Food and Drug Administration Memorandum: Recommendations regarding license amendments and procedures for gamma irradiation of blood products. July 22, 1993. Rockville, MD: CBER Office of Communication, Training, and Manufacturer's Assistance, 1993.
202. Rosen NR, Weidner JG, Boldt HD, Rosen DS. Prevention of transfusion-associated graft versus-host disease: Selection of an adequate dose of gamma radiation. Transfusion 1993;33:125-7.
203. Pelszynski MM, Moroff G, Luban NL, et al. Effect of gamma irradiation by limiting dilution analysis: Implications for preventing transfusion-associated graft-versus-host disease. Blood 1994;83:1683-9.
204. Drobyski WW, Thibodeau S, Truitt RL, et al. Third party mediated graft rejection and graft-versus-host disease after T-cell depleted bone marrow transplantation as demonstrated by hypervariable DNA probes and HLA-DR polymorphism. Blood 1989;74:2285-94.
205. Rock G, Adams GA , Labow RS. The effects of irradiation on platelet function. Transfusion 1988;28:451-5.
206. Read EJ, Kodis C, Carter CS, Leitman SF. Viability of platelets following storage in the irradiated state. Transfusion 1988;28:446-50.

In: Kickler TS, and Herman JH, eds.
Current Issues in Platelet Transfusion Therapy and Platelet Alloimmunity
Bethesda, MD: AABB Press, 1999

11

Platelet Transfusion Therapy: Future Considerations

CHARLES A. SCHIFFER, MD

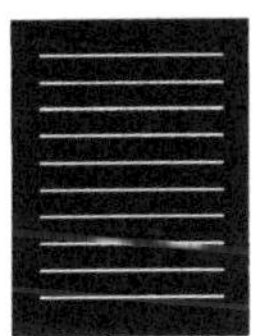

THE WIDESPREAD AVAILABILITY OF PLATELET TRANSfusions for the treatment and prevention of hemorrhage in patients with marrow failure has dramatically altered the morbidity level and the overall outcome for patients with leukemia and aplastic anemia. Thirty years ago, platelets had to be ordered from the blood center 3-4 days in advance, requiring an estimate of what the patient's future platelet count might be. Today, practitioners can choose the source of platelets (apheresis vs random donor), the type of platelets (volume-reduced, leukocyte-reduced), and the techniques used for histocompatible platelets. Whereas hemorrhage, often associated with gram-negative bacteremia, was a major cause of death in patients undergoing induction chemotherapy during the early 1970s, fewer than 1-2% of

Charles A. Schiffer, MD, Professor of Medicine and Oncology and Chief, Division of Hematology/Oncology, Wayne State University School of Medicine; and Director of Clinical Research, Barbara Ann Karmanos Cancer Institute, Harper Hospital, Detroit, Michigan

leukemia patients now succumb to hemorrhage; as a result, drug-resistant leukemia has replaced failure of supportive care as the major reason for patients not achieving complete remission.

Technical advances from a variety of disciplines have made these improvements possible. The development of supple plastics, which permitted the construction of unified blood collection sets to allow more convenient mass production of platelets, was an early critical step. Improvements in the permeability of the plastic bags, which allowed oxygen to enter more rapidly and thereby prevented anaerobic metabolism by the platelets, helped extend platelet storage to as long as 7 days.[1,2] Concern about bacterial proliferation with extended storage at room temperature, which had replaced 4 C as the standard storage temperature in the early 1970s,[1] reduced storage duration to the current 5 days.[3,4]

Apheresis technology developed in parallel, initially as part of a collaborative effort between the National Cancer Institute and the IBM Corporation.[5] Centrifugation technology, inspired by separation techniques used in the dairy industry, resulted in blood cell processors that used an intermittent batch collection technique.[6,7] The need for a rotating seal connecting the IV tubing to the separation chamber, a source of potential contamination because it was an "open" system, was obviated by technology borrowed from radar discs, which allowed full continuous circular rotation without "tangling" of the tubing or wires.[8,9] This in turn resulted in the continuous-flow apheresis devices used most commonly today, which allow the rapid processing of large volumes of blood.

The microchip revolution has permitted full automation of processes that previously had depended on operator decisions as to the best interface for cell procurement. Imaginative clinicians and investigators have used this technology in a variety of clinically important ways, ushering in the disciplines of therapeutic plasma exchange, therapeutic cytopheresis, and, ultimately, the entire field of autologous and allogeneic hematopoietic progenitor cell (HPC) transplantation. Biotechnology has produced cytokines enhancing the efficiencies of these procedures while the development of filtering technology and biocompatible fibers has permitted the efficient removal of leukocytes, resulting in a product that is less likely to cause alloimmunization[10] or infections from DNA-incorporated viruses such as cytomegalovirus (CMV).[11]

Still, the process is not perfect. Platelet transfusions are costly and associated with a number of side effects. Future research should be directed at extending these highly successful technological developments to make platelet transfusions even safer and more effective. This chapter addresses some of the issues deserving attention in the future.

Who Needs Platelet Transfusion?

Most platelet transfusions are administered to prevent rather than treat active hemorrhage. On the basis of relatively little data, clinicians had traditionally used a cutoff of below 20,000 platelets/μL as the "trigger" for such prophylactic transfusions.[12,13] This decision was usually based on a platelet count performed in the morning, neglecting the obvious point that patients had these low platelet counts for many hours before the count was obtained and often for many hours before the prophylactic transfusion was administered. Yet, the mortality and serious morbidity from severe hemorrhage in leukemia patients are quite low. Indeed, given the observation that bleeding times are markedly prolonged in thrombocytopenic patients with counts below 50,000/μL,[14] the more interesting point is not that patients occasionally bleed, but that the overwhelming majority do not experience significant hemorrhage.

A number of randomized trials have been completed over the past few years in patients with acute leukemia. These trials have documented that a prophylactic platelet transfusion trigger of 10,000/μL is as safe as the 20,000/μL-level trigger, with appropriate caveats for transfusion at higher levels in patients with active bleeding, coagulopathy, or a need for a surgical procedure.[15-17] These studies have demonstrated an approximately 20% reduction in platelet usage in patients transfused at the lower counts. Furthermore, the occasional occurrence of severe hemorrhage has usually been unrelated to the platelet count, and in some patients, has been noted at counts well in excess of 20,000/μL. It is probable that lower thresholds for prophylactic transfusion would also be safe in many of these patients. Future trials should address whether these guidelines can be safely applied to patients following high-dose therapy with transplantation, which produces more severe mucositis. In addition, as clinicians become more comfortable with these lower counts, it is likely that the number of transfusions will be reduced in patients with chronic, severe thombocytopenia, such as occurs in patients with myelodysplasia or aplastic anemia. Although patients with these disorders obviously require platelet transfusions at times, they often receive inappropriate prophylactic transfusions currently because of concerns about the risks of catastrophic spontaneous hemorrhage.

It has also been recognized that individual patients receive disproportionate numbers of transfusions. These are usually alloimmunized patients in whom there are poor to absent posttransfusion increments and who receive repetitive, probably futile transfusions until the diagnosis of alloimmunization is made by serologic tests and attempts are begun to find histocompatible donors. It is likely that more routine application of leukocyte reduction by filtration will reduce the incidence of alloimmunization and also somewhat decrease overall usage as well.[10]

Counterbalancing these reasons for reducing platelet usage is increasing the use of high-dose therapies for a wider variety of disorders. Although the use of peripheral blood progenitor cell transplants rather than marrow transplants has markedly decreased platelet usage, the number of procedures, particularly for women with breast cancer, has increased markedly over the past few years. Whether this trend continues will in part be determined by the results of randomized clinical trials in both the adjuvant and metastatic disease settings that have recently been completed. "Positive" results in these trials will likely increase demand for platelet transfusions, whereas less promising results may at least temporarily result in overall decreased demands.

Leukocyte Reduction and Prevention of Alloimmunization

The recently published TRAP (Trial to Reduce Alloimmunization to Platelets) study has conclusively demonstrated that both leukocyte reduction and ultraviolet-B (UVB) irradiation can reduce the incidence of alloimmunization and refractoriness to platelet transfusion in patients receiving induction chemotherapy for acute myeloid leukemia,[10] and it is likely, albeit unproved, that filtration would have similar benefits for patients being treated for other cancers as well. There are, however, relatively few groups of patients who require repetitive, prolonged courses of therapy with the need for repeated multiple platelet transfusions. Thus, although this is probably already being done in practice, there is no compelling rationale for the routine filtration of platelets in patients undergoing high-dose chemotherapy with HPC transplantation. Such patients generally require only a few transfusions for the transplantation and do not have planned further chemotherapy afterwards.[18] Therefore, leukocyte reduction should be restricted to patients who are likely to require long-term transfusion support.

As an alternative to filtration of platelets or red cells after storage, removal of leukocytes just after blood collection (so-called prestorage leukocyte reduction) is likely to be advantageous because of accumulating evidence that most transfusion reactions are a consequence of cytokines elaborated by leukocytes during storage.[19-21] Other than alloimmunization, it is these febrile reactions that are most disturbing and dangerous to the patient. Effective leukocyte removal also reduces the risk of transmission of infectious agents such as CMV.[11] It is expected that leukocyte reduction will increase in the future, given its multiple clinical advantages.

Decreases in the appreciable costs associated with the "work-up" of transfusion reactions, which also often result in hospitalization for neutropenic patients, as well as in the costs of providing CMV-negative blood components, should offset the increased expense associated with use of leukocyte-reduced blood.

An additional consideration relates to the filtration and processing of platelets prepared from buffy coats of red blood cells (RBCs), a practice that is in widespread use in Europe. Studies have shown these platelets to have posttransfusion increments similar to those of platelets prepared by the platelet-rich plasma method, with a possibility that buffy-coat-prepared platelets might be more suitable for prolonged storage. Potential disadvantages include the necessity for filtration to reduce the high white cell content when platelets are prepared by some of the buffy coat techniques, some loss of red cells, and the need for a major retraining and retooling of the blood collection system.[22] Nevertheless, comparative studies of the two approaches would be of considerable interest.

The mechanism by which leukocyte reduction or UVB irradiation decreases immune responsiveness to histocompatibility antigens remains unclear. Although it is likely that reduction in either the number or the function of donor antigen-presenting cells is an important component, this does not readily explain the apparent persistent immune tolerance that develops in most recipients. Indeed, the majority of patients with acute myeloid leukemia never become alloimmunized despite continued long-term transfusions even without leukocyte reduction or other such manipulations. This suggests that there is an additional and sustained immunosuppressive effect of the initial chemotherapy administered to the recipient.[23] This clinical scenario has the potential to serve as an instructive model to evaluate mechanisms of humoral immune tolerance. One intriguing hypothesis is that patients develop anti-idiotype (anti-HLA) neutralizing antibodies, as has been shown in renal allograft recipients.[24] Another possibility, which could potentially be manipulated clinically, is that there is a specific time sequence between the initial antigen exposure from transfusion and the cytotoxic chemotherapy that produces this immune tolerance.

UVB irradiation devices are not yet approved by the Food and Drug Administration or commercially available, although the results from the TRAP study are convincing about the benefits of this approach. UVB irradiation represents a potentially simpler manipulation than leukocyte filtration. Filtration does have the additional advantage of preventing CMV infection, however, and it remains to be seen whether the UVB technology will be submitted for regulatory review and be widely used.

Transmission of Infectious Agents

With current multiple screening techniques, the rate of transmission of viral or bacterial infection from blood or platelet transfusions is extraordinarily low. Indeed, whereas hepatitis was a routine problem in patients with leukemia in the 1970s, often limiting the delivery of subsequent therapy, current screening for hepatitis B and C has now made this a very unusual problem. Although the specter of transmission of human immunodeficiency virus has received significant attention, it represents a rare event in the United States.

Nonetheless, any relatively simple and practical means by which such organisms can be reliably inactivated would be welcomed and might also provide savings in terms of a reduced need to screen blood products and donors. This may be particularly important in developing countries. Thus, there has been great interest in recent publications describing the effects of psoralen compounds, which, with appropriate UV exposure, appear capable of inactivating most known viral and bacterial organisms.[25] In addition, there is suggestive evidence that such in-vitro treatments could provide prophylaxis against graft-vs-host disease with the theoretical possibility of reduction in the need for irradiation of the product in certain subgroups of recipients.[24] Although it is likely that any such treatments would initially increase the cost of transfusion, the costs could be offset by reductions in the need for donor screening for prior viral infections.

Platelet "Substitutes"

There has been a flurry of presentations in the past few years related to the use of nonviable platelet substitutes in place of the traditional transfusion of intact platelets (reviewed in Alving et al[26]). Lyophilized platelets, initially evaluated more than 30 years ago, are under evaluation again,[27] as are freeze-dried platelets, platelet membranes,[28] and even erythrocytes to which subendothelial binding proteins[29] have been attached (thromboerythrocytes). The operative hypotheses underlying all these products is that the "substitute" will bind to exposed subendothelium, providing an adequate stimulus for the coagulation cascade and clot formation. Some of these products have been initially evaluated in an ear bleeding time model in thrombocytopenic rabbits,[30] while the platelet membranes have been used in Phase I trials in humans with anecdotal reports of improved hemostasis in bleeding patients.[31] The appeal of these approaches is the potential for a sterilized product with an essentially indefinite shelf life, providing a ready supply of platelets at all times.

Evaluating these different products clinically to demonstrate hemostatic effectiveness is a complex and difficult task. Prior modifications to platelet transfusion products have been evaluated by their ability to produce posttransfusion platelet count increments in thrombocytopenic recipients, sometimes by the correction of template bleeding times, with additional evidence of viability being assessed by the recovery and survival of radiolabeled autologous platelets. Obviously, some of these parameters are not applicable with the platelet substitutes, and proof of benefit will depend on the demonstration of a hemostatic effect. It is, however, extremely difficult to measure hemorrhage objectively in thrombocytopenic patients. Severe hemorrhage is rare, and gastrointestinal and urinary tract hemorrhage, which are somewhat quantifiable, are even less common. These subjective endpoints would most certainly require some sort of double blinding on the part of the clinical observers.

It might also turn out that these platelet substitutes will be of benefit in only selected situations. For example, it is quite possible that the platelet substitutes will serve as a nidus for the coagulation system only with the stimulation and participation of residual circulating platelets. Thus, there might be differences in efficacy in thrombocytopenic patients with somewhat higher counts, such as 30,000/μL, compared with those who have very low counts of perhaps less than 5000/μL. It is accepted that a certain fraction of circulating platelets is required to maintain epithelial vascular integrity, and it might be that nonviable platelets are inadequate for this task but could stimulate clotting with higher levels of circulating platelets. It is expected that these issues will be addressed in upcoming studies involving these products, but the first barrier will be to design a clinical trial in humans by which benefit can be determined objectively, remembering that an adequate and well-proved alternative—that is, viable stored platelets—is currently readily available. One possible model could focus on alloimmunized patients for whom histocompatible platelets cannot be identified. Certainly the field would benefit from an in-vitro model predictive of hemostatic capability in vivo, which at least could help screen new modifications of these platelet substitutes.

Thrombopoietic Agents

Thrombopoietin has been cloned and mass-produced for clinical trials, and it is currently under evaluation in a variety of clinical circumstances.[32-35] Although interleukin (IL)-11 was recently approved as a thrombopoietic agent, its overall effects are relatively modest, and its approval was limited to the relatively uncommon situation in which patients experience thombocytopenia with one course of therapy and the physician wishes to maintain "dose intensity" assisted by IL-11 with the next course of therapy.[36] The clinical benefits of dose intensity at these intermediate dosage ranges are unproved for patients with solid tumors or lymphomas. Furthermore, recent experiments with IL-11 "knockout mice" have shown that these mice have a perfectly normal hematopoietic system and platelet count, strongly suggesting that IL-11 is not primarily a thrombopoietic agent.[37]

Clinical trials with thrombopoietin itself or in a pegylated form (megakaryocyte growth and development factor) have shown that this agent reproducibly increases the platelet count in a dose-dependent fashion, although with a 4- to 6-day delay after administration of the thrombopoietin.[33,34] Elevations in platelet count occur after a single injection of thrombopoietin, and studies in cancer patients and normal volunteers have shown no significant side effects or any apparent increase in thrombotic events. Early clinical trials have shown that platelet count nadirs can be attenuated by the administration of thrombopoietin.[33-35] However, recent trials in patients with acute myeloid leukemia or in recipients of HPC transplants have not shown shortening of the duration of thrombocytopenia or reduction in the number of required platelet transfusions, perhaps in part because endogenous levels of thrombopoietin are already quite elevated during severe thrombocytopenia and the marrow may already be maximally stimulated.[38-40] Additional trials using different doses and schedules of thrombopoietin are in progress, as are trials in patients with marrow failure states such as myelodysplasia or aplastic anemia. It should be recalled, however, that the myeloid growth factors granulocyte colony-stimulating factor and granulocyte-macrophage colony-stimulating factor were not particularly effective in such patients, presumably because of the severe compromise in marrow function, which could not be overcome by exogenous cytokines.[41] Thus, there is no consensus yet on the eventual impact of thrombopoietin on the need for platelet transfusion, and we can assume continued demand for platelets for many years to come.

There has also been preliminary evaluation of the use of thrombopoietin to stimulate normal donors to increase the yield from each apheresis procedure.[42] However, use of thrombopoietin does not necessarily improve overall product availability because of the need for two visits per procedure (first to receive the thrombopoietin and 10-14 days later to donate), as well as the theoretic concern about increased risk of thrombosis at higher donor platelet counts. Recently, however, there have been reports of severe thrombocytopenia in normal donors receiving multiple doses of megakaryocyte growth and development factor who developed neutralizing antibodies against thrombopoietin. This will certainly limit the use of this compound in normal donors. In certain situations, however, such as might occur when there are few donors for an alloimmunized patient or when patients are providing autologous platelets for cryopreservation,[43] donor stimulation with thrombopoietin could be a consideration.

Conclusions

It is likely that platelet transfusion technology will evolve further in the next 3-5 years. Some techniques, such as prestorage leukocyte reduction and possibly the use of psoralen additives, may be applicable to most or all platelet products. Other techniques, such as the use of UVB-irradiated platelets, platelet substitutes, or autologous cryopreserved platelets, will likely have a more restricted audience. Successful analysis of the characteristic benefits and risks of the selection among the current and newer products available from the blood bank will demand close communication between the transfusion service and clinicians. This communication has been absent in many centers and cannot be provided by molecular biologic technology or new machines. Yet it may be as important as the fancier technologies described, and it should be encouraged and developed.

References

1. Murphy S, Gardner FH. Platelet storage at 22°C: Metabolic, morphologic and functional studies. J Clin Invest 1971;50:370-6.
2. Hogge DE, Thompson BW, Schiffer CA. Platelet storage for seven days in second generation CLX™ blood bags. Transfusion 1986;26:131-5.
3. Buchholz DH, Young VM, Friedman NR, et al. Detection of quantitation of bacteria in platelet products stored at ambient temperature. Transfusion 1973;13:268-75.
4. Braine HG, Kickler TS, Charache P, et al. Bacterial sepsis secondary to platelet transfusion: An adverse effect of extended storage at room temperature. Transfusion 1986;26:391-3.
5. Freireich EJ, Levin RH, Whang J, et al. The function and fate of transfused leukocytes from donors with chronic myelocytic leukemia in leukopenic recipients. Ann N Y Acad Sci 1964;113:1081.
6. Tullis JL, Eberle WG, Baudanza P, Tinch R. Platelet-pheresis: Description of a new technic. Transfusion 1968;8:154-64.
7. Latham A Jr. Early developments in blood cell separation technology. Vox Sang 1998;51:249-52.
8. Ito Y, Suaudeau J, Bowman RL. New flow-through centrifuge without rotating seals applied to plasmapheresis. Science 1975;189:999-1000.

9. Suaudeau J, Kolobow T, Vaillancourt R, et al. The Ito "flow-through" centrifuge: A new device for long-term (24 hours) plasmapheresis without platelet deterioration. Transfusion 1978;18:312-9.
10. The TRAP Study Group. Leukocyte reduction and UV-B irradiation of platelets to prevent alloimmunization and refractoriness to platelet transfusion. N Engl J Med 1997;337:1861-9.
11. Bowden RA, Slichter SJ, Sayers M, et al. A comparison of filtered leukocyte-reduced and cytomegalovirus (CMV) seronegative blood products for the prevention of transfusion-associated CMV infection after marrow transplant. Blood 1995;86:3598-603.
12. Beutler E. Platelet transfusions: The 20,000/μL trigger. Blood 1993; 81:1411-13.
13. Schiffer CA. Prophylactic platelet transfusion. Transfusion 1992;32: 295-8.
14. Harker LA, Slichter SJ. The bleeding time as a screening test for evaluation of platelet function. N Engl J Med 1972;287:155-9.
15. Rebulla P, Finazzi G, Marangoni F, et al. A multicenter randomized study of the threshold for prophylactic platelet transfusions in adults with acute myeloid leukemia. N Engl J Med 1997;337:1870-5.
16. Heckman KD, Weiner GJ, Davis CS, et al. Randomized study of prophylactic platelet transfusion threshold during induction therapy for adult acute leukemia: 10,000/μL versus 20,000/μL. J Clin Oncol 1997;15:1143-9.
17. Wandt H, Frank M, Ehninger G, et al. Safety and cost effectiveness of a 10×10^9/L trigger for prophylactic platelet transfusions compared with the traditional 20×10^9/L trigger: A prospective comparative trial in 105 patients with acute myeloid leukemia. Blood 1998;91: 3601-6.
18. Bernstein SH, Nademanee AP, Vose JM, et al. A multicenter study of platelet recovery and utilization in patients after myeloablative therapy and hematopoietic stem cell transplantation. Blood 1998;91: 3509-17.
19. Heddle JM, Klama L, Singer J, et al. The role of plasma from platelet concentrates in transfusion reactions. N Engl J Med 1994;331:625-8.
20. Aye MT, Palmer DS, Giulivi A, Hashemi S. Effect of filtration of platelet concentrates on the accumulation of cytokines and platelet release factors during storage. Transfusion 1995;35:117-24.
21. Muylle L, Peetermans ME. Effect of prestorage leukocyte removal on the cytokine levels in stored platelet concentrates. Vox Sang 1994; 66:14-7.

22. Murphy S, Heaton WA, Rebulla P. Platelet production in the old world—and the new. Transfusion 1996;36:751-4.
23. Dutcher JP, Schiffer CA, Aisner J, Wiernik PH. Long-term follow-up of patients with leukemia receiving platelet transfusions: Identification of a large group of patients who do not become alloimmunized. Blood 1981;58:1007-11.
24. Reed E, Hardy M, Benvenisty A, et al. Effect of anti-idiotypic antibodies to HLA on graft survival in renal-allograft recipients. N Engl J Med 1987;316:1450-5.
25. Lin L, Cook DN, Wiesehahn GP, et al. Photochemical inactivation of viruses and bacteria in platelet concentrates by use of a novel psoralen and long-wavelength ultraviolet light. Transfusion 1997;37:423-35.
26. Alving BM, Reid TJ, Fratantoni JC, Finlayson JS. Frozen platelets and platelet substitutes in transfusion medicine. Transfusion 1997;37: 866-76.
27. Read MS, Reddick RL, Bode AP, et al. Preservation of hemostatic and structural properties of rehydrated lyophilized platelets: Potential for long-term storage of dried platelets for transfusion. Proc Natl Acad Sci U S A 1995;92:397-401.
28. Chao FC, Kim BK, Houranieh AM, et al. Infusible platelet membrane microvesicles: A potential transfusion substitute for platelets. Transfusion 1996;36:536-42.
29. Coller BS, Springer KT, Beer JH, et al. Thromboerythrocytes. In vitro studies of a potential autologous, semi-artificial alternative to platelet transfusions. J Clin Invest 1992;89:546-55.
30. Blajchman MA, Lee DH. The thrombocytopenic rabbit bleeding time model to evaluate the in vivo hemostatic efficacy of platelets and platelet substitutes. Transfus Med Rev 1997;11:95-105.
31. Scigliano E, Enright H, Telen M, et al. Infusible platelet membrane (IPM) for control of bleeding in thrombocytopenic patients (abstract). Blood 1997;90(suppl):267.
32. Kaushansky K. Thrombopoietin: The primary regulator of platelet production. Blood 1995;86:419-31.
33. Basser RL, Rasko JE, Clarke K, et al. Randomized, blinded, placebo-controlled phase I trial of pegylated recombinant human megakaryocyte growth and development factor with filgrastim after dose-intensive chemotherapy in patients with advanced cancer. Blood 1997;89:3118-28.
34. Vadham-Raj S, Murray LJ, Bueso-Ramos C, et al. Stimulation of megakaryocyte and platelet production by a single dose of recombi-

nant human thrombopoietin in patients with cancer. Ann Intern Med 1997;126:673-81.

35. Fanucci M, Glaspy J, Crawford J, et al. Effects of polyethylene glycol-conjugated recombinant human megakaryocyte growth and development factor on platelet counts after chemotherapy for lung cancer. N Engl J Med 1997;336:404-9.
36. Tepler I, Elias L, Smith JW, et al. A randomized placebo-controlled trial of recombinant human interleukin-11 in cancer patients with severe thombocytopenia due to chemotherapy. Blood 1996;87:3607-14.
37. Nandurkar HH, Robb L, Tarlinton D, Barnett L, Köntgen F, Begley CG. Adult mice with targeted mutation of the interleukin-11 receptor (IL11Ra) display normal hematopoiesis. Blood 1997;90:2148-59.
38. Archimbaud E, Ottmann OG, Liu-Yan JA, et al. A randomized, double-blind, placebo controlled study using PEG-rHuMGDF as an adjunct to chemotherapy for adults with de novo acute myeloid leukemia. Early results (abstract). Blood 1996; 88(suppl):447a.
39. Schiffer CA, Miller K, Larson RA, et al. A double blind, placebo controlled trial evaluating pegylated recombinant human megakaryocyte growth and development factor (MGDF) as an adjunct to induction and consolidation therapy in patients with acute myeloid leukemia (AML). Blood 1998;92(suppl):312a.
40. Emmons RVB, Reid DM, Cohen RL, et al. Human thrombopoietin levels are high when thombocytopenia is due to megakaryocyte deficiency and low when due to increased platelet destruction. Blood 1996;87:4068-71.
41. Negrin RS, Nagler A, Kobayashi Y, et al. Maintenance treatment of patients with myelodysplastic syndromes using recombinant human granulocyte colony-stimulating factor. Blood 1990;78:36-43.
42. Kuter D, McCullough J, Romo J, et al. Treatment of platelet (PLT) donors with pegylated recombinant human megakaryocyte growth and development factor (PEG-rHuMGDF) increases circulating PLT counts (CTS) and PLT apheresis yields and increases platelet increments in recipients of PLT transfusions (abstract). Blood 1997;90(suppl 1):579a.
43. Schiffer CA, Aisner J, Wiernik PH. Frozen autologous platelet transfusion for patients with leukemia. N Engl J Med 1978;299:7-12.

Index

Page numbers in italics represent tables

A

B

C

D

E

F

G

H

I

K

L

M

N

P

R

S

T

U

V

W